access to
Clinical
education

If you would further details about learning support in connection with this book, please contact either of the following:

Jean Clayton
APL Manager
Wolfson School of Health Sciences
Thames Valley University
32-38 Uxbridge Road
London W5 2BS

Tel   0181 280 5230
Fax   0181 280 5125
e-mail   jean.clayton@tvu.ac.uk

Madeleine Flanagan
Principal Lecturer, Tissue Viability
Department of Post-registration Nursing
University of Hertfordshire
College Lane
Hatfield
Hertfordshire AL10 9AB

Tel   01707 285 233
Fax   01707 28 4954

If you or your university require any further information about the ACE series, please contact:

Ellen Green
Senior Commissioning Editor
Robert Stevenson House
1-3 Baxter's Place
Leith Walk
Edinburgh EH1 3AF

Tel   0131 535 1718 (direct line)
Fax   0131 558 3171
e-mail   elleng@edinburgh.rsh.pearson-pro.com

access to
Clinical
education

Wound
Management

For Churchill Livingstone:

Commissioning Editor: Ellen Green
Project Manager: Valerie Burgess
Project Development Editor: Mairi McCubbin
Designer: Judith Wright
Illustrator: Robert Britton
Copy-editor: Sue Beasley
Page Layout: Kate Walshaw
Indexer: Liza Weinkove
Sales Promotion Executive: Hilary Brown

access to
Clinical
education

Wound Management

Madeleine Flanagan

BSc(Hons) MA DipN(Lond) CertEd(FE) ONC RGN

Principal Lecturer, Tissue Viability, Dept of Post-Registration Nursing,
University of Hertfordshire, Hatfield, UK

Educational Consultant, Access to Clinical Education series
Diane Marks-Maran

BSc RGN DipN(Lond) RNT

Associate Director, Wolfson Institute for Health Sciences, and
Head of the Centre for Teaching and Learning in Health Sciences,
Thames Valley University, London, UK

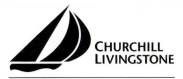

CHURCHILL
LIVINGSTONE

NEW YORK EDINBURGH LONDON MELBOURNE SAN FRANCISCO AND TOKYO 1997

CHURCHILL LIVINGSTONE

Medical Division of Pearson Professional Limited
Distributed in the United States of America by Churchill Livingstone Inc.,
650 Avenue of the Americas, New York, N.Y. 10011, and by associated
companies, branches and representatives throughout the world.

First edition 1997

ISBN 0 443 05531 9

British Library of Cataloguing in Publication Data
A catalogue record for this book is available from the British Library.

Library of Congress Cataloging in Publication Data
A catalogue record for this book is available from the Library of Congress

Medical knowledge is constantly changing. As new information becomes
available, changes in treatment, procedures, equipment and the use of
drugs become necessary. The editors/authors/contributors and the
publishers have, as far as it is possible, taken care to ensure that the
information given in this text is accurate and up to date. However,
readers are strongly advised to confirm that the information, especially
with regard to drug usage, complies with latest legislation and and
standards of practice.

The
publisher's
policy is to use
**paper manufactured
from sustainable forests**

Produced by Longman Singapore Publishers Pte Ltd
Printed in Singapore

Contents

Preface

Throughout history, numerous topical treatments have been applied to wounds, including boiling oil, honey, diluted wine and sea water. Unfortunately, the principles of wound management have often been neglected and, even today, are still poorly understood. Health professionals are often confused by competing philosophies of wound management. Too frequently they rely on practices aimed at providing a local environment that encourages healing, such as drying out the surface of the wound, removing exudate and applying topical antimicrobials; yet a growing body of theoretical evidence and practical experience demonstrates that such treatments are detrimental to tissue repair.

The purpose of this book is to provide clinically focused theoretical and practical information about the key concepts of wound management, across all clinical specialities and care environments. It adopts a practical approach based on the author's professional experience, both as a tissue viability clinical nurse specialist and as a specialist lecturer in wound management. The book has two fundamental aims:

- to increase understanding of contemporary advances in wound management and the delivery of tissue viability services
- to promote the application of research-based wound management practices.

Tissue viability services have developed considerably during the last 20 years, resulting in substantial improvements in the care of patients with wounds. The term 'tissue viability' is often misinterpreted. It literally refers to the preservation of healthy tissues, and, more broadly, to the prevention and management of tissue damage. It may include both acute and chronic wounds.

A growing number of nurses are involved in wound management and tissue viability. They may be employed in the community or hospital, public or private sector. No matter where they are working, they all share the need to increase their knowledge of developments in wound management. However, many nurses do not have access to specialised programmes of study. It is for this reason that this book has been written in a open learning format. It is part of a new series of open learning texts called 'Access to Clinical Education' (ACE) which allow nurses to study at their own pace and in their own time and—if they so desire—to get academic credit for their learning. (For more information about the series, see 'About the series' on page 1.)

The book is divided into the following sections:

Section 1 presents an overview of the historical perspectives of wound management and ritualistic practice, together with the contemporary political influences affecting the development of tissue viability services.

Section 2 focuses in detail on practical skills relating to wound assessment. It reviews the physiology of healing and the optimal environment for wound healing, then looks at the principles of nutritional support and the identification of clinically infected wounds. Specialist assessment methods relating to pressure sores and leg ulcers are briefly reviewed. (These topics are discussed in greater depth in other books in the ACE series.)

Section 3 examines the principles of wound management, including management of infected wounds, the principles of wound cleansing, and wound debridement techniques. This section encourages practitioners to define and prioritise specific wound treatment objectives.

Section 4 concentrates on the use of modern dressing materials. It considers recent technological advances in wound dressings, the cost implications of such treatments and factors influencing the selection of wound dressings. Also included is a review of currently available wound dressing materials.

Section 5 looks at management of complex wounds, focusing on frequently seen wounds that are difficult for the patient and carer to manage. This section examines both the general and specific principles of managing fungating wounds, non-healing leg ulcers, sinus, fistulae and diabetic ulcers.

Section 6 considers the impact of wounds on quality of life, emphasising the patient's perspective. It looks at the psychological aspects of wounding, including body image, patient compliance and the principles of health promotion.

Section 7 puts into context the developments in wound management services by examining legal and professional issues within the multidisciplinary team, and the contribution of tissue viability nurse specialists to this rapidly evolving clinical specialty.

The number of specialist textbooks on wound management has increased considerably in recent years, reflecting the growing body of research and practical experience within this developing field. However, to my knowledge, this is one of the first texts to focus on clinically relevant topics for practitioners and to adopt an open learning approach. I hope that sharing my own experiences in this way will help demystify current approaches to the management and treatment of wounds and thereby improve the quality of care for patients with compromised tissue viability.

Hatfield, 1997   M. F.

Acknowledgements

The author is grateful to her Wound Care Society colleagues, her students and the many tissue viability specialist nurses who have shared with her the issues that they face in everyday practice; and to Edward for his encouragement and support throughout this project.

The publishers would like to thank Ms Andrea Nelson, University of Liverpool, and Dr Moya Morison, Perth, for acting as Critical Readers for this book; and the Community and District Nursing Association for their assistance in field testing the books in the ACE series.

We are also grateful to the following for permission to reproduce the following articles in the Reader:

ConvaTec Ltd for Reader 8—Caring for your legs: an expert guide for people living with leg ulcers. February 1996

Ink Press International for Reader 1—Ellis T 1994 Training the wounded: Galen or Nightingale? Primary Intention 2(1): 14–19

Journal of Tissue Viability for Reader 7—Nelson A 1995 Compression bandaging for venous ulcers. Journal of Tissue Viability 5(2): 57–61

Macmillan Magazines Ltd for: Reader 2—McLaren S M G 1992 Nutrition and wound healing. Journal of Wound Care 1(3): 45-55; Reader 3—Lawrence J C 1993 Wound infection. Journal of Wound Care 2(5): 277-280; Reader 6—Moore D 1992 Hypochlorites: a review of the evidence. 1(4): 44–53

Mark Allen Publishing Ltd for Reader 4—Vowden K 1995 Common problems in wound care: wound and ulcer measurement. British Journal of Nursing 4(13): 775–779

Wound Care Society for Reader 5—Flanagan M 1995 Pressure sore risk assessment. Educational leaflet 3(4).

We are also grateful for permission to reproduce the following material:

Mrs J A Waterlow for The Waterlow Scale, in Reader 5.

About the series *Diane Marks-Maran*

This learning package has been designed to enable nurses to improve their specialist knowledge and understanding of an important area of clinical practice. To help you to make the most of this learning package, we have designed this introductory section as a guideline for those of you who are new to open and distance learning.

Who is this learning package for?

This learning package is for nurses in either hospital or community settings, or in the private sector, who provide wound care to a variety of patients or clients and who want to take the opportunity, through this learning package, to ensure that their knowledge and skills are up to date and that their practice is evidence based.

What is the best way for me to use this learning package?

This depends upon what you want to gain from completing the package. At one level, this package is an excellent way to update your clinical knowledge and skill through open learning. Open learning means that you complete the package in your own time and at your own pace, taking as long as you like, reading selectively from the text and focusing on those aspects that are important to you. You complete no assessment and merely complete the activities within the package for your own interest.

At another level, in addition to updating clinical knowledge and skill, you may wish to complete this learning package as part of fulfilling your PREP requirements. In this case, you will need to show evidence in your professional portfolio of how this package has improved your clinical practice.

At a third level, as well as updating your clinical knowledge and skill, you may be planning to undertake further study at your local university to gain, for example, a post-registration qualification and a further academic award. In this case, completing this package and successfully passing the written assessment at the end of the package may be used to gain academic credits towards your planned academic award if the university of your choice has approved this programme of study.

What do the learning outcomes mean?

More and more, colleges and universities are aware of the need to make explicit the exact requirements for completing a module or programme successfully. Learning outcomes are one way of doing this.

Learning outcomes indicate the specific knowledge, skills and understandings you will be exposed to in the learning package. They also tell you what your assessment will entail. Additionally, if you are planning to use this learning package towards achieving your PREP professional requirements, you may find the learning outcomes a useful basis for submitting evidence of learning within your personal professional profile.

What do I need to do to complete this learning package for my PREP requirements?

Completing this learning package can be used towards fulfilment of your PREP requirements to show evidence of your continued learning. The UKCC has sent you a package of information entitled 'PREP and You' which explains how to complete a personal professional profile to show evidence of learning and improvement in practice. If you have not received this information, the UKCC will be happy to send you the package. In addition, issue 17 of the UKCC magazine *Register* (Summer 1996) gives a comprehensive guide to writing your personal professional profile. Completing the written assessment at the end of this learning package provides one piece of evidence you can include in your profile even if you do not submit it for marking to gain academic credits; recording your reflection on learning as a result of completing this package is another form of evidence to include in your profile.

What do I need to do if I want to gain academic credits for completing this learning package?

Some universities have accredited this learning package at both diploma level (level 2) and degree level (level 3). Accreditation has been awarded on the basis of the expected learning outcomes for the package and for the written assessment at the end of the package. You can only receive academic credits for completing the written assessment and achieving a pass grade for that assessment. You can receive academic credits at level 2 if you successfully pass the associated assessment and achieve the level 2 learning outcomes; you will receive level 3 credits if you successfully pass the level 3 assessment at the end of the package and achieve the associated learning outcomes. This means that you can use this package towards your future study to gain a Diploma in Higher Education in Nursing or a BSc in nursing.

Prior to undertaking the assessment, you should find out from the university of your choice whether they will accredit this learning pack. If they have done so, you will be able, for a registration fee, to submit your assessment for marking. If you successfully pass the assessment, you will get the credits that your university has chosen to award this learning package. Thames Valley University (TVU) and the University of Hertfordshire (UH) have already accredited this package and would be willing to undertake this service for you. Other universities will follow shortly. The university of your choice may, however, accept the credits awarded you by institutions such as TVU and UH through their APL/APEL process. A visual illustration of how to use this learning package is given in Figure 1.

What exactly does level 2 study mean?

When we talk about a package or course being at level 2 or level 3 it means that the work expected of you is assessed at a certain level. Level 2 normally equates to the second year of a full-time degree programme, at the end of which students would achieve a Diploma in Higher Education. However, modern education allows students to take various routes, including part-time and distance learning modes.

At level 2 you are expected to:

- demonstrate good understanding of relevant concepts and issues
- make appropriate use and application of relevant research
- demonstrate the ability to solve problems
- analyse a range of information and apply this knowledge to practice
- demonstrate the ability to construct arguments and evaluate the relevance of issues to your professional practice.

Level 2 means that you are expected to demonstrate the ability to collect information and apply that information to solve a simple but unpredictable problem or a complex but predictable problem in your practice. Level 2 also means that you are expected to manage care within broad guidelines for

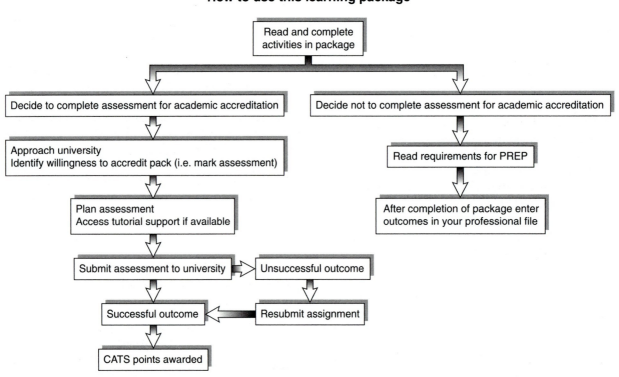

How to use this learning package

Fig. 1 How to use this learning package.

defined activities and to demonstrate knowledge and understanding of the subject and the variety of ideas and frameworks which may be applied to this subject. A level 2 student is one who also demonstrates the ability to analyse a variety of types of information with minimum guidance, can apply major theories of discipline and can compare alternative methods or techniques for gathering data. Within a level 2 learning package you will show that you can use a range of ideas and information towards a given purpose, such as solving a particular patient problem or situation, and can select appropriate techniques of evaluation, demonstrating that you are able to evaluate the relevance and significance of information you have collected.

In addition, when given a complex task to undertake, a level 2 student should demonstrate that she or he can choose an appropriate set of actions in sequence to complete the task, and can evaluate individual performance in terms of strengths and weaknesses. Level 2 students can challenge received opinion, adopt flexible approaches to study, identify their own learning needs and undertake activities to improve their own performance. At level 2 you are expected to demonstrate that you can study autonomously in completing straightforward study tasks. In tackling problems you should demonstrate that you can identify the key elements of a problem and choose appropriate methods for resolving problems.

What does level 3 study mean?

Level 3 study refers to a range of more advanced academic skills and equates to the third year of a full-time degree course. In addition to level 2 skills you are expected to:

- demonstrate a comprehensive and detailed knowledge of a major subject area
- critically analyse new or abstract information and relate this to your professional practice
- design creative solutions to problems
- critically evaluate evidence which supports conclusions or recommendations
- demonstrate the ability to sustain analytical argument whilst being aware of controversies and critical standpoints
- demonstrate the ability to develop a constructive, independent and original line of thought.

At level 3, you are expected to be able to demonstrate that you can work with complex and unpredictable situations, apply a wide range of innovative and standard techniques and demonstrate autonomy in planning and managing resources within broad guidelines. Your written assessments at level 3 should show that you can incorporate awareness of personal responsibility and a critical ethical dimension into

your written work. A level 3 student demonstrates a comprehensive and detailed knowledge of a major subject area with the ability to demonstrate specialisation and yet realise that knowledge within a specialism is always growing and changing. A level 3 student can analyse new and/or abstract data without guidance and can transform abstracted data and concepts towards a given purpose with minimum guidance. In addition, a level 3 student can also design novel solutions to problems and can critically evaluate evidence which supports conclusions or recommendations. The students can select appropriate responses to a situation from a repertoire of actions and can evaluate their own performance and the performance of others.

In addition, people who are working at level 3 can manage their own learning using a wide range of resources, can seek and make use of feedback and can apply their own criteria for judging their performance. Problem solving at level 3 involves demonstrating confidence and flexibility in identifying and defining complex problems and applying appropriate knowledge and evidence to their solutions.

I have never studied using an independent method before. How can I get help in developing the study skills I need to work in this way?

Studying independently through open and distance learning is very different from taking a course at a college or university. It affords nurses the opportunity to study at their own pace, in their own environment and in their own time. Distance learning is especially beneficial for nurses who do not have access to a university-based course, owing to geographical, work or domestic constraints or situations. However, studying through open or distance learning does require good study skills and time-management skills to make the most of the learning package. We would recommend that you read one of the many guides to study skills which are available for students. This will give you practical advice on how to get the most out of learning packages such as this one. We particularly recommend the following two books:

- Goodall C 1995 *A Survivor's Guide to Study Skills and Student Assessments*. Churchill Livingstone, Edinburgh
- Parnell J, Kendrick K 1994 *Study Skills for Nurses*. Churchill Livingstone, Edinburgh.

In addition, study skills packs may be available from the university accrediting the package; tutorial support may also be offered. Thames Valley University and the University of Hertfordshire are able to provide learning support in the form of feedback, tutorial support and advice to nurses undertaking this learning package. Details of the type of learning and tutorial support available from TVU and UH, as well as the amount and cost are available from:

Jean Clayton
APL Manager
Wolfson School of Health Sciences
Thames Valley University
32–38 Uxbridge Road
London W5 2BS
Tel: 0181 280 5230
Fax: 0181 280 5125
e-mail: jean.clayton@tvu.ac.uk

Madeleine Flanagan
Principal Lecturer, Tissue Viability
Department of Post-registration Nursing
University of Hertfordshire
College Lane
Hatfield
Hertfordshire AL10 9AB
Tel: 01707 285233
Fax: 01707 284954

What types of learning activities will I be undertaking in this learning package?

In order to make this learning package interesting and varied, the authors have included a wide range of activities for you to complete. One type is reading activities. These are interesting and informative parts of the package which are designed to give you important information and knowledge about the subject. Sometimes a reading activity will request that you read an article from a journal on a particular subject or aspect of care. This article can be found in the Reader at the back of the learning package. Reading activities are often followed by self-assessment questions (SAQs). SAQs are designed to enable you to test your understanding of what you have read and draw together some of the important points in the reading you have just completed. Sometimes SAQs are included to assess your prior learning (e.g. one SAQ might ask you to write your own definition of a wound) or are in the form of short true/false questions.

Another type of activity in the package is that which asks you to describe something that currently happens in your own practice. You may be asked to reflect on some previous experience or patient. This may be followed by a feedback section where the author enables you to analyse your practice or previous experience against the literature, research and evidence. Another activity may ask you to look at a photograph and make certain observations. This will be followed by some kind of feedback to check your observations with those of the author. Other activities may include completing a chart or diagram, followed by feedback from the author of the package.

As you can see, undertaking a learning package is not the same thing as reading a book! It involves you in a wide variety of activities to find information, use information, analyse information and make clinical judgements. You will always be given some sort of feedback from the activities within the package.

You mentioned a Reader at the end of this package. What is it?

The Reader is a selection of articles from various professional journals about the subject you are studying in the learning package. We recognise that some nurses are undertaking distance learning study because they do not have easy access to a college or university in their geographical area and therefore may not have access to some of the journals which specialise in the subject of this learning package. For this reason, we are including a Reader within the learning package. Some of the learning activities within the package ask you to read certain articles from the Reader and answer questions about those articles. Other articles are just related to the subject and are useful for you to have as reference material and to help you complete your written assessment.

There seem to be a lot of terms used in this learning package. How can I be sure that I am understanding these terms in the way I am supposed to?

To help you understand the terminology in this learning package the following glossary will be helpful.

Critically analyse: To critically analyse something means to look at a wide range of information about a subject or issue, to identify the strengths and weaknesses of the arguments for or against something, draw conclusions based on the diverse information available to you and defend your conclusions with reference to the widest possible sources of information. At level 2, students should be able to analyse a range of information with minimum guidance, apply major theories of a discipline and compare alternative methods or techniques for obtaining data (SEEC 1996). Level 3 critical analysis means that students can analyse new and/or abstract data and situations without guidance using a wide range of techniques appropriate to the subject being studied (SEEC 1996).

Define: When you are asked to define something in a learning activity, what you are being asked to do is to write the meaning of something, e.g. a wound is ....

Demonstrate knowledge: Demonstrating knowledge involves showing that you know relevant facts, principles and concepts and that you can select these appropriately to make a clinical decision and justify that decision. Knowledge is demonstrated by defining, naming, listing or identifying parts of a whole as well as interpreting information through explaining and describing facts and applying facts to solve a problem or to give an example of a situation.

Describe: When you are asked to describe something, you are being asked to interpret information. This means that you must first show that you have the information and then give your interpretation of it.

Evaluate: Evaluating involves assessing or re-assessing a situation, criticising it, identifying strengths and weaknesses, discriminating or judging something. In nursing, evaluation often involves making a judgement of care given as compared to evidence or research.

Reflect: Reflection is thinking in a structured way in order to learn something from your experiences as a nurse and to make a decision or take an action as a result of your thinking. There are a number of frameworks for reflection, each of which offers structured questions to think through a situation and learn from it. At the end of structured reflection is some sort of learning which points you in new directions for the way you practise as a nurse.

When I complete the activities in this learning package and write my assessment, how should I reference my essay?

It is important to cite references appropriately. There are a number of ways of referencing and, so long as you select a recognised method and are consistent in your approach, it does not matter which one you use. You should seek guidance from the university who will be marking your assessment about their preferred referencing system. Details of some approaches to referencing can be found in the two study skills books which were identified earlier.

REFERENCE

SEEC 1996 Guidelines on levels and generic levels descriptors. South East England Consortium/Wales HE CATS

Introduction

This learning package has been designed to provide practitioners with a specialised study programme relevant to the rapidly expanding speciality of wound management and tissue viability. It uses a problem-solving approach that incorporates clinically relevant themes associated with wound management and good clinical practice.

The speciality of wound management has developed rapidly over the last 30 years as a response to increased multidisciplinary research activity. During this time, wound management has emerged as a dynamic, complex and demanding speciality. This book has been designed to facilitate the integration of theoretical concepts and clinical practice and is flexible enough to allow learners to work at their own pace. It is focused around the key concepts of wound management and as such cuts across the traditional clinical speciality divisions. It should therefore meet the needs of a wide variety of practitioners from different backgrounds, whilst covering current philosophies of wound management relevant to all.

At the end of this open learning package you should be able to:

- demonstrate an awareness of the current political and professional influences affecting delivery of tissue viability services
- describe currently identified physiological and biochemical processes associated with normal wound healing
- describe the optimal environment for local wound management, relating each aspect to the concept of moist wound healing
- distinguish between different methods of wound assessment, identifying how to improve the reliability of wound assessment in clinical practice
- discuss the management principles of caring for patients with clinically infected wounds
- critically examine prevalent wound cleansing practices, discussing the merits/demerits of each
- describe a range of factors that influence the selection of wound dressings
- review a wide range of wound management treatments and evaluate their application to clinical practice
- recognise the many potential difficulties encountered when managing patients with complex wounds
- analyse those factors that may contribute to non-compliance in a patient with compromised tissue viability
- discuss the psychological and social impact that trauma has on individuals and their families
- discuss the ethical and legal issues relevant to management of patients with wounds
- outline contemporary advances in wound healing, discussing their clinical significance and nursing implications.

Learning outcomes

LEVEL 2 LEARNING OUTCOMES

At the end of this package nurses will demonstrate that they can:

1. identify the physiological aspects which influence wound healing
2. explore current research and technological advances in wound dressings and their application to patient care
3. analyse the process of wound assessment, examining how assessment influences wound management and the role that assessment takes in the provision of comprehensive wound management services.

LEVEL 3 LEARNING OUTCOMES

At the end of this package nurses will demonstrate that they can:

1. critically evaluate wound management practices in their place of work, taking into account national and local guidelines, technological advances and research evidence
2. appraise the role of the tissue viability specialist nurse and explore his/her role in advancing wound management.

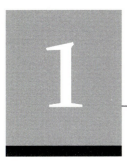

The developing speciality of tissue viability

Introduction

Wound management is a rapidly expanding and dynamic speciality that can be expensive to provide and difficult to evaluate. Levels of knowledge and delivery of good practice vary greatly and range from specialist wound care units to those areas where the availability of specialist advice is severely restricted. All practitioners responsible for the care and management of patients with wounds have, at some time or other, experienced frustration due to the lack of available resources or the failure to implement research-based practice, which for many patients results in inappropriate care and prolonged suffering. This section aims to introduce you to some of the important factors influencing our ability to change wound management practices.

LEARNING OUTCOMES

When you have completed this section, you should be able to:

- describe the effect that historical influences exert upon current wound management practices
- recognise the role that myth and ritualistic actions have in wound care and how they create a barrier to the implementation of research-based practice
- consider the implications that recent health care reforms have had on the delivery of wound management services.

1.1 HISTORICAL PERSPECTIVES OF WOUND MANAGEMENT

Introduction

Since time began man has used a variety of different treatments in an attempt to manage wounds. Treatments were based upon knowledge and beliefs available at the time and were dependent on the development of technological advances, many of which took place in times of major conflict and war.

Early times

Prehistoric wound management basically aimed to control bleeding using pressure and to cover the wound with dressings that were freely available such as mud, leaves, lichen and bark. Evidence suggests that larger wounds were held together with twine and thorns; such traditional practices are still seen today in African tribes.

The early civilisations of ancient Egypt left detailed medical records describing intricate wound care practices. They greatly favoured the use of topical applications for wound management which included the use of animal dung, honey and resins to stop bleeding. Frankincense and myrrh were used to deodorise offensive wounds, whilst mercury was used as an antibacterial agent. Both water and milk were extensively used to cleanse wounds. Commonly used dressings were pads of linen coated in goat's grease and a primitive form of adhesive bandage which consisted of linen strips soaked with gum; both of these treatments have parallels in wound management practice today. The ancient Egyptians generally considered that wounds were a punishment from god, so that treatments were a mix of religion, medicine and magic and involved many complex rituals devised by healers who combined the roles of high priests, doctors and astronomers. Such healers occupied important positions in society and were rarely challenged, enabling suggested treatments to be quickly incorporated into superstition and folklore.

The influence of Greek medicine

The Greek civilisations developed further some of these practices. Homer in the *Iliad* (800 BC) describes the use of hot irons as a method of cautery together with the chanting of incantations after the dressing of battle wounds. Wine was also used as a widely available antiseptic agent. But it was Hippocrates (460–377 BC) who advocated a much gentler approach to healing and expanded medical knowledge. His care was based upon sound management principles including cleansing wounds carefully with warm water, vinegar or wine, bringing the wound edges together and covering the wound with wool boiled in water. He argued that hands should be kept as clean as possible and fingernails short; although these practices could be seen as the origins of asepsis, at this time the concept was not understood.

The Roman Empire

Celsus, a Roman physician (25 BC–AD 50) described the classical signs of wound infection and recommended against the use of aggressive methods of wound treatment. However, it was the teachings of Galen (AD 130–200) late in this period that were to have a profound effect upon the management of wounds over the following centuries. Galen was a much respected physician to the Roman gladiators and athletes and wrote many medical textbooks. Among the remedies that he advocated were the use of salt water and wine for wound cleansing. Oil, bread and wheat were used as poultices and popular dressings for cavity wounds included sea sponges soaked in oil and wine, the use of which is documented in the Bible. Galen wrote over 300 books and was respected throughout the civilised world. The teachings of Galen focused around his 'laudable pus theory' in which he concluded, owing to the large numbers of infected wounds seen at this time, that the formation of pus was essential for the process of normal wound healing. Foreign bodies would be driven into any wounds that were not showing signs of suppuration in an attempt to stimulate pus formation. If this did not produce results, wounds were traumatised using hot irons or boiling oil, methods that effectively caused infection. This theory was accepted and slavishly followed until the late 1800s, when discoveries by Lister and Pasteur began to challenge these well-established practices.

After the fall of the Roman Empire, the Arabs dominated medical teachings. They added new topical applications to their treatment regimes which included the use of turpentine, lizard dung and pigeons' blood (Forrest 1982). Cautery using hot irons was still recommended for the majority of wounds. Wounds were covered with an increasing array of salves, ointments and cleansing lotions with the common aim of encouraging suppuration as the concept of 'laudable pus' was still very much in favour.

The Renaissance

Among those who disputed the teachings of Galen was Henri De Montville (AD 1260–1320) who observed that wounds heal faster and better without pus formation and was quoted as having said: 'many more surgeons know how to cause suppuration than to heal a wound.' The protective function of wound exudate was not generally recognised until the work of Holn et al in 1977, yet Paracelsus (AD 1493–1541) believed that 'surgeons should not interfere with nature's natural balsam which is produced and deposited on the surface of open wounds and ulcers.' There were few advances in the management of wounds during the 16th and 17th centuries, just an ever increasing plethora of topical ointments and home remedies of dubious efficacy. Pare (1510–1593) was a military surgeon who challenged the 'laudable pus' theory, preferring instead to rely on cleanliness and good nutrition to assist in the healing of his patients' wounds. He is attributed with being one of the first to introduce the use of suturing rather than cautery to control haemorrhage and discovered by chance that the use of clean dressings and simple salves promoted healing more effectively than the use of hot irons and boiling oil!

From antiseptics to antibiotics

During the 19th century a number of bizarre and positively harmful wound management treatments persisted as large numbers of patients continued to die from wound sepsis. Wound management focused on the use of topical agents, many of which were extremely painful and toxic to tissue. The use of antiseptics started at the beginning of the last century with compounds such as silver nitrate, yet the reason why antiseptics improved healing rates was not yet understood. The Industrial Revolution and its subsequent technological advances and social reforms brought rapid and far-reaching changes to wound management practices that had previously remained static for hundreds of years. The mechanisation of the textile industry in the north of England meant that, for the first time, large amounts of cheap material suitable for dressing wounds was readily available. The main dressings produced were gauze and lint. Until this time linen, old cloths, rags and oakum (shredded fibres from old rope) had been used for covering wounds. They were dirty before use and were washed, dried and reused in an attempt to make them more absorbent. It was not until the late 19th century that a surgeon called Gamgee used cotton wool as a surgical dressing. He combined it with a fine open-weave gauze to form one of the first absorbent surgical dressings which he sometimes soaked in antiseptic agents. He published widely in *The Lancet*, describing the need for gentle wound handling and infrequent changes of dressings. Semmelweiss, a Hungarian obstetrician, first demonstrated the value of handwashing with chlorine-based antiseptics in 1847. He was able to drastically improve maternal mortality rates by introducing strict handwashing practices for medical staff, but unfortunately his views were not shared by mainstream medical opinion until after his death.

Louis Pasteur discovered anaerobic bacteria in 1860 and went on to develop the process of heat sterilisation, but his work was applied to the suppuration of wounds and the development of septicaemia by Joseph Lister. In 1867 Lister published his now classic paper *The Antiseptic Principle* in which he described the use of carbolic acid spray during surgery, together with frequent handwashing and the use of clean dressings, all of which dramatically reduced his risk of surgical wound infection. Unfortunately Lister's ideas were vehemently opposed by his medical peers, which resulted in wound management in England, France and America continuing much as before. It took until the First World War for his ideas to become widely accepted, as a result of the mass mortality of wounded servicemen who, in particular, were dying of gas gangrene. During this period there was an increased use of antiseptics in order to minimise wound infection. Popular cleansing agents included carbolic, phenol, iodine and chlorine. The particular chlorine solution used by Lister in his operating theatres became so popular that it was known as Edinburgh University solution of lime which was later abbreviated to Eusol. This antiseptic enjoyed over a century of popularity until the work of Brennan & Leaper in 1985 caused its undignified fall from grace and the recognition that the routine use of antiseptics was no longer necessary. However, it must be remembered that the use of antiseptics before the advent of antibiotics represented a successful approach to the treatment of wound infection which was a major cause of patient mortality at this time. During World War I, hyperchlorite solutions such as Eusol, Dakin's solution and Milton were extensively used to combat wound sepsis and gas gangrene. At this time further advances in dressings occurred; a French military surgeon called Lumière developed 'tulle gras' dressings by dipping gauze pads into paraffin, which became the first low-adherent dressing.

World War II saw the development of the specialities of plastic and reconstructive surgery and also saw the introduction of blood transfusions. Penicillin was discovered in 1928 by Fleming, but was not used on blitz victims until 1941 and only became commercially available in 1946. Colebrook demonstrated considerable success in treating burn victims suffering from streptococcal infections with sulphonamide. The publication of this work in 1936 marked the beginning of the antibiotic era.

Modern developments in wound management

The development of modern wound dressings has slowly evolved since the 1940s, when Bull described the development of a dressing with a semipermeable window, which is now considered to be the foundation upon which semipermeable film dressings were developed in the early 1970s (Thomas 1990). The work of Winter in 1962 using pigs demonstrated that epidermal migration across the surface of superficial wounds took place more rapidly in moist conditions than in dry and stimulated interest in the development of modern wound dressings that could maximise this effect. Also in 1962, Norton et al developed the first pressure sore risk assessment scale for use with elderly patients. This has since been modified, adapted and applied for use in a variety of clinical settings. In 1973, skin barriers that were capable of protecting the skin became available as Stomahesive wafers and were subsequently developed into the range of dressing products known today as hydrocolloids.

During the last 20 years there has been an upsurge of interest in both the physiological process of wound healing and in the management of wounds. Research has focused on the development of new dressings technologies and has begun to question some of our more traditional wound management practices. Rapid advances in wound management have led to the recognition that this area is a speciality in its own right. The emergence of tissue viability nurse specialists is an important development, as they are ideally placed to challenge outdated rituals and to promote research-based practice.

Self-assessment 5 MINUTES

List five topical applications that have been used to manage wounds throughout history.

● ●

FEEDBACK

There are too many to list, but common ones are given in Box 1.1.

● ●

1.2 RITUALISTIC PRACTICE, MYTHS AND SUPERSTITIONS

Introduction

From the beginning of time, all civilisations have struggled to manage wounds appropriately and have relied heavily on superstition and ritualistic practice to guide their actions. Throughout history, innovators have tended to work in isolation and

Box 1.1 Topical applications that have been used in wound management

Natural materials
- Leaves
- Bark
- Mud
- Honey
- Egg white and oxygen

Antiseptics
- Eusol
- Mercurochrome
- Hydrogen peroxide
- Povidone-iodine
- Chlorhexidine
- Potassium permanganate

Antibiotics
- Fusidic acid
- Bactroban
- Cicatrin

Miscellaneous
- Sea water
- Vinegar
- Animal dung
- Boiling oil

Activity — 10 MINUTES

List the two types of dressing that were most commonly used when you were a student nurse and briefly describe the common wound care practices at that time.

FEEDBACK

The time period between your nurse training and the present day will be relatively short. Even if you have recently completed your nurse training, you should be able to report significant differences in the approaches used to manage wounds then and now. The answers obviously depend on when and where you trained as a nurse, but the general points in Table 1.1 were probably noted.

were usually shunned and often persecuted for their beliefs. Each medical and nursing advance must be reviewed within the context of the time period in which it took place, in order to appreciate its overall contribution to our understanding. Attitudes are notoriously difficult to change, particularly once a particular practice has become firmly embedded into our traditional customs and professional culture.

Nursing practice has been steeped in ritual for hundreds of years with many examples deriving from the care of wounds. Ritualistic action implies the performance of a task without thinking, and doing something because it has always been done that way (Walsh & Ford 1992). Historically, nurses have taken their instructions from others, be it the medical staff, the ward sister or the procedure book. Ritualistic practice is characterised by a reluctance to make decisions and to take professional responsibility for one's own actions, which clearly has no place in nursing today. However, despite a plethora of research related to wound management and an increased availability of accessible published material, many practitioners continue to fail to implement research-based wound care.

Table 1.1 Summary of changes in wound care during the last 30 years

Decade	Dressings commonly in use	Common wound care practices
Late 1960s–1970s	Gauze, Gamgee—dry pads, tulle-gras (often impregnated with chlorhexidine), introduction of film-membranes	Changing wound dressings daily, cleaning with antiseptics (Eusol, hydrogen peroxide, etc.). Massaging skin with methylated spirit, use of topical applications (egg white + oxygen, antibiotic powders). Exposing wounds so that they dried out
1980s	Introduction of hydrocolloids, low-adherent dry pads, introduction of alginate and foams dressings	Packing cavity wounds tightly with ribbon gauze soaked in antiseptics/paraffin. Collection of routine wound swabs. Continued use of topical antiseptics and other oddities —honey, yoghurt, soap-flakes. Use of salt in postoperative baths
1990s	As before. Introduction of hydrogels, increased use of interactive dressings	Increased use of moist wound dressings. Dressings changed as infrequently as possible. Use of compression therapy for venous leg ulcers. Avoidance of antiseptics for wound cleansing. Routine use of saline/water for wound cleansing

Rituals relating to the prevention of wound infection can perhaps be traced back throughout history when considerable confusion reigned because of a lack of understanding of the basic principles of asepsis. The teachings of Galen are a prime example of the widespread adoption of a principle that that was never substantiated by empirical evidence. Not even Florence Nightingale was convinced at first about Lister's observations and experiments relating to microorganisms and Lister continued to experience great difficulty convincing his medical colleagues that bacteria were responsible for wound infection and septicaemia. Lister's subsequent introduction of antiseptics for wound cleansing during the late 19th century eventually became so firmly established in medical practice that their use has become the subject of bitter professional debate that still continues today.

It is worth remembering that resistance to change has always existed and that it takes time to establish new practices and ways of thinking. However, today it is the responsibility of the accountable professional to critically evaluate new approaches to care, to implement research-based practice and to challenge outdated customs.

Activity   15 MINUTES

Think back to the first time that you used a modern dressing, e.g. Op-site, Granuflex, etc. Describe the first impressions that you and your colleagues had of this type of dressing. Have your attitudes to this type of dressing changed in subsequent years?

FEEDBACK

Again this answer depends on which dressing type you chose to review. The following general description outlines views and misconceptions commonly held about interactive dressings, especially when first used.

• The use of such dressings will encourage wound infection.
• A collection of fluid and exudate at the wound surface will delay wound healing.
• These dressings cause an unacceptable odour.
• These dressings will not stay in place and adequately absorb exudate.
• These dressings are too expensive.
• These dressings will not be acceptable to patients.

Ritualised practice is characterised by routine, i.e. tasks are performed because they have always been done in a particular way. Thus over time these practices become established and difficult to change. In contrast, practice which is based upon research questions the validity of established practices and challenges the ways in which we care for patients. Research-based practice is particularly threatening when it challenges strongly held beliefs as it has over recent years in wound care.

Activity   15 MINUTES

List four examples of ritualised wound management practices which may still be used today. Then list three examples of research-based wound care practices.

FEEDBACK

There are many examples of ritualised wound management practice. The types of activities you may have identified are:

• application of dry, adherent dressings to open wounds that potentially traumatise tissue when removed
• cleansing wounds with antiseptics or topical antimicrobials
• packing of cavity wounds with ribbon gauze
• routine collection of wound swabs in the absence of signs of clinical infection
• use of salt postoperatively in patients' baths to encourage healing
• massaging methylated spirits into the skin of patients prone to pressure damage.

In contrast to the practices described above, the following would be examples of research-based practice:

• application of interactive dressings that promote the principle of moist wound healing in open wounds
• gentle cleansing of the wound surface with warmed normal saline
• lightly filling cavity wounds with absorbent, atraumatic dressings that encourage free drainage
• application of sustained graduated compression for patients with venous leg ulcers.

1.3 POLITICAL INFLUENCES AND TISSUE VIABILITY SERVICES

Introduction

In recent years, an increased awareness of the high cost of providing care for those patients with compromised tissue viability has meant that health care professionals caring for this vulnerable group of patients have to be politically aware in order to maintain a comprehensive range of supportive patient services.

Health economics

The high costs of wound care which are estimated by Bennett & Moody (1995) to be in the region of £1 billion per annum in the UK are notoriously difficult to define accurately. These costs, particularly relating to the management of chronic wounds, are increasingly becoming a concern for both purchasers and providers of health care as they represent a massive drain on resources. There is, however, evidence that a significant cost saving could be made in relation to wound management without a reduction in quality (Thomas 1995).

Health economics is based on the principle that health care resources will always be scarce relative to needs, which inevitably means that resource allocation choices will always have to made. Nowhere is this more apparent than within the community nursing services. Decreased length of hospital stay has resulted in the discharge of increased numbers of debilitated patients, who are either at increased risk of tissue breakdown or have large chronic wounds. Community nursing services in most countries have limited resources for caring for patients with wounds, which can severely restrict treatment options and result in a lack of continuity of care for the patient. It is widely predicted that numbers of available hospital beds will diminish in the future. The effects of this upon tissue viability services can already be seen, for the numbers of community clinics, many of which are nurse led, are increasing all the time. Another factor responsible for inconsistencies of care is the rapid pace of technological developments within the speciality of wound management, which serves to widen the gulf between what can actually be achieved for patients and what constraints on resources actually allow to be done in clinical practice.

Provision of health care

The demographic changes affecting society are already resulting in increased numbers of frail elderly within the population, who live alone and who have increasing levels of disability. These individuals have an increased vulnerability to tissue breakdown and the development of chronic wounds and will in future make even greater demands on health care services.

Changes in the provision of health care services has increased competition for resources, so that allocation of resources is now dependent upon clinical effectiveness, cost–benefit analysis, key quality indicators and identified patient outcomes. Nurses are in an ideal position to be able to identify the challenges that primary care led purchasing introduces and as patient advocates have a responsibility to negotiate for improved patient services.

Of late, nurses at all levels have begun to play a significant part in determining the range of services that ought to be available for patients with wounds and have influenced the allocation of available resources by purchasers and providers of health care. The development of the role of the clinical nurse specialist within tissue viability has greatly influenced the political involvement of nurses within the rapidly developing but under-resourced speciality of wound management.

Activity   40 MINUTES

Read Article 1 in the Reader (p. 134), in which Ellis describes the influences that history and politics have on wound management today.

Identify two factors that may help to explain why changes in wound management practice are sometimes difficult to achieve.

● ●

FEEDBACK

The reasons why changes in wound management practices are sometimes difficult to achieve include:

• a general lack of assertiveness and negotiating skills exhibited by nurses
• the historical, professional relationship between doctors and nurses, in which the balance of power in the past has been traditionally with the medical staff
• prevalent social and professional stereotypes of nursing until recently supported the notion that nurses should be unquestioning and passive
• in the past, nursing has lacked a distinct knowledge base and has relied upon ritual, intuition and folklore to guide its actions.

● ●

Conclusion

Throughout this package, you will find practical information relating to the management of patients with many different types of wounds. This section has briefly introduced you to the concept that both historical and political influences have direct influence on your ability to practice effective and appropriate wound management today.

As you continue working through the rest of this pack the following issues should be kept in mind and related to your own personal experiences.

- If nurses are to provide best wound management practice, they need to be aware of the difficulties involved in changing attitudes and beliefs, recognising that for many individuals change is a threatening experience that may lead to resistance to new ideas.
- New ideas and research need to be based upon a sound methodological approach and be critically evaluated and not merely accepted at face value.
- Effective management of change requires a major commitment from the organisation at all levels ranging through governments/politicians, clinicians, industry and education.

In the next section you will begin to look at the practical aspects of wound care management, including the physiological aspects of wound healing and the environment in which it is taking place.

REFERENCES

Bennett G, Moody M 1995 Wound care for health professionals. Chapman Hall, London

Brennan S S, Leaper D J 1985 The effect of antiseptics on the healing wound: a study using the rabbit ear chamber. British Journal of Surgery 72: 780–782

Forrest R D 1982 Development of wound therapy from the dark ages to the present. Journal of the Royal Society of Medicine 75: 268–273

Holn D, Pounce B, Burton R 1977 Antimicrobial systems of the surgical wound. American Journal of Surgery 133(5): 597–600

Norton D, McLaren R, Exton-Smith A N 1962 An investigation of geriatric nursing problems in hospital. National Corporation for the Care of Old People, London

Thomas S 1990 Wound management and dressings. The Pharmaceutical Press, London

Thomas S 1995 The cost of wound care in the community. Journal of Wound Care 4(8): 350–354

Walsh P, Ford P 1992 Nursing rituals. Research and rational actions. Butterworth Heinemann, Oxford

Winter G 1962 Formulation of the scab and the rate of epithelialisation of superficial wounds in the skin of the domestic pig. Nature 193: 293–294

SUMMARY

In this section you have learned that:

- Wound management is a rapidly expanding and dynamic speciality that can be expensive to provide and difficult to evaluate.
- Throughout history the treatment of wounds has been based upon knowledge and beliefs available at the time and was dependent on the development of technological advances, many of which took place in times of major conflict and war.

- Rapid advances in wound management have led to the recognition that this field is a speciality in its own right.
- The emergence of tissue viability nurse specialists is an important development, as they are ideally placed to challenge outdated rituals and to promote research-based practice.

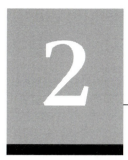

Wound assessment

Introduction

Wound assessment has traditionally been the responsibility of nursing staff and has had a tendency to be subjective, often relying on anecdotal evidence which frequently fails to report accurate information. If as nurses we are to be accountable for our actions, we need to base our delivery of care on informed and rational decisions. It is difficult to monitor the rate of wound healing or the effectiveness of prescribed care without using a holistic approach to wound management. This approach facilitates the assessment of the relationships between the patient, the wound and the treatment. Accurate wound assessment is dependent on an understanding of the physiology of healing and those factors that delay the process as well as the optimal conditions required at the wound surface to maximise healing. This section explores in some depth the complex activity of wound assessment and identifies the most important issues that need to be taken into consideration when assessing a patient's wound.

LEARNING OUTCOMES

When you have completed this section, you should be able to:

- describe the structure and function of the skin
- describe the normal physiological process of wound healing
- identify the optimal conditions required to promote wound healing
- describe the intrinsic and extrinsic factors that may delay wound healing
- evaluate the role of adequate nutritional support for patients with wounds
- discuss criteria for identifying clinical signs of infection in patients with both acute and chronic wounds
- describe the relevance of wound classification models in relation to clinical practice
- explain the relevance of specific wound assessment techniques for particular types of wounds
- discuss a variety of different methods of measuring and documenting wound healing rates.

2.1 THE PHYSIOLOGY OF THE SKIN

Introduction

The skin is the largest organ in the body. The skin of the average adult covers an area almost equivalent to 2 square metres, accounts for 15% of body weight and receives one-third of the body's circulating blood volume. Protection is one of its major homeostatic functions as the skin is constantly exposed to the external environment. The average pH of the skin is 5.5 (Roth & James 1988). Maintaining skin integrity is a complex process and one that is often taken for granted until damage occurs.

Self-assessment   2 MINUTES

How would you define a wound?

● ●

FEEDBACK

You should have said that a wound is an injury causing tissue damage, which may or may not result in loss of skin integrity.

Wounds are often classified depending on which structures of the skin are involved. Before considering wounds in more detail, we need to look at the skin itself and find out how it is structured.

● ●

Structure of the skin

The skin is divided into three layers of tissue (Fig. 2.1):

- epidermis
- dermis
- subcutaneous layer.

Epidermis

The epidermis is the outer layer of the skin; it is avascular and receives nutrients from the dermis directly underneath it. Despite having an average thickness

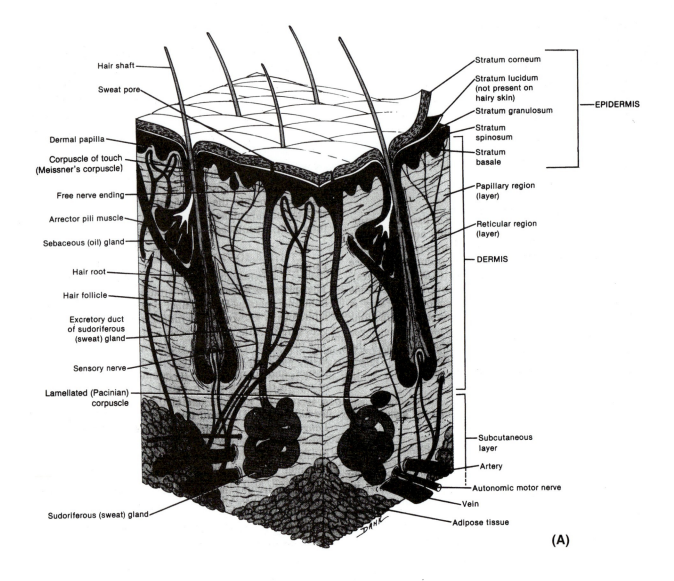

Hair shaft

Sweat pore

Dermal papilla

Corpuscle of touch
(Meissner's corpuscle)

Free nerve ending

Arrector pili muscle

Sebaceous (oil) gland

Hair root

Hair follicle

Excretory duct
of sudoriferous
(sweat) gland

Sensory nerve

Lamellated (Pacinian)
corpuscle

Sudoriferous (sweat) gland

Stratum corneum

Stratum lucidum
(not present on
hairy skin)

Stratum granulosum

Stratum
spinosum

Stratum
basale

EPIDERMIS

Papillary region
(layer)

Reticular region
(layer)

DERMIS

Subcutaneous
layer

Artery

Autonomic motor nerve

Vein

Adipose tissue

(A)

Hair shafts

EPIDERMIS

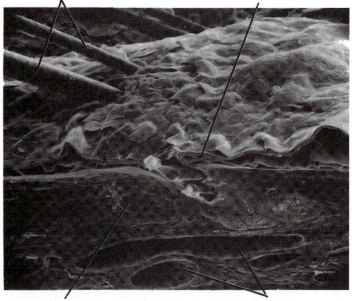

DERMIS

Blood vessels

(B)

Fig. 2.1 Skin: (A) structure of the skin; (B) scanning electron micrograph of the skin and several hairs at a magnification of × 260. (Reproduced with kind permission from Kessel R G, Kardon R H 1979 Tissues and organs: a text-atlas of scanning electron microscopy. In: Tortora G J, Anagnostakos N P 1987 Principles of anatomy and physiology, 5th edn. Harper & Row, New York, Fig 5.1)

of only 0.1 mm, the epidermis contains five different layers:

- the horny layer—stratum corneum
- the clear layer—stratum lucidum
- the granular layer—stratum granulosum
- the prickle cell layer—stratum spinosum
- the basal layer—stratum germinativum.

The horny layer

This is the surface layer of the skin composed of dead keratinocytes. These are thin, flattened cells filled with keratin, an insoluble protein that is resistant to changes in pH and temperature. This uppermost layer of cells constantly flakes off as a result of daily wear and tear caused by washing, scratching and friction.

The clear layer

This layer is only present in those areas of the body where the epidermis needs to be thicker, such as the palms of the hands and the soles of the feet, and serves a protective function. This layer is translucent and is made up of dead cells with no visible nuclei.

The granular layer

This layer lies directly beneath the clear layer if the latter is present; if not, it lies immediately underneath the horny layer. It is made up from dead granular cells that have not yet become flattened out.

The prickle cell layer

This layer contains living cells which replenish the cells of the layers above.

The basal layer

This is a single layer of living cells. The prickle layer and the basal layer together form the germinative layer that constantly produces new cells by the process of mitotic division. Once formed, these cells migrate upwards until they are eventually shed by the horny layer; in this way the entire epidermis is replaced approximately every 3 weeks in young adults. Melanocytes are also found in this layer. The size and distribution of these cells determine skin pigmentation.

The dermis

The dermis is firmly attached to the epidermis. It also can be divided into two layers:

- the papillary layer
- the reticular layer.

The papillary layer

This is primarily made up of connective tissue containing capillary loops, fine lymph vessels, nerve endings, temperature and touch receptors. Sebaceous glands, sweat glands and hair follicles are all specialised epidermal structures which lie within the dermis. Collagen and elastic fibres form a network giving the skin its tensile strength and elasticity. Some cells are able to move around the dermis within the confines of a gelatinous fluid matrix. These cells include fibroblasts and macrophages which play a major part in the process of wound healing (see p. 24).

The reticular layer

This is the base of the dermis. There is no clear division between the reticular and papillary layers, the main differences being that the size of the collagen fibres gradually increases and the vascular supply becomes more dense in the reticular layer.

The subcutaneous layer

This is the thickest layer and provides the main support for the skin. It is made up of adipose and connective tissue and blood vessels and forms a protective layer for the organs beneath.

Self-assessment   5 MINUTES

1. Name the two layers of the epidermis that are composed of living cells.
2. What is the name often given collectively to these two layers?
3. What is the main function of this collective layer?

FEEDBACK

1. You should have said that: the two layers of the epidermis composed of living cells are the prickle cell layer and the basal layer.
2. These two layers are often collectively termed the germinative layer.
3. The germinative layer continuously produces new cells, which are then pushed into the layers above where they die and are eventually sloughed off and replaced.

Functions of the skin

The skin has to perform many different functions which is why its structure is so complex. The functions of the skin are summarised in Box 2.1.

Box 2.1 Functions of the skin

Protection against
- Bacteria and viruses
- Cold, heat and radiation
- Chemical substances
- Mechanical damage
- Dehydration

Thermoregulatory control
- Secretion and evaporation of sweat
- Circulatory mechanisms—vasodilatation and constriction
- Insulation by adipose tissue and hair

Sensation
Nerve receptors are sensitive to:
- Pain
- Temperature
- Touch
- Pressure and vibration

Metabolism
- Synthesis of vitamin D
- Synthesis of melanin

Communication
- Facial expression
- Alterations in skin colour—blushing, pallor
- Secretion of pheromones
- Sensation of touching

- extremes of temperature
- invasion by microorganisms
- dehydration
- mechanical damage
- arterial insufficiency
- use of alkaline soaps.

The effects of ageing

There are many changes that occur as a result of ageing; those with the most significance in relation to wound healing are described below.

- The time taken for epidermal regeneration is increased from approximately 21 days in young adults to 40 days for those in their mid-30s.
- The barrier function of the skin is reduced.
- The inflammatory response is weakened. This and the preceding factor increase the likelihood of invasion by microorganisms and subsequent infection.
- Vascularity of the skin is diminished.
- Sensory perception is reduced.
- Elasticity and tensile strength of the skin is reduced.
- Sensitivity of skin can alter, increasing incidence of allergic contact dermatitis.

Causes of skin damage

Wound assessment must be underpinned with a thorough understanding of skin pathology, as wounding leads to a breakdown of the protective function of the skin. In addition you should be able to differentiate between different types of skin injury and relate this information to the appropriate treatment and prevention of skin damage.

2.2 Physiology of wound healing

Wound healing can be defined as the physiological processes by which the body replaces and restores function to damaged tissues. It is a complex series of events that are interlinked and dependent on one another. Appropriate wound assessment and subsequent management is based upon an understanding of the normal process of repair and the factors affecting this process.

Self-assessment   2 MINUTES

Suggest at least three factors that are known to damage the skin.

The process of wound healing

All tissues in the body are capable of healing. This occurs through two mechanisms.

- *Regeneration.* Damaged tissue is replaced by identical replication of cells. In humans complete regeneration is only possible in a limited number of cell types, e.g. epithelial, liver and nerve cells.
- *Repair.* Damaged tissue is replaced by connective tissue which then forms a scar. In man this is the main mechanism by which healing occurs.

FEEDBACK

There are many factors that damage the skin. You should have included some of the following:

- radiation, e.g. UV light
- chemicals

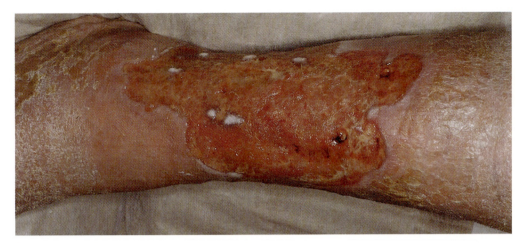

Plate 1 Venous leg ulcer (showing evidence of epithelialisation).

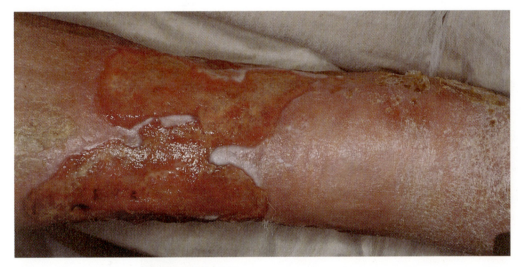

Plate 2 *(See Section 2, Self-assessment, p. 26.)*

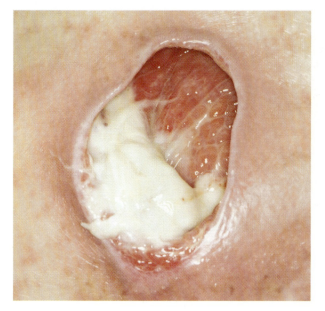

Plate 3 *(See Section 2, Activity, p. 36.)*

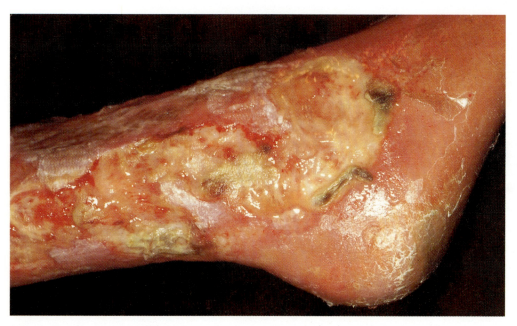

Plate 4 *(See Section 2, Activity, p. 36.)*

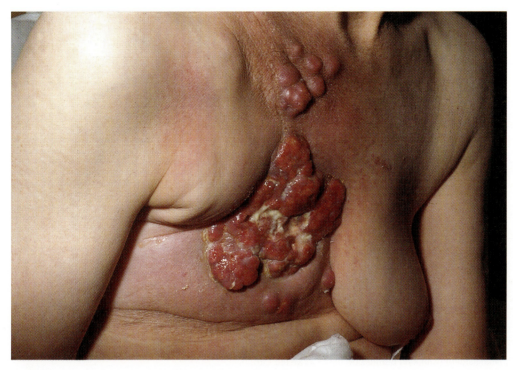

Plate 5 Mrs Williams: fungating breast wound.

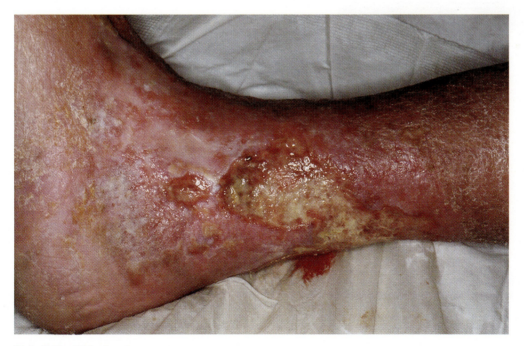

Plate 6 Mrs White: leg ulcer.

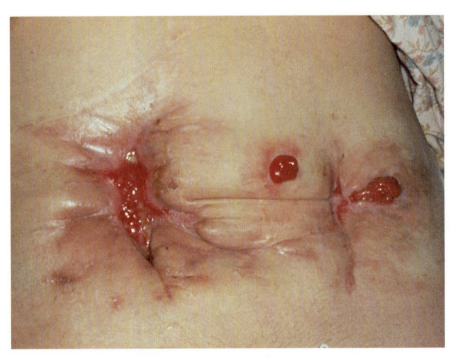

Plate 7 Mrs Edwards: abdominal fistulae (with kind permission from ConvaTec Ltd).

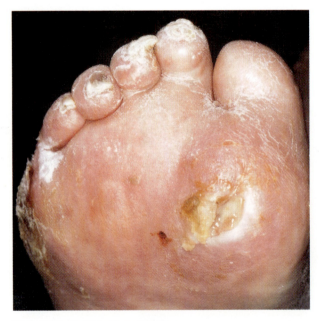

Plate 8 Mrs Patel: neuropathic ulcer.

In simplified terms, the process of wound healing can be divided into four phases:

- vascular response or homeostasis
- inflammation
- proliferation
- maturation.

These phases do not occur in isolation; there is considerable overlap between them and the time required by an individual to progress to the next phase is dependent on a multitude of factors (see Sect. 2.4). The stages of wound healing are illustrated in Figure 2.2.

The vascular response

Wounds involving anything more than the epidermis will immediately bleed. The damaged ends of blood vessels constrict seconds after injury in order to minimise blood flow and help to initiate the clotting process which is accelerated by platelet aggregation and the release of several growth factors required for wound repair. A blood clot is produced by a complex chain reaction called the coagulation cascade, which involves 13 different coagulation factors. The main constituent of a blood clot is a fibrin mesh which traps other blood cells. This gradually dries out to become a scab which temporarily closes the wound. At about the same time, vasodilatation of the vessels surrounding the wound begins to occur.

Inflammation

Tissue damage and the activation of clotting factors stimulate the release of various substances that cause local blood vessels to become more permeable and to dilate. This inflammatory reaction can be observed clinically by the presence locally of:

- erythema
- heat
- oedema
- discomfort
- functional disturbance.

These signs are due to increased blood flow to the area and the accumulation of fluid in the soft tissues. This eventually exerts pressure on sensory nerve endings, causing the wound to be uncomfortable. This combination of discomfort and swelling usually restricts the movement of the injured part. Inflammation is part of the normal protective response to injury and, although the clinical signs are similar, should not be confused with infection (see Sect. 2.6).

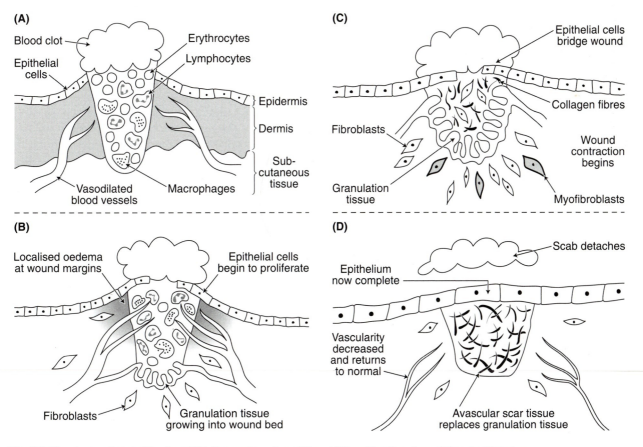

Fig. 2.2 The stages of wound healing: (A) inflammatory stage; (B) and (C) proliferation stage; (D) maturation stage.

Neutrophils are the first type of white blood cell to be attracted to the wound, usually arriving within a few hours of injury. They have a short life span, but provide initial protection against microorganisms as they are phagocytic and so engulf and digest foreign bodies. Monocytes are the second type of white blood cell to be attracted to the wound, owing to the release of growth factors. They too are capable of phagocytosis. As monocytes mature they develop into macrophages and play a vital role in the process of wound healing.

Macrophages produce a variety of substances that stimulate healing, including:

- transforming growth factors (TGF-α), TGF-β)—promote formation of new tissue and blood vessels
- tumour necrosing factor—facilitates the breakdown of necrotic tissue and tumours, stimulates growth of new tissues
- fibroblast growth factor—stimulates production of fibroblasts
- prostaglandins—promote the inflammatory response
- complement factors—mark invading foreign bodies.

The activity of macrophages and lymphocytes essentially cleanses the wound bed. The macrophage is usually present during all stages of wound healing. Studies have shown that absence of these cells at any phase significantly impairs healing rates (Riches 1988). In clean wounds the inflammatory phase lasts approximately 36 hours; in necrotic or infected wounds this process is prolonged.

The inflammatory phase is a vital stimulant to subsequent stages of wound healing. Patients who are immunosuppressed are often unable to produce a typical inflammatory response and therefore may fail to activate the normal process of healing.

Self-assessment   2 MINUTES

Identify two different reasons why patients may be immunosuppressed.

FEEDBACK

Reasons are many and varied, but can be summarised under the following groupings:

- immunological diseases—HIV, AIDS, rheumatoid diseases, e.g. rheumatoid arthritis, systemic lupus erythematosus

- immunosuppressive drugs—corticosteroids, non-steroidal anti-inflammatory drugs, transplant suppressors, cytotoxic drugs, e.g. methotrexate
- cancer treatments—radiotherapy
- advancing age.

Formation of new tissue in the wound bed will not occur until the macrophages have stimulated the release of growth factors and the wound bed has been cleaned by the inflammatory process.

Proliferation

During this phase the wound is filled with new connective tissue. The main processes involved are:

- granulation
- contraction
- epithelialisation.

Granulation

Granulation or angiogenesis is the term given to the formation of new capillary growth in the wound bed which in turn supports the development of new connective tissue. Angiogenesis is activated by tissue hypoxia resulting from the disruption of blood flow at the time of injury. Formation of new capillaries from the vessel walls of existing capillaries starts to occur within 36 hours of initial damage. Growth factors released by macrophages stimulate endothelial cells lining the walls of capillaries close to the wounded area, which then divide and branch out to form new capillary loops. This process continues until newly formed granulation tissue joins up with existing non-damaged blood vessels to form a network of vessels that fill the wound bed. Granulation tissue is so called because the appearance of healthy granulation tissue in the base of a wound is granular and slightly uneven. The condition of granulation tissue is often a good indicator of how the wound is healing. Table 2.1 summarises characteristics of healthy and unhealthy granulation tissue.

At the same time as granulation tissue formation, new connective tissue is produced. Fibroblasts

Table 2.1 Healthy and unhealthy granulation tissue

Healthy granulation tissue	Unhealthy granulation tissue
Bright red	Dark red or bluish discoloration or very pale
Moist	Dehydrated
Shiny	Dull
Does not bleed easily	Bleeds easily

> **Box 2.2** Types of healing
>
> **Primary intention**
> The edges of the wound are brought together and held in approximation by a variety of methods including; sutures, skin tapes, clips or staples. Suitable wounds are clean, simple wounds that have minimal tissue loss. They usually heal quickly without complications.
>
> **Secondary intention**
> This describes wounds in which it would be difficult to bring the skin edges together successfully, i.e. wounds with extensive tissue loss or large surface areas. These wounds are left open and heal more slowly through the combined processes of granulation, contraction and re-epithelialisation.

attracted by the release of fibroblast growth factor start to divide and collect at the wound margin. Fibroblasts are stimulated to produce collagen fibres, a process that is dependent on an adequate intake of vitamin C, iron and copper from the diet. Newly formed collagen fibres have a gel-like consistency and gradually mature to form cross-links which eventually provide tensile strength to the wound.

In wounds healing by primary intention (Box 2.2), collagen formation usually reaches its peak at approximately 6 or 7 days, although collagen production will continue for some time after this. In sutured wounds only a small amount of collagen is actually required to repair the wound. Collagen is produced at the same time as new epithelial cells are formed along the surface of the wound. Granulation occurs deep within the wound and is not visible because the wound edges are already closed. In open wounds healing by secondary intention (Box 2.2), a great deal more collagen is required to fill the wound defect. The more tissue that has been lost and the larger the wound, the longer it will take for this process of repair, which is particularly dependent on the patient's nutritional and vascular status.

Contraction

After the process of connective tissue production is complete, fibroblasts transform into either myofibroblasts or fibrocytes. Myofibroblasts congregate around the wound margin and are able to contract, pulling the edges of the wound together so that the size of the wound area is reduced. The amount of contraction possible in a particular wound depends on its anatomical location and the degree of mobility of the surrounding tissue. Sacral pressure sores occur in mobile areas that are usually well supported by the presence of subcutaneous tissue, but wounds situated over bony prominences such as the trochanter are not able to contract easily and will require the growth of more granulation tissue in order to heal satisfactorily. Contraction does not occur in sutured wounds where there is minimal tissue loss, but does play a significant part in the healing of large open wounds healing by secondary intention.

The process of contraction speeds up the healing of wounds because it reduces the amount of scar tissue required to fill the defect.

Epithelialisation

The growth of new epithelial cells across the surface of the wound occurs during the final stages of healing. This process is very delicate and is dependent on a variety of preconditions (see p. 27). In wounds healing by primary intention, stimulation of new epithelial cell growth takes place at the same time as collagen synthesis and in open wounds once the formation of granulation tissue has begun to fill the wound bed. In wounds healing by secondary intention, only when the surface of the wound bed is filled with newly formed, healthy granulation tissue and is approximately level with the surrounding non-damaged skin, will the process of re-epithelialisation begin. This explains why a cavity wound can take several months to fill with granulation tissue, its circumference remaining relatively constant until the wound bed becomes shallow when suddenly, owing to rapid epithelialisation, the wound can quickly reduce in size and heal. New epithelial cells originate from either the wound margin or from remnants of hair follicles, sebaceous or sweat glands because these structures are lined with cells which are capable of regeneration. They divide and migrate along the surface of the granulation tissue until they form a continuous layer of cells and close the wound. Newly formed epithelial cells have a translucent appearance and are usually whitish-pink in colour. They can often be seen on the surface of open, clean, granulating wounds at the wound margin and/or as small islands on the wound surface, originating from hair follicles or similar skin structures (see Plate 1, between pp. 22 and 23). The optimal conditions for epidermal migration are described on page 27.

In full-thickness wounds, epidermal regeneration only occurs from the wound margin because hair follicles and sweat glands have already been destroyed. If the wound is large, this presents additional difficulties as there is a limit to the extent that epithelial cells can migrate; for these reasons large wounds healing by the process of secondary intention often require skin grafting.

Maturation

This is the final stage of wound healing. It begins when the wound has been closed by connective tissue and epithelialisation and continues in some instances for up to 1 year or longer. At first the scar is raised and is reddish in colour. Remodelling of the scar is stimulated by macrophages and results in the reorganisation of collagen fibres to form a scar with maximum tensile strength. The tensile strength of scar tissue is never more than 80% of that of non-wounded skin. Remodelling can be influenced to some extent by the application of compression, which can reduce build-up of scar formation and produce better cosmetic results. This phase will be severely disrupted by either hypoxia or malnutrition which may result in wound breakdown. As the scar tissue matures, its blood supply decreases; as a result the scar becomes flatter, paler and smoother. Mature scar tissue is avascular and contains no hairs, sebaceous or sweat glands. The formation of keloids and hypertrophic scars are abnormalities of this stage of healing. They are thick mounds of scar tissue characterised by excessive production of collagen. Keloids differ from hypertrophic scars in that they continue to grow and spread for years after initial scar formation and are able to invade the surrounding healthy skin beyond the wound margin. Hypertrophic scars occur soon after trauma, whilst the onset of keloids is usually gradual. Those with darker pigmented skin are more susceptible to both keloid and hypertrophic scar formation than fairer skinned individuals.

Self-assessment | 5 MINUTES

Make a list of the different ways in which the macrophage helps in the process of wound healing.

FEEDBACK

Macrophages control the process of wound healing by producing:

- prostaglandins which promote the inflammatory response
- transforming growth factors which stimulate new tissue and capillary formation
- tumour necrosing factor which breaks down devitalised tissue
- fibroblast growth factor which stimulates the production of fibroblasts
- complement factors which help to inactivate foreign bodies.

They also:

- cleanse the wound surface by digesting bacteria and cellular debris
- stimulate the remodelling of scar tissue.

The normal process of wound healing ensures that the majority of wounds heal quickly and without complication. However, our nursing skills are often challenged by those patients with non-healing chronic wounds which can have a profound effect on the lives of the individuals, their families and friends. Application of our knowledge of wound healing to the practical problems encountered when caring for patients with complex wounds will maximise the effectiveness of treatment interventions.

Self-assessment | 10 MINUTES

Carefully examine the wound illustrated in Plates 1 and 2 (between pp. 22 and 23). Using only your observation skills, decide whether this wound is healing healthily or not. Justify your decision.

FEEDBACK

This leg ulcer demonstrates signs of healthy healing (see Plates 1 and 2).

- The granulation tissue appears to be moist and red with no evidence of fresh bleeding.
- The wound bed is clean and free from necrotic tissue or areas of dry eschar.
- There is evidence of active epithelialisation seen as whitish-pink areas at the wound margin and as small islands of tissue on the wound surface.

Clinical observation skills play a fundamental part in the process of wound assessment. A great deal of information can be gained about the status of wound healing and will vary depending on the type and location of a particular wound and the amount of experience that the observer has.

Activity | 10 MINUTES

What else may you be able to tell about the progress of healing by careful observation of the wound at dressing change as part of your regular reassessment of the patient's condition?

FEEDBACK

Careful observation of a wound at each dressing change can help to identify subtle changes which may indicate the presence of:

- prolonged inflammatory response
- wound infection
- necrotic tissue
- unhealthy granulation tissue
- delayed epithelialisation
- skin maceration
- skin sensitivities and allergies.

2.3 PROVISION OF OPTIMAL ENVIRONMENT FOR HEALING

Introduction

There are many factors locally at the surface of the wound that directly influence the rate of healing.

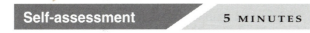

Self-assessment   5 MINUTES

Describe the four stages of wound healing.

FEEDBACK

The normal mechanism for healing consists of the following stages: the vascular response, the inflammatory phase, the proliferative phase and the maturation phase.

Environmental influences on wound healing

The rate at which a wound heals is dependent on two main factors:

- local conditions
- general conditions.

We will look at local conditions in the rest of this subsection.

Local conditions for optimal wound healing

The provision of a supportive microenvironment at the wound surface is known to be of utmost importance when trying to maximise the healing potential of a wound (Winter 1962). The maintenance of a controlled set of local conditions that is able to sustain the complex cellular activity present in wound healing is one of the fundamental aims of wound management. In recent years it has been widely acknowledged that control of these factors can significantly reduce the time that it takes a wound to heal. The methods used by health professionals to manage wounds should not interfere with or disrupt the delicate physiological process of wound healing. Wound cleansing and dressing techniques therefore must maintain as close an optimal environment as possible in order to maximise the wound's healing potential.

Provision of a moist environment

Delicate epithelial cells remain viable for longer and are able to migrate more easily across the surface of a moist wound environment (Winter 1962). The work of Winter demonstrated for the first time that moist wounds healed more rapidly than those that were left exposed to the air or covered with traditional dry dressings. The progress of epithelial migration is significantly slowed in the presence of either necrotic or desiccated tissue, as epithelial cells are forced to burrow underneath the scab or eschar which forms a mechanical obstruction in the wound bed. Eaglstein (1985) reported a 40% increase in epithelial migration rates in wounds which were kept moist. Wound exudate contains a variety of nutrients and growth factors that facilitate wound healing and also has antimicrobial properties (Holn et al 1977). Exudate production, which is most prolific during the inflammatory phase of healing, bathes the wound with these nutrients and actively cleanses the wound surface. However, excessive exudate production can cause skin sensitivities in susceptible individuals and may cause maceration of the surrounding skin. Figure 2.3 illustrates the fine balance between moisture and dehydration at the wound surface required to optimise healing.

Provision of a warm environment

The phagocytic and mitotic activity of cells within a wound is sensitive to fluctuations in temperature and is significantly slowed down at extremes of temperature. Following wound cleansing it can take up to 40 minutes for the wound to reach its optimal temperature and a further 3 hours for mitotic and leukocyte activity to return to normal (Myers 1982).

The actions described below are all known to affect the temperature of the wound bed:

- cleaning the wound with cold cleansing solutions
- exposing the wound for longer than necessary when applying a new dressing

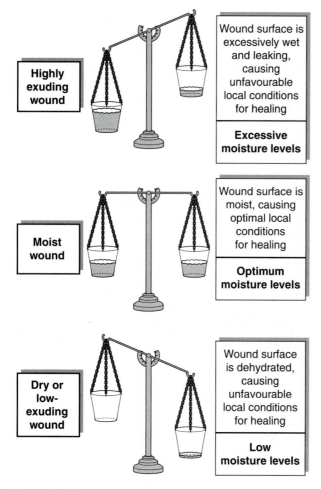

Fig. 2.3 Relationship between moisture levels at the wound surface and potential healing rates.

- changing the dressing more frequently than necessary
- leaving the wound exposed and without the protection of a dressing.

Provision of an oxygenated environment

The role of oxygen in wound healing is complex and is not fully understood. It appears that the role of oxygen in the healing of epidermal and connective tissue may be significantly different (Silver 1972). Angiogenesis and the growth of new granulation tissue is stimulated by tissue hypoxia in the wound bed, whilst the division and replication of epithelial cells is increased in an oxygen-rich environment. Macrophages can function in both aerobic and anaerobic conditions, but are much less effective at destroying bacteria in a hypoxic environment. Further studies are required to determine the significance of this in clinical practice.

Provision of an acidic environment

Current evidence suggests that reducing the pH of wound exudate may help to improve healing rates and reduce likelihood of infection (Wilson 1979), possibly as a result of increased oxygen availability (Leveen 1973).

Answer true or false to the following statements. Briefly justify your decision.

1. Dry scabs effectively protect the wound and promote healing.
2. Epithelial migration proceeds faster in a moist environment.
3. The temperature of a wound affects the rate of wound healing.
4. Oxygen is always essential to stimulate the growth of granulation tissue.
5. Exudate production is always beneficial for wound healing.

FEEDBACK

1. False—dry scabs or necrotic material form a mechanical barrier on the wound surface causing newly formed epithelial cells to burrow underneath in an attempt to bridge the wound surface.
2. True—moisture facilitates this process by providing conditions in which epithelial cells can slide easily across the surface of the wound.
3. True—extremes of temperature at the wound bed will reduce the rate at which cells both divide and destroy bacteria by the process of phagocytosis.
4. False—a hypoxic environment stimulates the growth of new blood vessels in the base of a wound, whilst an oxygen-rich environment increases the rate of epithelial division.
5. False—excessive exudate production can prolong healing by causing skin sensitivities and maceration.

Provision of the optimal healing environment in the clinical setting

There are several practical considerations that need to be remembered when trying to provide the optimal environment for wound healing. The most significant have been related to the four stages of wound healing and are described below:

The vascular response. Wounds at this stage of healing require irrigating with a non-toxic cleansing solution and covering with a low-adherent dressing which should be applied using firm pressure. The rationale for these actions is to be able to visualise the wounded area and to remove surface contaminants. Application of a dressing helps to promote clot formation and vasoconstriction of bleeding capillaries.

The inflammatory response. During this phase of healing it is important to ensure that any dressing is not too constrictive and to consider patient analgesia as tissues can become very oedematous. Dressings require changing when their absorptive capacity has been reached in order to minimise skin maceration and potential wound infection. Dressings and swabbing materials should be avoided that leave fibres in the wound bed as foreign bodies prolong the inflammatory response and delay healing. Care should be taken to minimise time taken at dressing change and warm cleansing solutions should be used as macrophages are sensitive to fluctuations in temperature.

The proliferative phase. The wound surface only requires cleansing if excessively sloughy, in order to minimise disturbances to granulation tissue. Application of a low-adherent dressing is required to provide favourable conditions for growth of granulation tissue. Warm cleansing solutions should be used and the wound kept covered in order to minimise temperature fluctuations at the wound surface.

The maturation phase. This phase occurs once the surface of the wound has closed over; therefore at this stage of healing the main requirement is for protection of newly formed epithelial tissue. Dressings may be used to provide extra protection particularly in those patients with fragile skin.

Self-assessment — 2 MINUTES

Answer true or false to the following statements.

1. Application of a dressing during the vascular response helps to promote clot formation and vasoconstriction of bleeding capillaries.
2. In the inflammatory response stage, cool cleansing solutions should be used as macrophages are sensitive to high temperatures.
3. The wound surface requires regular cleansing during the proliferative phase of healing.
4. In the maturation stage, wound margins and surrounding skin require protection against drying out in order to provide favourable conditions for epithelial migration and wound contraction.

FEEDBACK

Your answers should have been as follows:

1. true
2. false
3. false
4. true.

2.4 FACTORS AFFECTING WOUND HEALING

Introduction

Most wounds heal quickly and without incident, whilst a few for a variety of complex and interrelated reasons fail to heal. Research into the process of wound healing identifies many factors that significantly delay healing; in many instances the exact mechanism of delayed wound healing is not well understood and requires further study.

Nurses are in a unique position within the multidisciplinary team to assess patients' wounds and their rates of healing and need to take into account the subtle interrelationships between the physical and psychosocial influences affecting wound healing. A delicate balance must be maintained during the process of wound healing in order to promote the repair of damaged tissue. Wounds will be slower to heal when less than favourable conditions exist. Some of these conditions can be identified and corrected; some cannot.

Factors that delay healing

An awareness of the factors that influence wound healing is vital in order to develop realistic treatment objectives for individual patients' wounds.

Activity — 10 MINUTES

List as many factors as you can that you think influence wound healing. Try to think from as broad a perspective as possible. Two examples to start you off might be necrotic tissue and the location of the wound.

FEEDBACK

Now read through the rest of this sub-section which describes the many and varied factors that may delay healing. It starts by reviewing local factors which

Table 2.2 Local factors influencing the rate of healing at the wound site

Local influences	Rationale
Impaired blood supply	Disturbances to the peripheral blood supply will reduce tissue perfusion limiting the local supply of oxygen and other nutrients required for tissue repair
Oxygen deficit	Hypoxia stimulates angiogenesis, but adequate oxygenation is required at the wound margin. Reduced oxygen levels impair collagen synthesis and epithelial growth and lower tissue resistance to infection by lessening phagocytic activity of leukocytes
Temperature fluctuations	Mitotic activity of cells occurs most rapidly at body temperature. Extremes of temperature cause tissue damage
Dehydration	Epithelialisation, granulation and wound contraction all occur at a faster rate in a moist rather than dry wound environment
Wound location	Position of a wound affects its vascularity and will also determine the mobility of the wound site. Wounds on or close to joints are slower to heal
Age of wound	Chronic wounds by definition are slow to heal. Prolonged healing times always require further investigation
Mechanical stress	Mechanical stress delays healing by prolonging tissue damage. Pressure, shear and friction may be caused by poor lifting or bandaging techniques
Extent of tissue loss	Large, deep wounds with extensive tissue loss heal slowly. Healing by secondary intention requires more tissue regeneration than healing by primary intention or epithelialisation. Irregular, contused wound margins and the presence of a fistula or sinus in a wound delay healing
Local infection	Wound infection prolongs the inflammatory phase of healing, causes further tissue damage, delays collagen synthesis and epithelialisation
Type of tissue involvement	The presence of muscle, fascia, tendon or bone within a wound usually delays healing as these tissues have slower healing rates
Foreign bodies	Foreign bodies cause tissue irritation, prolong the inflammatory response and can potentiate infection. Commonly occurring foreign bodies include remnants of suture and dressing material, bone fragments and necrotic tissue.
Necrotic tissue	In addition to the effects described above, necrotic tissue, dry scabs and excess slough impede epithelial migration and impair the supply of nutrients to the wound bed
Skin maceration	If wound margins are exposed to excess moisture from exudate, sweat or incontinence, damage to the surrounding skin can occur. This may predispose to infection, skin sensitivities and irritation
Surgical technique	Excessive handling of tissues, tight skin closure materials and inadequate wound drainage can all delay wound healing

potentially prolong wound healing (Table 2.2) and finishes by exploring some of the psychological and lifestyle influences on healing rates. When you have finished check your original list, identifying any areas that you overlooked.

● ●

General physical condition

The general health status of individuals will obviously have a direct influence on their ability to heal quickly. Chronic diseases affect wound healing in a multitude of different ways. Conditions resulting in reduced tissue perfusion, metabolic disturbances or malabsorption syndromes will contribute to delayed healing and need to be anticipated when planning care. Ill health also has the cumulative negative effects of reducing appetite, increasing patient anxiety and increasing the possibility of taking drugs that may prolong wound healing.

There are many chronic disease processes that prolong healing rates. The most common are summarised in Box 2.3.

Self-assessment   **5 MINUTES**

List as many conditions as possible that delay wound healing by reducing the oxygen supply to a wound and give the reason for your choice.

Box 2.3 Chronic disease processes that prolong healing rates

Circulatory disorders
- Anaemias
- Peripheral vascular disease
- Arteriosclerosis

Respiratory disorders
- Chronic obstructive airway disease
- Bronchitis
- Pneumonia

Malabsorption disorders
- Crohn's disease
- Ulcerative colitis

Metabolic disorders
- Diabetes
- Renal and hepatic failure

Disorders of mobility and sensation
- Hemiplegia—CVA
- Paraplegia
- Neuropathy

Immune deficiency disorders
- Rheumatoid arthritis
- HIV, AIDS
- Malignancy

FEEDBACK

The most commonly occurring conditions that limit the amount of available oxygen to the wound bed are:

- all types of anaemia—owing to a reduction in the oxygen-carrying capacity of red blood corpuscles
- arteriosclerosis, peripheral vascular disease, rheumatoid arthritis, diabetes—owing to defective functioning of the peripheral circulation
- respiratory diseases (COAD, bronchitis, pneumonia, congestive cardiac failure) —owing to reduced efficiency of gaseous exchange
- shock and haemorrhage—owing to rapid peripheral shutdown and reduced tissue perfusion.

General factors that may prolong healing

The normal process of wound healing is a complex physiological activity. A variety of factors can have a detrimental affect on the rates of healing and include:

Nutritional state. Proteins, fats, carbohydrates, vitamins and minerals all play a fundamental role in the process of wound repair and are required to produce collagen and connective tissue.

Dehydration. Dehydration and resultant electrolyte imbalance impair cellular function and may be markedly increased if wound drainage is significant, e.g. burns, fistulae.

Body build. Extremes of body build can influence healing rates. Cachexia and anorexia are indicative of poor nutritional status. Obesity can exert considerable tension on the wound, reducing the effect of contraction and increasing the likelihood of dehiscence.

Systemic infection. Infection makes additional demands on the inflammatory response and disrupts fibroblast activity.

Stress. Anxiety causes the release of glucocorticoids, which have anti-inflammatory effects and inhibit fibroblasts, collagen synthesis and formation of granulation tissue.

Immunosuppressive agents. Consequences of radiotherapy and chemotherapy include inhibition of cellular division and suppression of cell growth. Irradiated skin is prone to loss of vascularity, ulceration and atrophy.

Drug therapy. Anti-inflammatory drugs, cytotoxic agents, immunosuppressive agents and anticoagulants all reduce healing rates by interrupting either cellular division or the clotting process.

Lack of sleep/rest. Tissue repair and rate of cellular division are enhanced by sleep. Healing of wounds particularly near joints will benefit from the reduction in tension and physical stress that occurs when resting.

Ageing. Increasing age reduces activity of fibroblasts. Wound contraction and epithelialisation is slower. The immune system becomes less efficient, reducing resistance to infection, and the likelihood of chronic disease increases.

Inappropriate wound care. Inaccurate assessment and diagnosis, inappropriate selection of wound management products, failure to evaluate care and inadequate pain control all result in delayed healing.

Factitious injury. Patients may cause further injury to their wounds for a variety of reasons including self-abuse, confusional states, lack of understanding, or extreme skin irritation.

Psychological influences on wound healing

The relationship between health and psychological status is well recognised. The patient's psychological well-being has both direct and indirect effects on the rate of wound healing. These factors can be particularly important when caring for patients with chronic or complex wounds such as fungating lesions.

Motivation. Motivation of patients and carers influences treatment compliance. Poorly motivated patients may lack the ability to continue with recommended treatments. Patient motivation is directly influenced by attitudes of carers; fear, guilt and denial all have powerful effects.

Compliance. Compliance is affected by many factors including the length of time the wound has been present, success of previous treatments, the patient's health beliefs and confidence in professional carers.

Attitudes of patients and carers. Chronic wounds are often associated with feelings of helplessness and low expectations. A positive attitude towards the wound and its treatment can do much to promote healing.

Knowledge and understanding. Knowledge of patients and carers directly influences both the acceptance of the wound and its subsequent treatment. Failure to implement research-based practice may be due to lack of awareness.

Body image. Distortions of body image can result from all types of wounds and affect people of all ages.

Lifestyle influences on wound healing

The presence of most wounds will affect a person's lifestyle in some way or other. At least, this may be a minor inconvenience; at most, the wound may severely disrupt daily activities of living. Another aspect of this problem is the influence that the patient's environment may have on the rate of wound healing.

Lifestyle. Working patterns can influence care, e.g. need for infrequent dressing changes. Hobbies, e.g. sport and exercise, make specific demands on types of dressings.

Care environment. Considerations include: whether care is in hospital or the community; access to members of the health care team; availability of support from professional or lay carers; availability of wound care products and equipment.

Financial status. This influences living conditions, e.g. provision of a balanced diet, and the ability to afford care and specific treatments, e.g. prescription costs. Worries about financial status and stress are directly interrelated.

Cultural/religious beliefs. These may have a direct influence on diet, fasting, washing and uptake of medical intervention and technologies.

Substance abuse. Smoking, alcohol and drug dependency can all negatively affect healing. Excessive abuse leads to an impaired general physical condition owing to inadequate nutritional intake. Nicotine narrows the peripheral circulation, reducing tissue perfusion of the wounded area. Smokers also often have a deficiency of vitamin C which is an essential factor required for tissue regeneration.

Major life stressors. Bereavement, separation and unemployment may have a cumulative negative effect due to anxiety, depression, lack of sleep and loss of appetite. Psychological stress has been shown to reduce healing rates by interfering with the body's immune system (Pediani 1992).

Activity   **45** MINUTES

Select a patient for whom you are currently caring. Read through his or her nursing and medical notes, identifying as many factors as possible that may potentially delay healing (allow 35 min).

When you have completed this activity, discuss this patient with your colleagues and add any factors that you had omitted (allow 10 min).

2.5 PRINCIPLES OF NUTRITIONAL ASSESSMENT

Introduction

Wound healing depends on adequate nutrition. When malnutrition occurs, the normal physiological process of healing is prolonged and a weaker wound is the end result. Patients with complex wounds are at great risk of malnutrition due to increased metabolic needs, increased loss of nutrients and inadequate dietary intake resulting from loss of interest and appetite. Patients at particular risk are those who have undergone major trauma with extensive tissue loss, or those with wounds producing excessive exudate such as fistulae and burns.

Activity   **25** MINUTES

After reading Article 2 in the Reader (p. 139), in which McLaren describes the role that essential nutrients have in the promotion of normal wound healing, complete the following table.

Local and metabolic effects of nutrition in injury	
Nutrients	*Effect on wound healing*
Glucose and carbohydrates	
Fats (fatty acids)	
Protein	
Zinc	
Iron	
Vitamin C	

FEEDBACK

The local and metabolic effects of nutrition in injured patients are given in Table 2.3.

Nutritional support

The general aims of nutritional support for wounded patients include:

1. to maintain the patient's body mass
2. to maintain the body's organ function

Table 2.3 Effects of different nutrients on wound healing	
Nutrients	*Effect on wound healing*
Glucose and carbohydrates	Provide energy after injury for the production of factors which stimulate fibroblast growth and collagen synthesis
Fats (fatty acids)	Important source of energy for cells. Are required for normal functioning of cell membranes and for formation of prostaglandins which have an anti-inflammatory action
Protein	Depletion delays collagen synthesis, markedly reducing tensile strength of wounds and interrupts normal formation of granulation tissue together with remodelling of scar tissue
Zinc	An essential cofactor for the activity of enzymes concerned with protein synthesis, carbohydrate and fat metabolism. Zinc has antibacterial properties. Deficiency will also depress the normal immune response, increasing likelihood of wound infection
Iron	Deficiency disturbs wound healing through reduced oxygen transport. Iron is also a cofactor for enzymes concerned with collagen synthesis
Vitamin C	Deficiency increases risk of wound dehiscence and increases the fragility of granulation tissue. Vitamin C is another vital cofactor for enzymes concerned with collagen synthesis and can help to limit tissue damage caused by the release of oxygen free radicals during the inflammatory response

3. to support and promote wound healing and tissue repair
4. to minimise or eliminate complications associated with malnutrition and delayed wound healing.

Activity   10 MINUTES

Refer back to Article 2 in the Reader and briefly summarise those factors that should be taken into consideration when planning nutritional support for an injured patient.

FEEDBACK

The planning of nutritional support should be from a multidisciplinary perspective and should consider the following:

- How nutritionally depleted is the patient?
- Assessment of the patient's nutritional requirements, which are dependent on metabolic status, extent and nature of injury, presence of systemic or localised wound infection.
- Assessment of the patient's fluid and electrolyte balance.
- How is nutritional support to be administered? This is dependent on the functional status of the gastrointestinal tract.
- How will nutritional content be monitored and evaluated throughout treatment?
- What is the patient's prognosis and capacity for recovery?

Assessment of nutritional state

Eating is a very important social, cultural and psychological experience which is influenced by a variety of factors. The impact of such influences should be borne in mind when attempting to make an assessment of nutritional balance. There is no single method of accurately determining an individual's nutritional status, so a combination of approaches is used, including collection of information from patient histories and physical examinations, anthropometric and biochemical data.

Activity   10 MINUTES

Referring once again to Article 2, list the most commonly used methods of assessing a patient's nutritional status.

FEEDBACK

Frequently used methods of assessing nutritional status are:

- dietary history and surveys
- physical examination
  —weight loss
  —muscle wasting
  —oedema
  —signs of vitamin deficiency
- anthropometric indices
  —skin fold thickness
  —limb muscle circumference
- biochemical analysis
  —plasma proteins, commonly albumin
  —nitrogen balance and creatinine clearance
  —full blood count—haemoglobin and lymphocyte counts.

Influences on the intake of nutrients

In the clinical setting there are many reasons why the nutritional intake of patients may be affected. Such reasons may be due to organisational constraints, psychological factors, or anorexia either resulting from the disease process or associated with particular treatment or therapy regimes.

Activity   10 MINUTES

List those factors in your own working environment that may influence the nutritional intake of your patients.

FEEDBACK

Some are general points irrespective of the care environment, whilst others are specific to the environment in which you work.

General factors influencing nutritional status

- Loss of appetite.
- Lack of interest in food.
- Lack of knowledge of adequate nutritional requirements.
- Lack of supervision of meal choices and intake.
- Inability to feed oneself.

- Badly fitting or absent dentures.
- Poor oral hygiene.
- Individual cultural/religious beliefs.
- Carers' lack of nutritional assessment skills.
- Failure to refer patients early for specialist advice.
- Shortage of available specialist advice.

Specific factors influencing nutritional status

- Community setting:
  —financial status of individual
  —inability to shop and prepare food
  —inadequate cooking and preparation facilities.
- Hospital/institutional setting:
  —budgetary allocation for meals
  —poor presentation of meals
  —treatment restrictions, i.e. nil-by-mouth.

Activity   5 MINUTES

Re-read the activity on page 32 and add any more factors which impair healing.

2.6 IDENTIFYING CLINICALLY INFECTED WOUNDS

Introduction

Wound infection prolongs the inflammatory phase of healing, often causes distress and discomfort for the patient and is a commonly occurring clinical problem contributing to delayed wound healing. However, evidence suggests that many health professionals experience difficulty when diagnosing wound infection. An objective approach is required to help differentiate between colonised and infected wounds.

The significance of bacteria within a wound

All chronic wounds contain large numbers of bacteria (Gilcrest & Reid 1989). Bacterial colonisation is not of any clinical significance and should not be confused with a clinical diagnosis of wound infection. The definition of surgical wound infection is that the wound contains more than 10^6 bacteria per gram of tissue (Robson & Heggers 1984); however, many chronic wounds contain much higher numbers of bacteria, up to 10^8 per gram of tissue without visible signs of infection (Lookingbill et al 1978). The presence of slough or bacteria in a wound therefore does not necessarily indicate that the wound is infected. Bacteria within a wound are transient and a single bacteriological sample alone is not able to indicate whether the bacterial count is rising or falling. Therefore the established practice of diagnosing wound infection by isolating bacteria in the wound bed from a single bacteriological swab is inadequate and misleading (Peel & Taylor 1992).

Ayton (1985) defines the significance of bacteria within wounds as follows:

- *Contamination:* the presence of bacteria without multiplication.
- *Colonisation:* the presence of bacteria with multiplication, but no host reaction.
- *Infection:* the presence of bacteria with multiplication and an associated host reaction.

The response of individual patients to the presence of bacteria within their wounds varies from person to person. Factors determining the effects of bacterial multiplication on the surrounding tissue are as yet unclear, but critical factors include the number, type and virulence of invading organisms. The term 'host reaction' describes the variety of different signs and symptoms that may occur in clinical practice once bacteria overwhelm the body's normal healing process.

Pathogenic microorganisms prolong wound healing in several ways.

- They are invasive and destroy cells by competing for available oxygen supplies within the wound.
- They release toxins that damage tissue locally, causing necrosis and pus formation.
- They release toxins into the bloodstream that cause toxaemia.

Infected wounds are often caused by a mixture of bacterial species, although one pathogen may predominate. If the infection is not immediately controlled by the immune response, exhausted phagocytic white blood cells, necrotic cellular debris and proliferating bacteria collect to form slough or pus, the characteristics of which are determined by the predominant pathogen. Pus formation is one of the many signs and symptoms commonly associated with a host reaction (Table 2.4).

Assessing wound infection

It is fundamental to establish whether or not the patient is responding clinically to the presence of a pathogen within the wound (Ayliffe et al 1992). Any factors causing immunosuppression will influence a patient's ability to respond classically to the presence of infective organisms. Elderly patients and babies may present with generalised septicaemia

Table 2.4 Clinical signs of bacterial infection of wounds			
Type of infection	Characteristics	Type of organism	Clinical signs
Pyogenic	Heavy pus formation	Staphylococci Streptococci Escherichia coli Pseudomonas aeruginosa	Creamy yellow pus Pus and extensive cellulitis Faecally offensive pus Blue/green offensive pus
Putrid	Cellular destruction	Proteus vulgaris	Tissue breakdown and production of offensive odour
Anaerobic	Production of highly potent life-threatening toxins	Clostridium tetani	Toxins rapidly cause skeletal muscle spasm and convulsions
		Clostridium perfringens	Rapid tissue oedema and necrosis Watery, offensive exudate

without any localised evidence of wound infection. Clinicians may also fail to discriminate between the normal inflammatory response and the presence of infection, which further complicates accurate assessment of clinical wound infections.

Self-assessment   5 MINUTES

List four reasons why the diagnosis of wound infection can be a difficult clinical decision to make.

FEEDBACK

You should have mentioned the following.

1. The normal signs of inflammation present in the early stages of wound healing may be confused with the clinical signs of infection.
2. The clinical significance of bacterial presence in a wound may not be fully understood, so that the distinction between colonised, contaminated and infected wounds is not made.
3. Patients with a low white cell count who are immunosuppressed may not demonstrate any of the classical signs of either inflammation or infection and have 'silent infections' which are difficult to detect.

Other reasons could include:

- lack of consensus as to what constitute criteria for determining wound infection
- overreliance on bacteriological swabs or misinterpretation of their results
- overreliance on the presence or absence of specific diagnostic criteria such as pus formation.

Activity   20 MINUTES

Referring to Plates 3 and 4 (between pp. 22 and 23), identify which of the wounds is infected. Give reasons for your decision.

FEEDBACK

The wound in Plate 3 is a sacral pressure sore which extends into the subcutaneous tissue. Approximately 50% of this wound is covered by a dense sloughy material, the remaining 50% is filled with clean, well-perfused, healthy granulation tissue.

From the evidence presented in this photograph, this wound is unlikely to be infected. The surrounding slough, although firmly adherent, is not impeding the growth of granulation tissue from the wound bed. In the absence of necrotic tissue or pus this wound is unlikely to be offensive, despite producing copious exudate which in itself is not a reliable indicator of infection. If a microbiological swab were taken, all it would demonstrate is that this wound is colonised with bacteria, which could be assumed without the additional expense of taking a swab. In conclusion, this wound is sloughy but not clinically infected.

The wound in Plate 4 is a venous leg ulcer which extends over the right lateral malleolus. The wound surface is covered by a combination of thick slough and pus. At various points across the surface of the wound are small areas of necrotic tissue. The wound is producing copious amounts of exudate which is evident from the wet, macerated tissue surrounding the wound margin. It would be likely that owing to the presence of pathogenic organisms in the wound at this time, the wound odour would have become more noticeable, to the point of being offensive.

Evidence of cellulitis can be seen at the wound edges together with areas of skin excoriation. The skin is red and inflamed and would be warm to touch. It would be usual for the patient to be complaining of increased pain and discomfort due to the presence of infection, which would be exacerbated by the application of compression therapy at this time. In conclusion, from the evidence presented by this photograph, this wound is likely to be clinically infected.

· ·

Taking a wound swab

A patient's wound should be carefully assessed at each dressing change for the signs described in Figure 2.4. Care needs to be taken to avoid either the under- or overestimation of wound infection. Only if infection is suspected should a bacteriological sample be taken. Many wounds are swabbed routinely if the presence of erythema and/or oedema is noted, despite the fact that these signs are normally seen during the inflammatory phase of healing. However, failure of a wound to heal or sudden unexplained deterioration may be indicative of 'silent infection'. Infection delays epithelial migration, so that any wound failing to improve with appropriate management should be investigated for 'silent infection' (Robson 1988).

Activity   20 MINUTES

Read Article 3 in the Reader (p. 150) and describe the correct procedure for taking a wound swab.

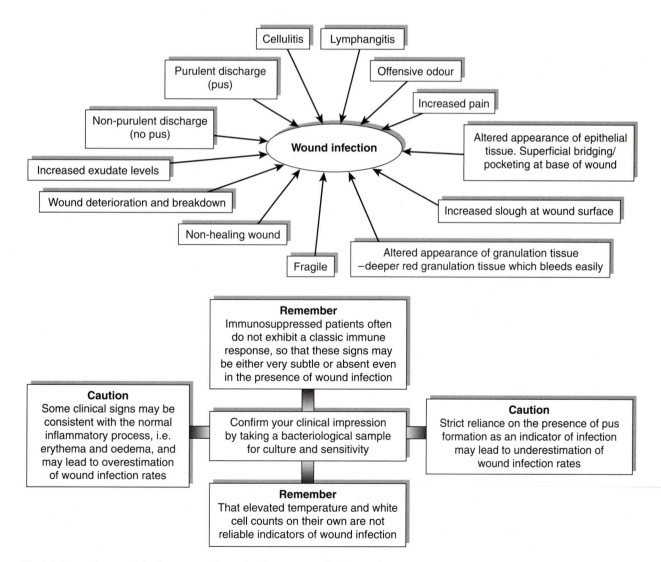

Fig. 2.4 Signs of wound infection: assess the patient for some or all of these signs.

FEEDBACK

The correct procedure for taking a wound swab is given in Box 2.4.

Box 2.4 Steps to be taken to obtain an accurate wound swab

- Use a serum-tipped swab in a sealed plastic tube.
- Moisten the swab in its own medium before use if the wound is dry.
- Rub the swab by zigzagging across the wound surface and rotate the swab between your finger and thumb at the same time.
- Replace swab tip into the tube and carefully label the pathology form with the patient's name and number, the wound site and the date.
- Keep swabs as cool as possible and return them to the laboratory as quickly as possible.

There is no consensus agreement on the term 'wound infection', which causes difficulties when trying to differentiate between colonised and infected wounds and also makes comparisons of wound infection rates for audit purposes misleading. A review of this problem by Mishriki et al (1993) suggests that the diagnosis of wound infection is likely to be most accurate if based upon the presence or absence of objective clinical signs and confirmed when possible by bacteriological analysis.

2.7 WOUND CLASSIFICATION MODELS

Introduction

Several methods exist to classify wounds. Unfortunately, owing to the many different types of wound and the complexity of the healing process, there is not one universally accepted approach, which can result in confusion and inconsistencies in practice.

The commonest methods of classifying wounds are:

- aetiology
- acute or chronic
- depth and extent of tissue damage
- clinical appearance.

Aetiological classification of wounds

This classification of wound type takes into consideration the origin of tissue damage (see Box 2.5). This method of classification can be an important predictor of healing rates.

Box 2.5 Aetiological classification of wounds

Traumatic wounds
- Blisters
- Bruises
- Abrasions
- Lacerations
- Bites
- Stab wounds
- Gunshot wounds
- Degloving injuries
- Crush injuries
- Compound fractures
- Amputations

Thermal injuries
- Burns
- Frostbite
- Electrical injuries

Chemical injuries
- Acid burns
- Alkaline burns

Iatrogenic wounds
- Radiation injuries
- Surgical incisions
- Laser treatment
- Diathermy
- Biopsies
- Split-skin grafts

Acute or chronic wounds

For management purposes this type of classification does not offer many practical benefits, apart from giving an approximate indication of the estimated length of time expected for the wound to heal. Wounds healing by primary intention where tissue loss is minimal take less time to heal; healing by secondary intention takes considerably longer. Wounds traditionally categorised as chronic are those associated with prolonged healing times.

The term 'acute wound' is usually reserved for wounds that are healing without complication. Such wounds heal quickly and with minimal intervention, e.g. a surgical incision on a healthy patient. Any wound can develop complications that result in delayed healing. An acute wound that does not heal within the expected time frame will require further investigation to determine the factors responsible for the extended healing time. If healing were severely prolonged, for example by the presence of wound infection and sinus formation, this incision could be redefined as a chronic surgical wound. This classification system is shown in Box 2.6.

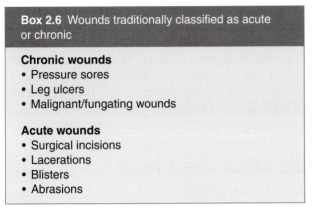

Box 2.6 Wounds traditionally classified as acute or chronic

Chronic wounds
• Pressure sores
• Leg ulcers
• Malignant/fungating wounds

Acute wounds
• Surgical incisions
• Lacerations
• Blisters
• Abrasions

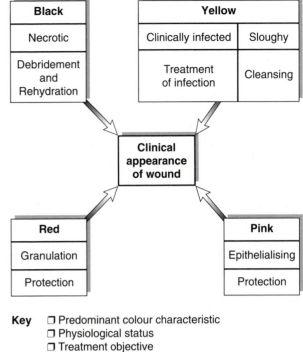

Key   ❐ Predominant colour characteristic
       ❐ Physiological status
       ❐ Treatment objective

Fig. 2.5 Classification model based on clinical appearance of wounds.

Depth and extent of tissue damage

Wound classification should include assessment of the type of tissue damage present, which may not always be easy to determine. This type of classification model relies heavily on an understanding of the anatomy and physiology of the skin and related structures. The terms 'partial thickness' and 'full thickness' have traditionally been used to describe the amount of skin loss within a wound. Partial thickness wounds involve damage to the epidermis and to some of the dermis and are relatively superficial. Damage in full thickness wounds is, however, more extensive, involving tissues in the subcutaneous layers or deeper. Clinical observation skills are required to determine which skin structures are damaged and the nature of any other type of tissue involvement, i.e. muscle, fascia or bone. Pressure sores are classified in this way, although there are a variety of different staging classification models available and a general lack of consensus as to which are the most appropriate.

Clinical appearance

A popular method of assessing wounds is by direct observation of the predominant colour characteristics of the wound surface (see Fig. 2.5). This approach can be criticised for its oversimplicity, but is quick and relatively easy and has minimal resource implications. It can also help to identify and prioritise treatment objectives so that the most appropriate management options can be selected. This type of classification requires careful observation of the wound at each dressing change; it is worth remembering that as wounds heal they may pass through each of the stages identified in Figure 2.5.

Black necrotic wounds

Necrotic areas are dehydrated dead tissue, easily recognisable by its black or brownish appearance. Necrotic tissue always prolongs healing and should

be removed (see Sect. 3.6). Necrotic eschar may completely cover the wound surface, or alternatively may present as small patches at the base or margin of the wound bed.

Yellow infected wounds

Infection prolongs the inflammatory response and often causes considerable distress for the patient. It can be difficult to identify wound infection (see Sect. 2.6) as not all wounds that are yellow are clinically infected. Signs of clinical infection vary between different wounds. The criteria included in Figure 2.4 may provide a useful guide.

Yellow sloughy wounds

Slough is formed when a collection of dead cellular debris accumulates on the wound surface. It is usually creamy yellow in colour owing to the large amounts of leukocytes present. Chronic wounds in particular may develop areas of fibrous tissue that cover the base of the wound; this often combines with slough making it harder to remove. Desloughing needs to be carried out with caution as it may cause unnecessary trauma and prolong the inflammatory response. It may also damage delicate granulation tissue. Unless excessive or clinically infected, slough should be left in the wound bed as it performs a useful protective function.

Red granulating wounds

Granulation tissue is bright red in appearance and should be moist. It is fragile, so careful handling is essential to avoid unnecessary trauma. Granulation tissue is normally slightly uneven in texture and may be raised in some areas of the wound. Unhealthy granulation tissue often looks pale and may bleed spontaneously which may indicate that the wound is ischaemic or clinically infected.

Pink epithelialising wounds

These are wounds in the final stages of healing, once a healthy bed of granulation tissue has grown across the wound bed. This is when the process of re-epithelialisation can begin. This process can be recognised by the presence of pinky-white tissue which migrates either from the wound margin or from the remnants of hair follicles within the dermis. In practice these small islands of cells can be difficult to identify, especially if they are hidden by slough, fibrous tissue or exudate. It is therefore important to be able to differentiate between slough and epithelial tissue. Delicate epithelial cells that are partly translucent can also be confused with macerated, wet skin sometimes seen at the wound margin as a consequence of either high levels of exudate or use of dressings with a high water content.

Assessment of wounds is a complex activity which aims to collect a large quantity of information so that appropriate treatment decisions can be made. All of the assessment methods described above should be used in combination, so that an objective and comprehensive assessment of each patient's healing potential can be determined.

Self-assessment   5 MINUTES

Name three types of wound in which it may be difficult to assess the amount of tissue damage present.

FEEDBACK

Wounds that are difficult to assess are commonly the following types.

1. *Local pressure damage to intact skin.* The extent of damage can not be seen, but can be determined—haematoma, blistering.
2. *Wounds covered with hard, necrotic eschars.* The full extent of the damage can not be seen and may extend deep into the tissues to involve muscle, tendon and bone. Damage can be determined following wound debridement.
3. *Chronic wounds which contain either undermining or the development of sinuses or fistulae.* The extent of these wounds can be determined following careful exploration of the wound using a probe such as a gloved finger.

2.8 MEASUREMENT AND DOCUMENTATION OF WOUND HEALING RATES

Introduction

It is vitally important to keep accurate nursing records of the progress of wound healing in order to determine whether progression or deterioration is occurring. Measurement of wounds can help to identify the efficacy of prescribed care and can assist as a means of predicting healing times. Studies of wound healing have in the past been hampered by a lack of objective methods of assessment that can be easily used in clinical practice. There are a variety of different methods available for measuring wounds, ranging from the very simple to the use of extremely sophisticated assessment systems. Choice of assessment tool is usually dependent on what resources are available, the wound type and location and the reason that wound healing rates are being monitored.

Measuring surface area

Simple measurement of surface area is more suited to superficial, shallow wounds and can be crudely estimated by measuring the widest and longest parts of the wound with a ruler. Although imprecise, especially for irregularly shaped wounds, such measurements do at least provide a baseline for objective evaluation of healing. Accuracy will be improved if the points from which the measurements are taken are marked so that reliability of results is improved. The circumference of the wound can be measured, after tracing the shape of the wound on to a transparent material such as acetate or plastic. Again this technique depends heavily on the clinical judgement of the user to determine exactly the perimeter of the wound. Tracings made in this way do not consider the three-dimensional aspect of the wound bed, but it is the relative change in wound size that is important to establish. Weekly tracings of a wound's circumference are usually sufficient, as measurements taken more frequently tend not to easily demonstrate changes in wound size. The wound margin should be carefully traced using a fibre-tipped pen. The outline can be then transferred on to graph

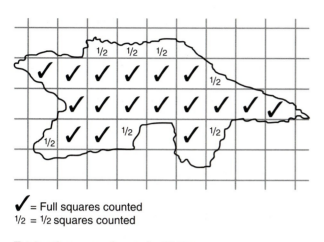

✔ = Full squares counted
1/2 = 1/2 squares counted

Total surface area of wound = 20.5 cm

Fig. 2.6 Calculating the surface area of a wound.

paper or a wound assessment chart and recorded. If graph paper is used, the surface area of the wound can be roughly calculated by counting each full square that falls within the perimeter of the wound tracing; half squares can be added up in the same way (see Fig. 2.6). This method can be both tedious and time consuming in practice, but the development of the Polaroid GridFilm, which superimposes a photograph of the wound on to a grid, speeds up the process of calculating wound area.

Activity   5 MINUTES

Briefly list up to four reasons why in clinical practice it may be difficult to obtain a high level of accuracy when trying to measure the surface area of a wound.

• •

FEEDBACK

Measuring the surface area of a wound on its own will only provide a limited amount of information about the status of wound healing. Problems associated with this type of measurement can be summarised broadly as follows.

• There may be slight discrepancies when defining and tracing the wound margin which will affect the final result.
• Wounds on curved surfaces such as the heel are difficult to measure in this way.
• Wounds in inaccessible areas such as the axilla may be difficult to reach.
• Irregular wounds with deep cavities make the tracing of the wound circumference problematic.

• Counting the squares on a piece of graph paper is subjective, especially when adding up incomplete squares.

• •

Measuring wound volume

Measuring wound depth, especially in irregularly shaped, deep wounds, has always been problematic from a practical point of view. Sophisticated methods of measurement such as stereophotography and structured light techniques are usually reserved for research purposes and are not generally suitable for everyday use. Use has been made of probes, sterile swabs, forceps and gloved fingers, all with varying degrees of accuracy. It is most important to establish which is the deepest part of the wound bed in order to achieve any degree of accuracy. Wounds with undermined edges and or sinuses will always be difficult to measure accurately in this way. It has been demonstrated that the evaluation of wounds with a probe consistently underestimates the size of the larger and more irregularly shaped wounds (Thomas & Wyscki 1990). It is always useful to describe sinus formation or undermining by associating the surface of the wound with a clock face, e.g. small sinus present at approximately 3 o'clock. Some success has been reported in measuring the volume of cavity wounds during clinical trials using alginate filling materials as casts (Covington et al 1989) and using saline to fill wounds covered with film dressings (Berg et al 1990). However, in everyday clinical practice neither method is particularly useful.

Activity   15 MINUTES

Read Article 4 in the Reader (p. 154) in which Vowden describes different wound measurement techniques. Briefly describe one three-dimensional wound measurement system using photographic imaging.

• •

FEEDBACK

You could have mentioned the structured light technique where the wound is illuminated by a set of parallel strips of light. Calculations are taken from the points where the wound surface intersects with the strips of light by a camera connected to an image-processing computer. From this a three-dimensional image of the wound surface is generated by the computer. This technique takes about 5 minutes but requires several hours of training. The cost of such equipment makes its use prohibitive for anything other than research purposes at the moment.

● ●

Increases in wound size

Deterioration in wound size may relate to various intrinsic factors associated with delayed healing. The usual reasons for sudden increases in size of a patient's wound include:

- development of wound infection
- development of ischemia
- development of pressure damage—constriction of bandages or dressings
- unrelieved pressure from patient support surface
- interference from the patient—scratching due to skin sensitivities
- treatment of the wound with dressings containing a high water content such as hydrogels and hydrocolloids—the overall size of the wound often appears to increase as necrotic tissue is debrided away.

Documentation of wound healing

Documentation of all parameters related to wound healing is the responsibility of accountable practitioners and failure to keep such records may be judged to be negligent practice. This highlights the need for accurate documentation and use of objective wound assessment techniques.

Following a nursing assessment of the patient's general condition and identification of those factors that may delay healing, the wound itself should be systematically assessed.

The following information needs to be accurately documented:

- type of wound
- location and position of wound
- grading/classification of wound
- wound dimensions—length, depth, breadth
- condition of surrounding skin
- clinical appearance of wound bed
- nature of wound drainage—serous, purulent
- levels of wound exudate
- amount of odour
- amount of patient pain/discomfort
- patient allergies or skin sensitivities
- previous treatments
- miscellaneous—type of wound closure, drains.

These details need to be reassessed at each dressing change. The most practical method of collecting all of this information quickly is to incorporate it into a wound assessment chart that takes into consideration the wound types that you commonly see. There are many examples of such charts (see Fig. 2.7). The most important criterion is to select an assessment chart which can easily be adapted to suit the specific needs of your particular patients.

In addition to these points, the following information should be clearly documented in the nursing care plan:

- objective of treatment
- type of cleansing solution
- type of dressings/bandages
- anticipated frequency of dressing change
- extra equipment required
- details of pain management.

Dressing regimes will alter as the condition of the wound changes. Therefore the care plan should include specific times and dates for re-evaluation. The amount of detailed information can be vast, especially if the patient's wound is a chronic, non-healing wound. Information trends can be difficult to pinpoint when described within more generalised nursing notes.

Documentation using photography

An increasingly popular method of documenting the progress of a wound is by taking photographs. However, this method is not without various problems. Availability of suitable cameras is an obvious difficulty, although the price and ease of use is improving all the time. When taking photographs for wound assessment, consistency of results will improve if the rules listed in Box 2.7 are observed.

Box 2.7 Rules for taking photographs for wound assessment

- Always obtain the patient's written consent.
- Select a camera capable of taking close-up shots of wounds.
- Never take a photograph which may identify the patient.
- Ensure that nothing other than the wound is in the photograph.
- Photograph the wound against a dark background which helps to absorb the flash and acts as a contrast to the wound.
- Always include a measurement scale in the photograph.
- Always try to take subsequent photographs from the same distance and angle, using the same magnification, exposure and lighting.
- Always try to use the same type of film as well as the same film processors.
- Ensure that the photographs are stored securely and are not published without patient permission.

INITIAL ASSESSMENT

NAMES

PATIENT NAME [   ]   AGE [   ]

GP/CONSULTANT NAME [   ]

DESCRIBE THE WOUND

TYPE OF WOUND [   ]

LOCATION OF WOUND [   ]

WOUND DIMENSIONS   MAX LENGTH [   ]   cm/mm (DELETE AS APPROPRIATE)

MAX WIDTH [   ]   cm/mm (DELETE AS APPROPRIATE)

DEPTH [   ]   cm/mm (DELETE AS APPROPRIATE)

LENGTH OF TIME WOUND PRESENT [   ]   DAYS/WEEKS/MONTHS/YEARS (DELETE AS APPROPRIATE)

RISK ASSESSMENT

PRESSURE SORE RISK ASSESSMENT SCALE USED [   ]   SCORE [   ]

$$\text{DOPPLER READING} = \frac{\text{ANKLE PRESSURE}}{\text{ARM PRESSURE}} \quad [\underline{\quad}] \text{ mm Hg} \quad \text{INDEX} \quad [\quad \bullet \quad]$$

CONDITION OF SKIN   GOOD/INTACT [ ]   FAIR/RED AREAS† [ ]   POOR/ BREAKS† [ ]

† DESCRIBE IN MORE DETAIL TOGETHER WITH ACTION TAKEN

[   ]

FACTORS THAT MAY DELAY HEALING

INFECTION [ ]   MEDICATIONS [ ]

DIABETES [ ]   ALLERGIES [ ]

ANAEMIA [ ]   NON-COMPLIANCE [ ]

IMMOBILITY [ ]   OTHERS

POOR NUTRITIONAL STATUS [ ]

REFERRAL REQUESTED

DATE

CLINICAL NURSE SPECIALIST [   ]

DERMATOLOGIST [   ]

VASCULAR SURGEON [   ]

DIETICIAN [   ]

CHIROPODIST [   ]

OTHERS [   ]

Fig. 2.7 Wound assessment chart (Flanagan 1994).   **(Cont'd)**

ONGOING ASSESSMENT

DATE OF DRESSING CHANGE (ENTER DATE OF VISIT)

USE 1 COLUMN PER VISIT									

WOUND DIMENSIONS (ENTER DIMENSIONS)

MAX LENGTH (cm/mm)									
MAX WIDTH (cm/mm)									
DEPTH (cm/mm)									

ARE DIMENSIONS... (TICK APPROPRIATE BOX)

INCREASING?									
DECREASING?									
STATIC?									

WOUND BED - APPROX. % COVER (ENTER APPROXIMATE PERCENTAGES. THEY SHOULD ADD UP TO 100%)

NECROTIC (BLACK)									
SLOUGHY (YELLOW)									
GRANULATING (RED)									
EPITHELIALISING (PINK)									

EXUDATE LEVELS (TICK APPROPRIATE BOX[ES])

HIGH ❶									
MODERATE									
LOW									
AMOUNT INCREASING ❶									
AMOUNT DECREASING									

❶ MAY INDICATE WOUND INFECTION.

WOUND MARGIN/SURROUNDING SKIN (TICK APPROPRIATE BOX[ES])

MACERATED ❶									
OEDEMATOUS									
ERYTHEMA ❶									
ECZEMA									
FRAGILE ❶									
DRY/SCALING									
HEALTHY/INTACT									

❶ MAY INDICATE WOUND INFECTION.

SIGNATURE/INITIAL

(Cont'd)

ONGOING ASSESSMENT

DATE OF DRESSING CHANGE (ENTER DATE OF VISIT)

USE 1 COLUMN PER VISIT											

PAIN❶ (TICK APPROPRIATE BOX)

CONTINUOUS											
AT SPECIFIC TIMES											
AT DRESSING CHANGE											
NONE											

❶ MAY INDICATE WOUND INFECTION.

IN ADDITION, SUSPECT WOUND INFECTION IF... (TICK APPROPRIATE BOXES)

GRANULATION TISSUE BLEEDS EASILY											
FRAGILE BRIDGING OF EPITHELIUM OCCURS											
ODOUR INCREASES											
HEALING IS SLOWER THAN ANTICIPATED											
WOUND BREAKDOWN											

ACTION TAKEN (TICK APPROPRIATE BOX)

SWAB SENT											
RESULT OBTAINED											

TREATMENT OBJECTIVE(S) (TICK APPROPRIATE BOX[ES])

DEBRIDEMENT											
ABSORPTION											
HYDRATION											
PROTECTION											

DOCUMENTATION - 7 TO 10 DAY INTERVALS - (TICK WHEN DONE)

TRACE WOUND CIRCUMFERENCE †											
PHOTOGRAPH											
EVALUATE PRESSURE RISK-ASSESSMENT SCORE											

† ATTACH TRACING TO PAGE 6

SIGNATURE/INITIAL											

(Cont'd)

Wound assessment is the first step in identifying appropriate treatment objectives for management of a patient's wound. Accurate wound assessment is within the reach of every practising nurse and represents one of the most positive contributions that nurses can make to the lives of those patients with chronic, non-healing wounds.

Activity   20 MINUTES

Use the wound assessment chart in Figure 2.7 to assess and plan the wound care of a patient that you are currently managing. Try to use this wound assessment chart throughout the patient's treatment period.

2.9 SPECIALISED ASSESSMENT METHODS—LEG ULCER ASSESSMENT AND PRESSURE SORE RISK ASSESSMENT

Assessment of leg ulcers

Studies in both Europe and the UK indicate that between 1 and 2% of the population develop leg ulcers at some time in their lives (Laing 1992). More than one-third of patients are below 50 years old at onset of their first period of ulceration, and more than two-thirds are below 65 (Callum et al 1987). However, the incidence of leg ulceration rises significantly with advancing age.

Leg ulcers have a significant impact on a patient's quality of life. They cause pain, restrict mobility, and may lead to depression, anxiety and hostility for many suffers. In excess of 80% of patients with leg ulcers are cared for at home by the community nursing services (Cornwall et al 1986).

Assessment is the key to effective management of leg ulcers. Recent studies demonstrate that significant improvements in healing rates can occur when services are rationalised and based upon research-based protocols (Moffatt et al 1992).

However, many leg ulcer patients have never been referred for specialist opinion, despite suffering from ulceration for many years, and consequently may not have ever had the aetiology of their ulcer correctly diagnosed (Lees & Lambert 1992).

Correct treatment of leg ulcer patients depends upon accurate diagnosis and differentiation between venous and arterial disease. The clinical signs are summarised in Table 2.5 and are intended as a framework to help identify the significance of the symptoms of vascular disease.

Many of the signs given in Table 2.5 are suggestive of one or other type of disease, but not specific to either. The use of simple vascular assessment methods such as Doppler ultrasound can increase the accuracy of patient assessment, since although approximately 75% of ulcers are of venous origin, it is recognised that many of these patients will have coexisting arterial disease. In the absence of Doppler ultrasound techniques, nurses have had to rely on the palpation of pedal pulses to determine the vascularity of the lower limb (Fig. 2.8) . This is a crude and unreliable method of assessment which can result in inappropriate care (Vydelingum 1990). The posterior tibial pulse on the foot is more reliable than the dorsalis pedis which is congenitally absent in approximately 10% of people. In addition, a further 10% of people have an impalpable dorsalis pedis.

Doppler ultrasound should be seen as part of an overall holistic patient assessment which aims to determine the differential diagnosis of leg ulceration. This procedure is used to record the resting pressure index (RPI), which is an indicator of arterial disease. The RPI compares the highest brachial systolic blood pressure with the highest ankle systolic

Table 2.5 Comparison of clinical signs and symptoms of venous and arterial leg ulceration

	Venous ulceration	*Arterial ulceration*
Previous medical history	Deep vein thrombosis, thrombophlebitis, varicose veins	Cerebrovascular accident, angina, peripheral vascular disease, hypertension, diabetes
Site/position	Often near the malleolus, may be anywhere on the leg	Usually on the foot, or close to the medial malleolus, may be anywhere on the leg
Appearance	Often large, shallow wounds producing copious exudate	Often smaller, deep wounds producing less exudate
Surrounding skin condition	Dark pigmentation, lipodermatosclerosis, atrophie blanche, eczema	Atrophic, shiny skin. Dusky pink feet turning pale when raised above heart. Trophic changes in nails
Pain/discomfort	Aching or heaviness in legs Localised pain, tenderness of ulcer	Intermittent claudication. Rest pain, severe, constant pain, often worse at night

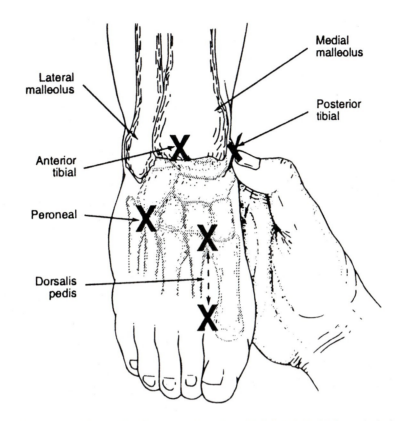

Fig. 2.8 Diagram showing the position of the pedal pulses (reproduced from Moffatt 1993 by kind permission).

blood pressure in order to determine the blood flow to the feet. It is now considered good clinical practice for all patients with leg ulcers to have their RPI calculated prior to commencement of treatment (Moffatt 1993).

Like any measurement of blood pressure, this reading is affected by many variables. The factors that may affect the accuracy of Doppler ultrasound include:

- inability of the patient to lie flat
- difficulty in palpating pedal pulses
- calcification of arteries
- noisy surroundings.

Other factors relate to lack of training and inconsistencies in method; commonly made mistakes include:

- incorrect transducer head size
- incorrect cuff size
- incorrect probe angle
- application of excessive pressure from probe
- deflating cuff too quickly
- calculation errors
- misinterpretation of results.

The approach described below attempts to minimise these variables in order to increase the accuracy of the reading.

Recording an ankle pressure index

- Any person performing a Doppler ultrasound assessment should have received appropriate training and supervision.
- The patient should, whenever possible, lie flat for 15–20 minutes prior to the procedure to ensure accuracy of results. During this time a full explanation should be given and the equipment prepared.
- The brachial blood pressure should be taken in both left and right arms using the doppler. These pressure measurements should be repeated and the highest of the readings recorded.
- The highest readings of both the ankle and brachial systolic blood pressure are required to calculate the ankle pressure index (RPI).
- The foot pulses should now be palpated on both feet. Identify the posterior tibialis and the dorsalis pedis. If these cannot be located, pulses may sometimes be located over either the lateral or medial malleolus or between the first and second toe. Palpation of foot pulses will depend on the location of any ulcers and areas of localised oedema.
- Using the doppler and electrode gel, the foot pulses should be identified. The probe head should be held at a 45° angle to the skin and

towards the direction of the blood flow within the vessels.

- If the ulcer is located around the gaiter area, it should be covered before the sphygmomanometer cuff is applied to the leg. The correct position for the cuff is approximately 5 cm above the malleoli.
- The sphygmomanometer cuff should now be inflated, so that the ankle systolic blood pressure can be identified. The systolic pressures in each foot should be taken twice, as described above.
- Taking the highest recorded systolic blood pressures in both the upper and lower limbs, calculate the resting pressure index ratio using the following equation:

$$\frac{\text{Highest systolic ankle pressure}}{\text{Highest systolic brachial pressure}} = \begin{array}{l}\text{resting} \\ \text{pressure} \\ \text{index (RPI)}\end{array}$$

The way in which different values of RPI are interpreted is shown in Box 2.8.

- Currently it is recommended that measurement of the RPI is repeated once every 3 months, as for many elderly patients rapid deterioration of the arterial blood supply can occur.

The use of Doppler ultrasound forms only part of the full assessment that patients with leg ulcers should receive. Care must be taken to ensure that all available information is considered before deciding to use compression therapy or not. Many factors can lead to inaccurate readings which should be taken into account at all times. If this procedure is rushed or compromised, results will be invalid. Doppler ultrasound is a useful diagnostic aid if performed correctly, but will in the majority of cases take approximately 45 minutes to perform.

Pressure sore risk assessment

Pressure sores increase patient morbidity and mortality (Davies et al 1991), prolong hospitalisation, waste valuable resources, require 50% more nursing time (Allman et al 1986) as well as causing immeasurable pain and suffering to patients and their families. The incidence of pressure sores is difficult to define as there remains lack of consensus on classification of pressure damage and on methodologies used to collect data.

The aetiology of pressure sores is complex and poorly understood, but if pressure sores are to be reduced, an individual's at-risk status must be determined so that predisposing factors can be minimised by early and appropriate intervention. A bewildering variety of scoring systems based on clinical assessment skills have been developed to identify those patients at high risk. Pressure sore risk assessment scales are based upon those factors known to predispose to pressure sore formation. The published literature shows no consensus on the relative importance of each predisposing factor (Berlowitz & Wilking 1989) which is reflected in the variation among the risk assessment scales currently used in clinical practice.

Box 2.8 Resting pressure index: interpretation of results

1 or above	indicates normal arterial blood flow
0.9	indicates a mild degree of arterial involvement
0.8	indicates that only 80% of arterial blood flow is reaching the foot, modified compression may be applied under supervision.
0.7 or below	indicates increasing arterial insufficiency; referral for a vascular opinion is required

---

Activity   15 MINUTES

1. Read Article 5 in the Reader (p. 158) which describes some of the more commonly used pressure sore risk assessment scales, and complete the following table.

Assessment scale	Year	Country of origin	Original practice setting

2. Which pressure sore risk assessment tool is currently used in your clinical setting?

3. Summarise the difficulties experienced by staff when trying to use this risk assessment tool in everyday clinical practice.

FEEDBACK

1. Your completed table should look like Table 2.6.

Table 2.6 Pressure sore risk assessment scales			
Assessment scale	Year	Country of origin	Original practice setting
Norton	1962	UK	Elderly care
Gosnall	1973	USA	Elderly care
Lowthian	1975	UK	Orthopaedics
Waterlow	1985	UK	Medical and surgical
Braden	1986	USA	Elderly care

2. Any one of the assessment tools in Table 2.6 may be used in your clinical setting. They all have their advantages and disadvantages, and you may find it interesting to compare the one that you use with the others mentioned in the article.

3. Some of the difficulties noted may be specific to the clinical environment in which you work. The following are common problems reported when using risk assessment scales in general.

- It does not consider the specific needs of patients in my clinical setting.
- Some staff do not know how to use it accurately.
- Some staff do not use it regularly to reassess patients when their condition changes.
- The scores obtained by different users for the same patient are subjective and vary, thus affecting its reliability.

- It appears to regularly under- or overestimate those patients at risk.
- Despite these limitations, it is used exclusively to select pressure-relieving support surfaces for patients.

Activity   20 MINUTES

Return to Article 5 in the Reader and select a scale that you have not previously used. Assess one of your patients using this tool, comparing the results with the risk assessment scale that you are currently using. Following this exercise would you consider changing your present method of risk assessment?

FEEDBACK

Your answer will depend on what you found. However, the criteria listed below should have influenced your decision.

- Is it easy to understand?
- Is it easy to use?
- Does it meet the needs of your specific patient group?
- Is it understood by all team members?
- Are consistent results obtained?
- Have the reliability and validity been tested?
- Is it research based?
- Does it assist in the decision to allocate resources?

Despite the limitations of pressure sore prediction scores, any method of assessment that can assist in the identification of vulnerable patients is valuable when planning care. No one score will ever be 100% accurate and choice will always be influenced by personal preference and the type of patient being cared for. Pressure sore risk assessment scales are not a substitute for sound clinical judgement and become a pointless exercise unless preventive measures are quickly implemented. However, many patients are nursed on inappropriate pressure-relieving systems for longer than necessary because risk status is not reviewed often enough, whilst others never benefit from such intervention owing to lack of resources.

SUMMARY

This section has explored the complex process of holistic wound assessment. In it you have learnt the importance of the following:

- The need to relate the anatomy of the skin and the physiology of healing to the assessment and observation of patients' wounds.

- The significance of identifying the multitude of factors both intrinsic and extrinsic that can prolong wound healing rates.

- The different methods of classifying wound types in order to be able to begin planning appropriate management and treatment.

- The advantages and disadvantages of measuring and documenting wound healing rates.

- The need for specialised wound assessment methods for the optimal management of leg ulcers and pressure sores.

REFERENCES

Allman R, Laprande C, Noel L B 1986 Pressure sores among hospitalised patients. Annals of Internal Medicine 105: 337–342

Ayliffe G A, Lowbury E J, Gebbes A M 1992 Control of hospital infection. Chapman & Hall, London

Ayton M 1985 Wounds that won't heal. Nursing Times 81(46)(Community Outlook Nov): 16–19

Berg W, Traneroth C, Gunnarsson A 1990 A method for measuring pressure sores. Lancet 335: 1445–1446

Berlowitz D, Wilking S 1989 Risk factors for pressure sores. Journal of the American Geriatrics Society 37(11): 1043–1049

Callum M, Harper D, Dale J, Ruckley C V 1987 Chronic ulcers of the leg: clinical history. British Medical Journal 294: 1389–1391

Cornwall J, Dore C, Lewis J D 1986 Leg ulcers: epidemiology and aetiology. British Journal of Surgery 73: 693–696

Covington J, Griffin J, Mendius R, Tooms R 1989 Measurement of pressure ulcer volume using dental impression materials: suggestions from the field. Physical Therapy 69(8): 690–693

Davies K, Strickland J, Lawrence V et al 1991 The hidden mortality from pressure sores. Journal of Tissue Viability 1: 18–20

Eaglstein W H 1985 The effect of occlusive dressings on collagen synthesis and re-epithelialisation in superficial wounds. In: Ryan T J (ed) An environment for healing: the role of occlusion. International Congress Series No. 88, Royal Society of Medicine, London, pp 31–38

Flanagan M 1994 Assessment criteria. Nursing Times 90(35): Journal of Wound Care Nursing Supplement

Gilcrest B, Reid C 1989 The bacteriology of chronic venous ulcers treated with occlusive hydrocolloid dressings. British Journal of Dermatology 121: 337–344

Holn D, Pounce B, Burton R 1977 Antimicrobial systems of the surgical wound. American Journal of Surgery 133(5): 597–600

Kessel R G, Kardon R H 1979 Tissues and organs: a text-atlas of scanning electron microscopy. W H Freeman, Oxford

Laing W 1992 Chronic venous diseases of the leg. Office of Health Economics, London

Lees T A, Lambert D 1992 Prevalence of lower limb ulceration in an urban health district. British Journal of Surgery 79: 1032–1034

Leveen H H 1973 Chemical acidification of wounds, an adjuvant to healing and the unfavorable action of alkalinity and ammonia. Annals of Surgery 178: 745–753

Lookingbill D P, Miller S H, Knowles R C 1978 Bacteriology of leg ulcers. Archives of Dermatology 114: 1765–1768

Mishriki S, Law D, Jeffery P J 1993 Surgical audit: variations in wound infection rates according to definition. Journal of Wound Care 2(5): 286–292

Moffatt C 1993 Assessing leg ulcers. Practice Nursing 21(Sept): 8–10

Moffatt C, Franks P, Oldroyd M 1992 Community clinics for leg ulcers and impact on healing. British Medical Journal 305: 1389–1392

Myers J A 1982 Modern plastic surgical dressings. Health Society Service Journal 4(18 March): 336–337

Pediani R 1992 Preparing to heal. Nursing Times 88(27): 68–70

Peel A G, Taylor E E 1992 Proposed definition for the audit of post-operative infection: a discussion paper. Surgical Infection 4: 1

Riches D 1988 The multiple roles of macrophages in wound healing. In: Clark R, Henderson P (eds) The molecular and cellular biology of wound repair. Plenum Press, New York

Robson M C 1988 Disturbances in wound healing, Annals of Emergency Medicine 17(12): 1274–1278

Robson M, Heggers J 1984 Quantitative bacteriology and inflammatory mediators in soft tissue. In: Hunt T, Heppenstall R, Pines E, Rovee D (eds) Soft and hard tissue repair. Praeger Publications, New York

Roth R R, James W D 1988 Microbial ecology of the skin. Annual Review of Microbiology 42: 441–444

Silver I A 1972 Oxygen tension and epithelialization. In: Mailbach H I, Rovee D T (eds) Epidermal wound healing. Year Book Medical Publishers, Chicago, pp 71–112

Thomas A C, Wyscki A B 1990 The healing wound: a comparison of three clinically useful methods of measurement. Decubitus 3: 18–25

Vydelingum V 1990 Leg ulcer assessment. Journal of District Nursing 2: 5–10

Wilson I A 1979 The pH of varicose ulcer surfaces and its relationship to healing. Vasa (Bern) 8: 339–342

Winter G 1962 Formulation of the scab and the rate of epithelialisation of superficial wounds in the skin of the domestic pig. Nature 193: 293–294

FURTHER READING

Moffatt C, Harper P 1997 Leg ulcers. (Access to Clinical Education Series) Churchill Livingstone, Edinburgh

Phillips J 1997 Pressure sores. (Access to Clinical Education Series) Churchill Livingstone, Edinburgh

3

Managing wounds

Introduction

This section aims to introduce you to the basic principles of wound management. Once these concepts are understood, they can be modified in order to effectively plan the care of patients with a variety of complex wound management problems. The principles discussed within this section will be reinforced and developed in Section 5 where consideration will be given to patients with specific types of complex wounds.

LEARNING OUTCOMES

When you have completed this section, you should be able to:

- discuss the general principles of wound management
- discuss the specific management of patients with infected wounds
- identify the clinical indications for cleansing wounds
- identify a range of commonly used wound cleansing practices
- evaluate the advantages and disadvantages of using topical wound cleansing solutions
- describe the principles of wound debridement.

3.1 GENERAL PRINCIPLES OF WOUND MANAGEMENT

Introduction

Wound healing is a delicate and complex physiological process that is affected by a multitude of factors (see Sect. 2.4). The principles of caring for wounds of all types are fundamentally similar and should be based upon comprehensive wound assessment which will facilitate the identification of specific management objectives (see Sect. 5). Wound assessment and the subsequent identification of specific treatment options is an activity which involves complex decision-making skills and experience.

The overall aims of wound management are:

- to identify those factors that may be responsible for prolonging healing
- to provide the optimum environment to maximise healing potential
- to implement appropriate supportive interventions
- to critically evaluate the effectiveness of wound management interventions.

It is always a priority to determine the aetiology of the wound, as this will help to determine the appropriateness of various treatment options. The control or elimination of all causative factors may not always be a realistic objective, e.g. achieving an increased blood flow to an ischaemic limb or cooperation in a non-compliant patient. Any factors identified as likely to prolong healing should then become wound management priorities and corrected if possible. If these principles are ignored, the net result will be the development of a non-healing, chronic wound in spite of the implementation of appropriate systemic and local interventions. The selection of appropriate wound dressings alone can not compensate for those unresolved systemic conditions known to impair rates of healing.

The ultimate objective of local wound management is to provide the optimum environment that supports and facilitates the process of wound repair (see Sect. 2.3).

Activity   5 MINUTES

Select from the following list those objectives which you think are inappropriate when managing wounds:

- removal of devitalised tissue and foreign bodies
- identification and control of wound infection
- maintenance of a warm, moist wound environment
- absorption of exudate production at the wound surface
- maintenance of free fluid drainage from the wound bed
- application of topical cleansers to the wound bed
- firm packing of 'dead space' and cavities with absorbent materials

- protection of the wound bed and the surrounding skin from trauma
- effective pain management to promote patient comfort.

FEEDBACK

Your answer should have identified the following as being inappropriate wound management objectives.

Absorption of exudate production at the wound surface

Although it is necessary to absorb excess exudate production to avoid dressing leakage or skin maceration, the presence of some exudate at the wound surface is vitally important to maintain the correct local environment necessary to support both the movement of leukocytes across the wound surface, which are responsible for wound cleansing, and the division and migration of epithelial cells. Overdrying the wound surface will considerably delay the rate of wound repair.

Application of topical cleansers to the wound bed

Topical cleansers come in a variety of forms (see Sect. 3.4) and should only be used in specific circumstances owing to concerns about probable cytotoxic effects on delicate healing tissue. The use of cleansing agents can prolong the acute inflammatory response by disturbing healing tissues; they could be used more appropriately to clean the skin surrounding the wound. If used at all, physiological saline 0.9% would be the recommended cleansing solution.

Firm packing of 'dead space' and cavities with absorbent materials

Cavities and areas of 'dead space' within a wound do need filling to encourage the development of healthy granulation tissue from the base of the wound. However, if any type of dressing material is tightly packed into such a cavity it will have a tendency to exert excessive local pressure on the developing capillary loops, resulting in ischaemia and tissue death. In addition, tightly packed wounds are usually painful for the patient, restrict the absorbent capacity of the dressing and may contribute to trauma when eventually removed.

3.2 MANAGEMENT OF INFECTED WOUNDS

Clinically infected wounds prolong healing, cause considerable patient distress and present a variety of management difficulties for practitioners. Wound infections also have considerable financial implications due to increased length of hospital stay, the additional cost of antimicrobial therapy and a higher incidence of related wound management complications. Consequently it has been recommended by the Department of Health, that hospital-acquired infection rates should be specifically identified in purchaser contracts (Sedgewick 1995). Section 2.6 discusses in detail the criteria for identifying the clinical signs of infection in both chronic and acute wounds, together with the importance of collecting accurate bacteriological samples.

The complete removal of bacteria from a wound is neither possible nor necessary in order to promote healing. Adequate healing rates are frequently observed in chronic wounds that are colonised by bacteria (Gilcrest & Reed 1989)

Self-assessment   **2 MINUTES**

Identify three reasons for taking a wound swab.

FEEDBACK

Your answer should have included the following points.

1. Wound swabs should be taken from wounds exhibiting the clinical signs of infection (see p. 37) in order to identify the pathogens that are responsible for causing a host reaction. They should only be taken if clinical infection is suspected so that appropriate antibiotic therapy can commence and never purely to see what is growing in the wound.

2. Exceptions to this principle include:
   a. the need to assess the effectiveness of antibiotic therapy once treatment for a wound infection has already begun
   b. the need to determine the presence or absence of epidemic strains of bacteria such as methicillin-resistant *Staphylococcus aureus* (MRSA).

Section 2.6 discusses in detail the criteria for identifying the clinical signs of infection in chronic wounds, together with the importance of collecting accurate bacteriological samples.

Specific treatment objectives for infected wounds

The early detection of wound infection will limit the amount of local tissue damage and minimise disruption of the healing process. The treatment objectives listed below have been discussed in greater detail elsewhere in the pack:

- to identify the infective organism (Sect. 2.6)
- to control and/or eliminate wound infection (Sect. 2.6)
- to remove devitalised tissue from the wound bed (Sect. 3.6)
- to cleanse the wound surface (Sect. 3.4)
- to absorb excess exudate production (Sect. 4.3)
- to protect the surrounding skin from the effects of maceration (Sects 5.2 and 5.4)
- to control patient pain/discomfort (Sect. 5.2).

Activity   15 MINUTES

Read Article 3 in the Reader (p. 150) and briefly describe the clinical significance of the wound swab results in Box 3.1.

Box 3.1 Microbiology report	
SITE	Leg ulcer
GRAM STAIN	No white blood cells seen Gram-positive bacilli +/– Gram-positive cocci +/–
CULTURE	No pathogens isolated after 24 hours
SUB-CULTURE (aerobic)	To follow if significant
SUB-CULTURE (anaerobic)	To follow if significant

FEEDBACK

These results indicate that:

- rod-shaped bacteria (bacilli) and spherical bacteria (cocci) are present
- less than 30 colonies of both types of bacteria were found in zone 1 of the agar plate, i.e. less than 10^5 bacteria per gram of tissue
- the wound is therefore heavily contaminated, but not infected
- the bacteria have not been specifically identified as, after a 24-hour incubation period, no pathogenic organisms have been isolated. No treatment is required.

Managing infected wounds

The principles of managing infected wounds should be aimed at providing an optimum healing environment. This can be achieved by removing necrotic tissue, pus and any excess exudate (see Sect. 3.6). Necrosis is caused by a lack of essential materials required for cellular activity, which can result from mechanical injury, extreme heat or cold, radiation damage, chemical toxicity or the release of bacterial toxins. The presence of devitalised tissue in wounds prolongs healing by:

- acting as a mechanical barrier on the wound surface which impedes wound contracture, epithelialisation and the cleansing activity of leukocytes
- providing an optimum environment for bacterial multiplication
- prolonging the inflammatory phase of healing.

It is important to remove necrotic and sloughy tissue from a wound before taking a wound swab as the presence of devitalised tissue within a wound may harbour anaerobic bacteria which are often difficult to isolate. Bacteria present at the surface of the wound are unlikely to be responsible for producing the localised clinical signs of infection. Swabs should therefore be taken from deeper within the tissues and preferably from clean areas of the wound.

Management of infected closed surgical wounds

There are a number of factors that influence infection rates in surgical wounds (Cruse & Foord 1973, 1980, Mishriki et al 1990), which are summarised in Figure 3.1. Those factors relating to duration of hospital stay have been minimised by the increased development of day surgery units and the overall trend for early postoperative discharge. However, many community nurses report an increase in postoperative wound complications such as sinus, abscess and haematoma formation, wound breakdown and dehiscence.

Self-assessment   5 MINUTES

Identify two possible reasons why early postoperative discharge may decrease the incidence of surgical wound infection and two reasons why this may contribute to infection rates in surgical wounds.

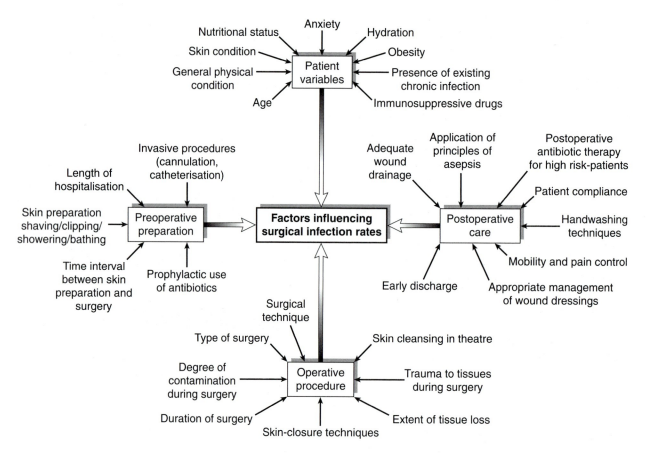

Fig. 3.1 Factors influencing infection rates in surgical wounds.

FEEDBACK

Your answer should have considered the following issues:

1. reasons for potential decreases in postoperative infection rates after early discharge:
   - the patient is exposed to fewer multiresistant microorganisms, so the potential for cross-infection is reduced
   - patient anxiety levels are decreased, so the effects of stress on the immune system are minimised.

2. reasons for potential increases in postoperative infection rates after early discharge:
   - patients may not comply with wound care advice and may contaminate their wounds
   - patients are likely to be more active and may fail to rest adequately, which may exert undue stress at the wound incision.

Most surgical wounds can be dressed with a simple low-adherent dressing, which can be left undisturbed unless exudate strikes through the dressing.

If wound drains have been inserted it is important to check their patency in order to encourage free drainage of fluid from the wound site. Fluid collecting at the wound site increases the risk of infection and exerts increased pressure on the incision line which may result in wound breakdown. The presence of wound drains themselves may increase the risk of wound infection as they act as a foreign body and can stimulate localised tissue reactions. Infected surgical incisions need to be encouraged to drain freely and should be lightly filled with an absorbent dressing material such as alginates or foam cavity dressings which are capable of encouraging drainage of infected exudate (see Sect. 4.3).

Topical treatments for infected wounds

The use of topical treatments for the management of infected wounds remains a contentious issue. Topical antimicrobials are still used for the management of some types of infected wounds, although in order to achieve a sustained therapeutic effect they should be used as an adjunct to systemic antibiotics. Antiseptics are chemical solutions that are used to reduce infection in living tissues. Unfortunately they need to be applied in high concentrations in order to effectively destroy invading pathogens. The use of antiseptics will be considered in greater detail on page 59.

Antibiotics

All wound infections should be treated systemically using appropriate antibiotic therapy; pathogenic organisms should be identified as quickly as possible following the collection of specimens for culture and sensitivity (Greenwood 1995). Topical antibiotics are widely considered to have no place in the management of wounds. There are no controlled trials demonstrating the superiority of topical antibiotics over antiseptics. The use of antibiotic powders is unjustified and in many cases has led to the development of bacterial resistance (Lowbury 1981). Currently, there are only limited exceptions to these statements. Mupirocin ointment is appropriate for the treatment of skin infections as its absorption through broken skin can be significant (Ashurst 1994) but its effectiveness is severely compromised when used on wounds covered with thick slough or necrotic tissue. This has implications for the management of wounds infected with methicillin-resistant staphylococcus which are often treated with mupirocin prior to removal of devitalised tissue. Metronidazole gel 0.8% can effectively control smell in malodorous wounds (Bower et al 1992) and silver sulphadiazine (Flamazine) cream has a role in the prevention of infection for severe burns (Hoffman 1984). Allergic reactions to topical antibiotics are common; the commonest causes of sensitivity reactions include: neomycin, framycetin, gentamicin and sodium fusidate (Bajaja & Gupta 1986). In wounds that are slow to heal, it is advisable to screen for pathogenic bacteria known to significantly prolong healing such as β-haemolytic streptococci, *Escherichia coli* and *Pseudomonas* species. Systemic antibiotics are the treatment of choice for clinically infected wounds where a positive bacteriological culture has been identified and appropriate advice sought from a microbiologist. The risks of toxicity, sensitisation, and bacterial resistance far outweigh any potential benefits that the use of topical antibiotics have in the treatment of wound infection.

Wound dressings for infected wounds

Wound dressings should primarily be selected for their ability to absorb high levels of exudate and to facilitate debridement (see Sects 3.6 and 4.3). Dressings can play an important role in minimising bacterial spread. The use of traditional dry cellulose dressing materials affords little protection from external contamination once 'strike through' has occurred and does little to contain bacteria within a wound. Studies by Lawrence et al (1992) have demonstrated that the use of occlusive dressings such as hydrocolloids can significantly reduce airborne dispersal of bacteria during dressing change. For further details about the use of dressings with infected wounds see Section 4.3.

Handwashing

For the management of wounds, effective handwashing is the single most important method of achieving infection control. Studies indicate that social handwashing tends to miss important areas such as the fingertips and thumbs and that despite continuing education, basic handwashing is still not performed effectively in the clinical setting (Willis 1995).

Activity   20 MINUTES

Refer to Article 3 in the Reader (p. 150) and briefly describe the recommended method of effectively disinfecting hands.

FEEDBACK

In your answer you should have described the following procedure.

- The cleansing solution should be rubbed between the palms of the hands.
- Fingers should be interlaced and the right palmar surface rubbed over the left dorsum; repeat with the left palmar surface over the right dorsum.
- The fingers should be then interlaced palm to palm and rubbed together.
- The knuckles of each hand should be worked into the palm of the opposite hand.
- Care should be taken to ensure that each thumb is rubbed by the palm and fingers of the opposite hand and that all fingertips are rubbed into the opposite palm.
- This procedure should be repeated three times before rinsing and carefully drying to ensure effective hand hygiene. If alcoholic solutions are used, this sequence should be repeated until the hands are dry and the alcohol has evaporated.

Following the introduction of universal precautions in recent years, it has been suggested that the increased use of gloves may compensate for poor handwashing techniques. However, the warm, moist conditions that exist when wearing gloves provide an ideal environment for the multiplication of bacteria. The wearing of gloves should therefore in no way be a substitute for effective handwashing (Gould 1994).

Methicillin-resistant *Staphylococcus aureus* and wound management

Many organisms acquire the ability to develop resistance to antibiotics. In particular *Staphylococcus aureus* has quickly developed a resistance to methicillin which was first introduced in 1959. *Staphylococcus aureus* is a skin commensal present in 30% of the general population and is the most common pathogen infecting wounds. Today large numbers of methicillin-resistant *Staphylococcus aureus* (MRSA) strains are resistant to an increasingly wide range of other antibiotics (Duckworth 1993). MRSA has been found to be the causative organism for approximately 50% of all staphylococcal wound infections and has been shown to significantly prolong healing and increase length of inpatient stay (Esuvaranathan & Kaun 1992). Regional variations of antibiotic resistance patterns will always exist and include the following: penicillin, gentamicin, cephalosporins, erythromycin and streptomycin. Bacteriological sampling and laboratory analysis is required to establish the extent of antibiotic resistance of MRSA and to identify the individual strain of the organism. This is particularly important as new resistance patterns are constantly evolving.

It is important to establish as quickly as possible if the wound is infected or colonised with MRSA (see Sect. 2.6). Colonisation with MRSA for many patients will not prolong healing, but these wounds remain a source of a potentially pathogenic organism (Longfield & Townsend 1985). If the wound is infected, the patient will require systemic antibiotics. Advice should always be sought from a microbiologist in order to identify the most appropriate antimicrobial therapy. Advice concerning the general management of these patients varies and should be available from local infection control teams who will also provide guidance concerning screening of patients and staff. The most significant mode of spread of MRSA is by direct contact, usually due to ineffective hand hygiene. The use of 4% chlorhexidine detergent or alcohol hand rub is still recommended before and after patient contact (Duckworth 1993, Simpson 1992). Topical antimicrobials for the management of wounds colonised or infected with MRSA are widely used but still remain a contentious issue.

Infection control activities can cause considerable distress to both patients and their families, may compromise general wound management principles and may be ineffective at eradicating MRSA from clinical practice (Faoagali & Thong 1985). However, every effort must be made to contain MRSA and to identify realistic, patient-centred goals.

Self-assessment   5 MINUTES

Define the following terms: antimicrobial, antibiotic and antiseptic.

FEEDBACK

Much confusion exists surrounding the use of these terms, which are often used interchangeably.

- Antimicrobial agent is a general term to describe substances used to treat infections and includes antibiotics, disinfectants and antiseptics.
- The term antibiotic should be reserved for substances that are capable of destroying or inhibiting pathogens and are either derived from microorganisms or synthetically manufactured. Antibiotics are able to selectively target bacteria rather than viable tissue, so can be used in low concentrations and are less toxic than antiseptics.
- Antiseptics is yet another general term used to describe chemical cleansing solutions used to limit infection in living tissues; they are toxic to viable tissue as, unlike antibiotics, they are not able to act selectively. They need to be used in high concentrations in order to destroy invading pathogens.

All those involved in caring for patients with wounds require a basic understanding of bacteriology and the principles of infection control in order to minimise the discomfort, psychological distress and social isolation commonly experienced by patients with infected wounds

3.3 PRINCIPLES OF WOUND CLEANSING

Introduction

Wounds have been cleansed using a bewildering variety of techniques since the beginning of time, in an attempt to actively promote healing. The principles of wound cleansing have often been misinterpreted and poorly understood, resulting in the inappropriate and often ritualistic use of cleansing solutions. In the past, many practices have concentrated on drying out the surface of wounds and the removal of exudate, despite evidence provided by

Holn et al in 1977 that wound exudate contains active antimicrobial substances that naturally cleanse the wound bed. Critical evaluation of the effectiveness of commonly used wound cleansing agents is long overdue as evidence to support claims of improved healing rates is generally lacking.

The inappropriate use of cleansing agents is not only time consuming for both patient and nurse, but may also prolong the healing of the wound. The following questions should be answered prior to the cleansing of any wound.

- What is the purpose of wound cleansing?
- Do the advantages of cleansing outweigh the disadvantages?
- What method of wound cleansing would be most appropriate?
- Does the wound require cleaning at each dressing change?
- Which type of wound cleansing product would be most appropriate?

Self-assessment   5 MINUTES

Refer back to Section 2.2 in which the process of wound healing is described. Identify which phase of healing is predominantly responsible for naturally cleansing the surface of a wound and briefly describe how this process occurs.

● ●

FEEDBACK

The inflammatory phase of healing is part of the protective response to injury. Neutrophils which are phagocytic are immediately attracted to the wounded area and provide initial protection against invading microorganisms. Macrophages release tumour necrosing factor which is responsible for breaking down any cellular debris, fibrin, blood clots and necrotic tissue present at the wound's surface. The continued presence of necrotic tissue will actively prolong the inflammatory response and thus delay healing. One of the main functions of lymphocytes and macrophages is to cleanse the wound bed by digesting bacteria and releasing proteolytic enzymes to destroy foreign bodies and cellular debris. This process is hindered if the migration of lymphocytes across the surface of the wound is interrupted by the presence of dehydrated eschar or devitalised tissue. Wound exudate production is increased during the inflammatory phase of healing in an attempt to facilitate wound cleansing and to provide the optimal local environment required to maximise healing (Alvarez 1988).

● ●

The purpose of wound cleansing

Much confusion still surrounds the clinical indications for wound cleansing. The routine cleansing of clean granulating wounds with antiseptic solutions is a practice that still persists in some clinical areas today. However, cleansing practices are beginning to change, as many nurses question the need to routinely cleanse wounds at each dressing change.

Self-assessment   2 MINUTES

List a minimum of four reasons why a wound may benefit from cleansing.

● ●

FEEDBACK

Both acute and chronic wounds may require cleansing for a variety of reasons. The main functions of a wound cleansing agent are summarised below:

- to remove debris from the surface of the wound, including devitalised tissue, foreign bodies and dressing residue
- to rehydrate the surface of a wound in order to provide a moist environment
- to keep the skin surrounding the wound clean and free from excessive moisture
- to facilitate wound assessment so that the size and extent of the wound can be visualised
- to minimise wound trauma when removing adherent dressing materials
- to promote patient comfort and psychological well-being.

● ●

It is important to achieve the correct balance between the beneficial effects of wound cleansing as indicated above and the potential harmful effects of unnecessarily disturbing the delicate equilibrium that naturally exists at the wound surface.

The ultimate aim of wound cleansing is to remove both organic and inorganic debris whilst maintaining the optimum local environment to facilitate wound healing.

The decision to cleanse a wound should be based upon the following:

- the size, shape and location of the patient's wound
- the condition of the wound bed and stage of healing
- the availability and effectiveness of different methods of cleansing

- the availability and effectiveness of different cleansing agents
- the patient's perceptions and needs.

3.4 WOUND CLEANSING TECHNIQUES

Introduction

In the past, wound cleansing has been associated with ritualistic practice and many myths still surround this practice today. Advances in wound care technology have in recent years provided practitioners with alternative methods of cleansing wounds, which do not necessarily involve the use of traditional cleansing solutions. The use of interactive wound dressings have in many instances effectively replaced the need to routinely cleanse the wound at each dressing change. Advances in dressing technology in recent years have been responsible for the widespread acceptance of dressings as an alternative method of safe, effective wound cleansing. For these reasons, increasingly large numbers of practitioners are questioning the continued use of potentially toxic antiseptics as wound cleansing agents.

The relative merits of different methods of cleaning wounds are still debated. Thomlinson in 1987 was able to demonstrate that no one method of swabbing wounds was significantly more effective in reducing the bacterial count at the wound's surface. Swabbing from clean to dirty areas, top to bottom, or inside to outside merely resulted in the redistribution of bacteria across the surface of the wound. Swabbing the wound surface may mechanically dislodge loose, devitalised tissue but does not actively remove pathogens from the wound. Vigorous cleansing has the additional detrimental effect of causing further trauma to healing tissue, which may be uncomfortable for the patient and in many cases can actively prolong the inflammatory response. If foreign bodies are present in the wound, swabbing may only serve to drive them deeper into the tissues where they can act as a focus of infection. Traditional wound swabbing materials such as cotton wool or gauze are known to shed fine, fibrous particles on to the surface of the wound, which can be responsible for foreign body reactions, a prolonged inflammatory response and an increased risk of wound infection (Wood 1976). The Surgical Materials Testing Laboratory (1992) recommend that the use of non-woven swabs or non-filamented cotton wool is more appropriate for wound cleansing procedures, as they shed less fibres than traditional gauze swabs. However, evidence suggests that significant numbers of hospital nurses are still using traditional cotton wool balls to routinely wipe over the surface of wounds (Russel 1993). The same study indicated that nurses preferred to use gloves rather than forceps when dressing wounds. From a practical point of view, it can be difficult to apply some of the new-generation dressing products using forceps, especially those which have an adhesive backing or are presented as a gel.

Wound irrigation

Wound irrigation can be performed using a variety of methods including syringes, spray canisters, semi-rigid ampoules or showering. Irrigation under pressure is an effective method of cleansing wounds that are infected or heavily contaminated (Madden & Edlich 1971). High pressure irrigation using a 30 ml syringe and an 18–20 G needle lowers the infection rates in contaminated wounds (Chisholm 1992). Optimal pressures for effective wound irrigation are reported as being between 10 and 15 pounds per square inch; evidence suggests that achieving the correct pressure is more important than the type of cleansing solution chosen (Fergason 1990). High pressure wound irrigation is usually achieved using syringes and needles, and care is required to avoid the risk of needlestick injuries in both patient and carer. Consideration also should be given to the possibility of splash back and the dissemination of microorganisms into the surrounding tissues and possible contamination of the practitioner. The adoption of universal precautions is necessary to minimise the risks of cross-infection with hepatitis B virus or with HIV (human immunodeficiency virus) and refers to the practice of wearing gloves at all times when handling body secretions. The availability of sterile saline in semi-rigid ampoules and pressurised canisters allows practitioners to irrigate wounds without the risk of needlestick injuries. Advantages of using pressurised canisters over traditional methods of irrigation include speed, ease of use, cost-effectiveness and the absence of reports of significant differences in wound infection rates (Lawrence 1994). Disadvantages include unreliability of the canisters and difficulty in warming the contents to a consistent temperature.

Irrigation at high pressure can, however, cause damage to delicate granulation and epithelial tissue and may cause discomfort for some patients. The use of lower pressures is recommended for the irrigation of clean granulating wounds and higher pressures should be reserved for infected wounds. Cleansing of acute traumatic wounds is particularly important to remove dirt and soil from the wound bed, which provide the necessary conditions for the multiplication of microorganisms (Rodeheaver 1974).

Bathing and showering

It is becoming increasingly common practice for chronic wounds such as leg ulcers to be cleansed in the bath, shower or a bucket of lukewarm tap water (Morison & Moffatt 1994). As well as cleaning the wound and the surrounding skin, this practice can be of great psychological benefit to the patient. Patients with wounds in areas that are likely to be heavily contaminated with bacteria, such as perineal wounds, sacral pressure sores, pilonidal sinuses or rectal abscesses will greatly benefit from being given the opportunity to allow adherent dressings to soak free. Bathing also facilitates thorough cleansing of these wounds and allows patients to attend to their own personal hygiene needs. Care should be taken not to soak wounds for long periods of time, as open tissue has a tendency to absorb water which increases the amount of exudate produced over the following few days and often necessitates more frequent dressing changes. Chrinz et al (1989) were able to demonstrate that allowing surgical patients to remove dressings and shower on the first post-operative day did not increase wound infection rates. However, bathing facilities are not always safe and easily accessible in patients' homes and some cultures and religions prohibit bathing in non-running water.

3.5 WOUND CLEANSING SOLUTIONS

Introduction

Wound cleansing is a general term often used to describe the combined processes of wound cleansing and disinfection. Rodeheaver (1988) urges practitioners to separate these two actions, by cleansing the wound first and then, if necessary, disinfecting the wound using an antimicrobial. Not all wounds will require cleansing at each dressing change and even fewer will require disinfecting. If this principle were followed, the indiscriminate use of antimicrobials would be limited and far less tissue damage would occur.

Antiseptics

Since the introduction of topical antiseptics by Lister in the 1860s, a wide range of antimicrobial agents have been used in an attempt to prevent and treat wound infections. For many years it has become established practice to rely on the use of antiseptic agents for both the cleansing and debriding of wounds. During the last 25 years much conflicting research has emerged regarding the effectiveness of antiseptics on open wounds. Interpretation of findings is difficult, as sample sizes are often small, methodologies inconsistent and many studies are carried out using either animal models, or in vitro and in vivo techniques. The significance of these results for human tissue and implications for clinical

practice is still unclear and is fiercely debated (Rodeheaver 1988, Moore 1992). Bacteria do cause local inflammation, delay wound contraction, reduce wound tensile strength and are leukocytotoxic. It is therefore important to balance the cytotoxicity of bacteria against the potential cytotoxicity of antiseptics. Problems associated with the use of hydrogen peroxide and sodium hypochlorite (Eusol) have meant that in recent years the continued use of antiseptics for the routine cleansing of wounds has been widely questioned by practitioners.

Table 3.1 summarises the evidence that collectively indicates the potential damage that these antiseptics may have on healthy tissue. Currently the literature reveals a lack of consensual findings, but suggests that the use of these antiseptics for wound management should be confined to specific clinical indications.

Activity   35 MINUTES

Read Article 6 in the Reader (p. 170).

1. List the detrimental effects that are attributed to the use of hypochlorite solutions when used for cleaning wounds.
2. Briefly summarise any weaknesses in the arguments presented above.

FEEDBACK

1. For the last 20 years the use of hypochlorite solutions for wound management has been fiercely debated and has resulted in many differences of opinion. In her extensive and comprehensive review of the literature Moore identified the following objections to the use of hypochlorites.

- Action of hypochlorites is reduced in the presence of organic matter.
- Hypochlorites are cytotoxic—fibroblasts, keratinocytes, leukocytes.
- Hypochlorites can prolong the inflammatory response.
- Hypochlorites can cause capillary shut-down.
- Hypochlorites can cause acute renal failure and hypernatraemia.
- Hypochlorites damage granulation and epithelial tissue.
- Hypochlorites reduce collagen synthesis and decrease wound tensile strength.
- Hypochlorites are irritant to local tissues and cause localised oedema.

Table 3.1 Antiseptics commonly used for infected wounds

Antiseptic	Action	Adverse effects
Hypochlorite solutions (Eusol)	Effective against Gram-positive/negative bacteria, some spores and viruses	Cell toxicity Reduced capillary blood flow Toxic to granulation tissue Prolongs the inflammatory response Skin irritation, discomfort and pain Localised oedema (Moore 1992)
Hydrogen peroxide	Mechanical cleansing action, reacts with catalase in wounds, releasing oxygen which removes some contaminants	Toxic to fibroblasts (Linweaver et al 1985) Irrigation into closed cavities can cause air emboli and surgical emphysema (Sleigh 1985) Effects are short lived Causes pain on contact Irritates surrounding skin (Morgan 1993)
Acetic acid	Effective against *Pseudomonas aeruginosa* in superficial wounds as a result of altering the pH of the wound	Efficacy is short lived, requiring twice-daily dressings Can cause overgrowth of *Staphylococcus aureus* and *Proteus* (Sloss et al 1993) Causes severe stinging on contact with wound (Morgan 1993)
Povidone-iodine	Has the broadest spectrum of any antiseptic	Extensive reviews suggest use should be avoided in larger, open wounds owing to delay in wound healing and iodine toxicity May increase infection rates in contaminated wounds (Rodeheaver 1988)
Cetrimide	Broad spectrum antiseptic	Marked fibroblast toxicity (Morgan 1993) Can cause skin sensitivities Less effective against pseudomonas

- Hypochlorites cause some patients pain on contact.
- Hypochlorite usage is both costly and time consuming.

2. Although most practitioners would now agree that it is not necessary to expose patients to the potential or actual risks of hypochlorite toxicity, it is interesting to consider how this decision was reached in the light of the following points.

- There is a lack of consensual findings reported in the literature regarding the effects of hypochlorites on wound healing.
- Much of the research has methodological weakness.
- Some studies are descriptive and anecdotal.
- Studies reporting life-threatening side-effects document single cases only.
- Many studies make use of animal wound models; the relevance of these findings to clinical practice remains uncertain.
- Only limited studies have been conducted using humans.
- There has been a tendency for nursing literature to refer to these studies without adopting a critical stance.

- There is still a body of medical opinion that prescribes and supports the use of hypochlorites.

However, Moore reminds us that on a 'balance of probabilities' the continued use of hypochlorites is too risky, especially in the light of the development of alternative methods of wound cleansing that are safe, effective and easy to use.

• •

The principles of using any antiseptics should always be carefully considered and rigorously applied in order to safeguard patients.

Principles of using antiseptics

Careful consideration should be given to the advantages and disadvantages of their use.

- Antiseptics should not be indiscriminately used for the cleansing of clean, granulating wounds.
- Prior to cleansing with an antiseptic, hard eschar should be removed.
- Antiseptics should only be used as an adjunct to systemic antibiotic therapy.

- Antiseptics should only be used for limited periods of time and should be reviewed at regular intervals.
- Following cleansing with an antiseptic, the wound area should be liberally flushed with saline to minimise potential toxicity.

General disadvantages of antiseptics

- Antiseptics are rapidly deactivated by the presence of organic material within wounds—pus, slough, necrotic tissue (Rodeheaver 1988, Morgan 1993).
- Antiseptics do not penetrate tissue or exudate (Rodeheaver 1995).
- At low concentrations antiseptics only act as an irrigant solution; at high concentrations they can reduce bacterial counts but can damage tissues (Thomas 1990).
- Antiseptics require sufficient contact time to be effective (Zamora 1986).
- Many studies question the cytotoxicity of commonly available antiseptics (Linweaver 1985, Rodeheaver 1988).
- Some antiseptics are known to cause allergic contact dermatitis (Bajaja & Gupta 1986).

Practical disadvantages of antiseptics

- Chemical instability results in a limited shelf life.
- Availability is restricted in many practice areas.
- Use can be associated with leakage and skin maceration.
- Leakage may stain the patient's skin, clothes and bedding.
- Effective use of antiseptics requires frequent dressing changes.
- Use of antiseptics makes dressing changes more time consuming.
- Use of antiseptics can increase patient pain and discomfort.
- Antiseptics are not cost effective when additional resources are considered.
- Use of antiseptics raises issues related to professional accountability.
- There are other more effective cleansing agents available.

If antiseptics are to be used, careful consideration should be given to ensuring that their beneficial effects are maximised and side-effects limited. In most instances, the principle of allowing sufficient contact time between the antiseptic and the wound surface is ignored in clinical practice. The practical disadvantages of using antiseptics, described above, challenge the validity of the continued use of antiseptics for the management of the majority of wounds. The use of topical antibiotics has previously been discussed in Section 3.3.

Saline or water?

For those wounds that are not grossly contaminated, an isotonic 0.9% saline solution, applied at room temperature, is currently the cleansing agent of choice. There are no reports of any adverse effects on healing tissue, it is easy to use, inexpensive, widely available and as such fulfils the requirements of an ideal cleansing solution. For similar reasons, the use of tap water for wound cleansing is becoming an acceptable alternative for the cleansing of both acute traumatic soft tissue wounds (Angeras & Brandbard 1992) and chronic wounds such as leg ulcers (Cullum 1994). Water has been used for centuries without any reported detrimental effects and has always been used in first aid situations to clean wounds. Any fears concerning bacterial contamination from non-sterile water supplies and subsequent effects on wounds appear to be unfounded (Angeras & Brandbard 1992). Microbiologists recommend the running of tap water for a few minutes prior to wound cleansing to flush out any potentially high levels of bacteria. However, bacterial cultures grown from wounds cleansed with tap water were never isolated from the tap water (Angeras & Brandbard 1992). Immersion of ulcerated legs in water for any length of time should be avoided as contact with non-isotonic cleansing fluids will allow water to pass across the semipermeable cell membranes of the tissues causing them to swell and eventually rupture. This can be observed after soaking patients' leg ulcers for relatively short periods of time when a slight increase in the overall circumference of the wound can be seen.

The continuing trend of early postoperative discharge and the increased use of day-surgery units inevitably means that patients can be back in their own homes within hours of surgery. The management of patients' wounds within their home environment has to be more appropriate to the philosophy of self-care and should make use of readily available resources such as tap water or normal saline.

Temperature of cleansing solutions

The temperature of a wound directly affects the rate of healing. Lock (1979) demonstrated that phagocytic and mitotic cellular activity is significantly decreased at temperatures below 28°C. The application of cool cleansing solutions can have similar local effects. It can take as long as 40 minutes for a wound to regain its original temperature after cleansing and up to 3 hours for cell division and leukocytic activity to return to normal (Myers 1982). Cleansing solutions should therefore be stored at room temperature or can be warmed if cold, by immersing sachets in warm water.

The method of application of a wound cleanser is of as much significance as the selection of which type of cleanser to use, together with the frequency of its use and justification of a supportive rationale. Optimum wound healing is achieved by using only non-toxic solutions for cleansing.

Self-assessment   5 MINUTES

Briefly describe four undesirable consequences of wound cleansing.

. . . .

FEEDBACK

In your answer you should have discussed the following main points.

- Removal of exudate may reduce the healing potential of the wound, as exudate has bactericidal properties which help to naturally cleanse the wound during the inflammatory stage of healing. Exudate production also helps provide the moist environment that is required to support the migration of phagocytic leukocytes across the wound bed.
- The unnecessary removal of slough should also be avoided, as slough has a protective function at the wound surface. In practice, newly formed epithelial cells are difficult to distinguish from slough and fibrous tissue and are often removed accidentally in an attempt to clean the wound bed. Small areas of slough will not significantly impair wound healing and can be safely ignored.
- The application of cold cleansing lotions can significantly impair the rate of healing by slowing down the rate at which cell division occurs. This effect will be exacerbated if dressings are changed frequently and the wound is routinely cleaned on each occasion.
- The application of some cleansing solutions such as antiseptics may have undesirable side-effects on healing tissues making their use questionable.
- Various cleansing techniques such as swabbing and use of high pressure irrigation can cause additional mechanical trauma to the delicate tissues within the wound.
- The process of wound cleansing may be extremely painful for some patients and may greatly exacerbate feelings of fear and anxiety.

. . . .

For the reasons described above, it is not necessary to routinely cleanse a patient's wound. The decision to cleanse a wound should be carefully considered after a detailed assessment of the patient's circumstances and the condition of the wound has been made. There are many valid justifications for wound cleansing. If after careful consideration the decision to cleanse is made, thought should then be given to which is the most appropriate method of achieving this and the cleansing solution with the least toxic effects should be selected.

3.6 METHODS OF WOUND DEBRIDEMENT

Introduction

Wounds are frequently covered by a combination of sloughy or necrotic tissue, fibrin and exudate which harbour bacteria and contain inflammatory mediators. The presence of this mixture of devitalised tissue increases the risk of wound infection and can actively delay wound healing by prolonging the inflammatory response. Slough and necrotic tissue act as an effective bacterial culture medium, as well as a mechanical barrier limiting the phagocytic activity of scavenging leukocytes which have the ability to destroy invading microorganisms. One of the fundamental principles of effective wound management is to facilitate the process of debridement in order to promote healing and reduce the risk of infection.

The term wound debridement is usually reserved to describe the removal of either devitalised tissue, which in many instances is firmly adherent to the wound bed, or foreign bodies, which may be firmly embedded in the tissues.

Selecting an appropriate method of wound debridement

There are several methods of debriding wounds which may be used in a variety of different clinical circumstances. The choice of an appropriate method of debriding wounds is a complex one that can sometimes provoke controversy. The main treatment options include:

- surgical excision
- hydrogel dressings
- hydrocolloid dressings
- alginate dressings
- polysaccharide pastes
- enzymatic cleansers.

The use of dressing products to debride wounds is discussed in greater detail in Section 4.3.

There is a variety of different methods that can be used to successfully debride wounds. Selection of a particular method of wound debridement should be carefully considered and is dependent on a combination of factors.

Wound debridement— clinical considerations

- The type of injury and potential contamination.
- The aetiology of the wound.
- The location of the wound.
- The extent of tissue damage and type of tissue involvement.
- The size of the wound and extent of devitalised tissue.
- The amount of exudate production.

Wound debridement— practical considerations

- Time available.
- Availability of resources.
- User skill, knowledge base and professional accountability.
- Cost-effectiveness.
- The care environment—hospital or community.
- The patient's wishes.

The degree of potential contamination by microorganisms is an important factor to be considered when selecting an appropriate method of debridement. Traumatic wounds differ from surgical or chronic wounds in a number of ways and are contaminated by various combinations of dirt, oil, foreign bodies, bacteria, fungi or spores. This type of injury requires thorough cleansing and debridement of the wound and surrounding skin, which is best achieved using large volumes of saline or tap water. Decontamination of traumatic wounds should be carried out quickly, as the organic and inorganic components of soil have a detrimental effect on exposed tissue, providing the necessary conditions for the multiplication of microorganisms (Rodeheaver 1974). Following thorough wound cleansing, surgical debridement is required in order to facilitate the thorough removal of devitalised tissue and foreign bodies. This can be performed under local or general anaesthetic depending upon the extent of contamination and tissue damage. The use of laser therapy for debridement is becoming more widespread; it has the additional benefits of instant haemostasis and can be performed on an outpatient basis. All traumatic wounds, however superficial, require careful exploration in order to exclude the possibility of even the smallest foreign body such as grit, splinters, glass or grease remaining within the wound where they are likely to prolong healing by acting as foci for infection. The continued presence of grit in a wound may lead to the development of permanent 'tattooing' of the skin . The overall aim of surgical wound debridement is to remove gross contaminants with the minimum of pain to the patient and trauma to the tissues. For minor traumatic wounds, asepsis is unnecessary until all gross contamination is removed.

Self-assessment   10 MINUTES

Consider the similarities between the processes of wound cleansing and wound debridement.

FEEDBACK

Your answer should have included the following points.

Essentially the processes of wound cleansing and debridement are similar in that they both aim to rid the wound of surface contaminants. Wound cleansing is a more general term used to describe methods of removing stale exudate and loose debris.

The aetiology of a wound will influence the choice of different methods of debridement. It is well recognised that early surgical excision of devitalised tissue is the treatment of choice for a diabetic patient with a necrotic or sloughy foot ulcer, owing to the increased risk of infection associated with such wound types. Conservative methods of achieving debridement using moisture-retentive dressings may not always be appropriate in such circumstances.

The location, size and amount of devitalised tissue present in the wound influence selection of particular debridement methods. Smaller areas of slough or necrotic tissue can be quickly and safely removed using dressing products such as hydrogels, hydrocolloids, alginates, polysaccharide pastes or enzymatic preparations. These types of dressing effectively enhance the body's ability to debride devitalised tissue by the process of autolysis. Autolytic debridement facilitates the breaking down and liquefying of devitalised tissue. The maintenance of a moist wound surface helps to promote rehydration of slough and necrotic tissue, whilst allowing leukocytes and enzymes present in exudate to break down avascular tissue (Alvarez 1988). The speed of this process is dependent on a number of factors including the size of the wound and the general physical condition of the patient; in many instances significant improvement can be observed within 3–4 days. Surgical debridement remains the quickest method of removing larger areas of necrosis.

Care needs to be taken to determine the extent and type of tissue involvement present in the wound. The presence of tendon, muscle or bone necessitates specialist referral before the decision to debride further should be taken. Surgical management may be necessary, although conservative treatment in some circumstances may be a more appropriate option. This would generally involve the use of moisture-retentive dressings which facilitate autolytic wound debridement whilst preventing dehydration of the exposed deeper structures.

Finally the amount of exudate produced by the wound is also an important consideration when deciding which method of debridement is most suitable. Wet, viscous, slough in a wound can be difficult to remove surgically at the bedside when compared with the removal of a hard, dry eschar. The use of alginate dressings for the management of highly exudating, sloughy wounds is effective, as they form a hydrophilic gel at the surface of the wound which absorbs exudate and promotes autolytic debridement. Enzymatic preparations are another useful alternative method of debriding exudating wounds as they are able to quickly penetrate softer, devitalised tissue. The use of either alginates or enzymatic debriding agents is not successful on hard, dehydrated eschar as they are not active in a dry environment. Conversely, the use of hydrogels and hydrocolloids is not appropriate for debriding highly exudating wounds owing to their restricted ability to absorb large amounts of fluid; they are better suited to wounds that produce less exudate.

In addition to the clinical factors already discussed, there are other practical considerations to be taken into account when debriding a wound. The availability of resources is often determined by the care environment. Access to members of the multidisciplinary team who possess the appropriate technical skills to safely, surgically debride a wound, is usually more limited in the community setting and in such instances the use of more conservative debridement methods may be a more realistic alternative. However, the length of time taken to achieve debridement is an important variable when considering the overall cost-effectiveness of treatment. The patient's wishes should at all times be taken into consideration when deciding how best to manage a sloughy or necrotic wound as cooperation with treatment obviously influences the final outcome.

Self-assessment 2 MINUTES

Suggest a suitable method of debriding the wound of a patient with a hard, dry, necrotic pressure sore on the heel, justifying your choice.

FEEDBACK

Although there are a variety of treatment options available, the most effective method of debriding this type of wound would be surgically. Excision of necrotic tissue should always be dependent on the availability of an appropriately qualified practitioner, i.e. someone who has received specific training and supervision and who has the appropriate knowledge base in order to take responsibility for the consequences of his or her actions. In the absence of such circumstances, conservative methods of debridement would be appropriate. Selection of a moisture-retentive dressing capable of donating fluid to the dehydrated wound bed, e.g. a hydrocolloid or hydrogel, is essential to encourage autolytic debridement.

Methods of wound debridement to be used with caution

- Wet-to-dry saline soaks.
- Antiseptic solutions.
- Antiseptic creams.

The use of wet-to-dry saline soaks to achieve wound debridement remains common practice in some clinical environments (Bryant 1992). This method of achieving debridement uses saline-soaked gauze which dries out on the wound surface facilitating the mechanical removal of devitalised tissue at dressing change. This technique is usually painful for the patient and carries the additional risk of damaging healthy tissue on removal. Frequent dressing changes are usually required and in practice this technique can encourage the tight packing of wound cavities, which compromises capillary blood flow, causes additional patient discomfort and prolongs wound closure. For these reasons this method of debridement should not be used. The use of antiseptics in various formats has already been fully discussed in Section 3.5.

Myiasis (maggots)

No discussion of wound debridement would be complete without mentioning myiasis. Infestation of open wounds with maggots is commonly seen in tropical countries and becomes a more frequent occurrence in temperate countries during warm summers—in 1995 anecdotal reports of wound infestation dramatically increased in the UK. Although usually treated with repulsion and disgust by both patient and carers alike, maggots generally only digest necrotic tissue, slough and bacteria, leaving the wound bed clean; this encourages the rapid growth of granulation tissue (Morgan 1995) making them an effective, if less popular, method of debriding wounds. Disadvantages of maggot therapy are obvious and include aesthetic reasons and local discomfort and itching sometimes caused by their use. Removal of maggots from a wound can be achieved either surgically or by using various antiseptic solutions. The general use of maggots has declined since the 1940s with the introduction of antibiotic therapy, but is set for a revival as breeding of appropriate species of flies in a sterile environment becomes a viable, commercial proposition.

Contraindications for surgical wound debridement

Not all types of wound are suitable for surgical debridement. The following would be unsuitable for localised excision of necrotic tissue by nurses and should be referred to a member of medical staff:

- friable wounds with an increased tendency to haemorrhage, e.g. fungating wounds
- wounds with firmly adherent devitalised tissue where the difference between viable and nonviable tissue is difficult to distinguish
- wounds in which there is the possibility of damaging associated structures, e.g. blood vessels, nerves, tendons
- hand wounds—these should *always* be referred to an appropriate surgeon
- ischaemic wounds which have an increased risk of infection and susceptibility to additional tissue trauma, e.g. diabetic patients with ulcers.

Self-assessment   10 MINUTES

What clinical and professional issues should be taken into consideration by nurses when debriding a wound using a scalpel?

FEEDBACK

The clinical and professional issues relating to the use of local surgical debridement are summarised below:

Clinical considerations

- The need for informed patient consent.
- Thorough wound assessment and identification of devitalised tissues.
- The use of extreme caution at all times, especially at the wound margin which is usually superficial.

- The need for the use of local anaesthetic.
- The need for patient reassurance and support.
- The need for adequate time and appropriate resources, e.g. the use of sharp, sterile blades.

Professional considerations

- Possession of the appropriate knowledge base.
- Specific training and adequate supervised practice.
- Individual acceptance of professional accountability.

Debridement is necessary to remove devitalised tissue from the wound bed in order to facilitate the natural process of wound cleansing. There is a variety of different methods of achieving wound debridement which depend on availability of resources, practical skills and user experience (see Sect. 7.1). The fundamental principle when attempting to debride a wound, is to remove any necrotic areas as quickly as possible without causing additional trauma to the underlying viable tissues.

SUMMARY

This section has highlighted some of the complex issues related to wound management and has emphasised the need to identify treatment objectives when planning care. Practitioners require a good understanding of the principles of wound management in order to make informed clinical decisions based upon an accurate assessment of their patient's circumstances.

In this section you have learnt that:

- The application of basic wound management principles supports clinical decision making and will help to justify the use of selected treatment interventions.
- Early identification of patients with infected wounds is essential if appropriate treatment is to be implemented.
- The aim of wound cleansing is to gently remove contaminants from the surface of the wound without disturbing the delicate granulation tissue present on the wound bed.
- Normal saline or water are the recommended wound cleansers of choice.
- Involvement of patients in the decision-making process is likely to improve both compliance with and acceptability of their treatment.
- Multidisciplinary collaboration is of fundamental importance when planning care of patients with compromised tissue viability.

REFERENCES

Alvarez O 1988 Moist environment for healing: matching the dressing to the wound. Ostomy/Wound Management 6(Winter): 64–83

Angeras A D, Brandbard A 1992 Comparison between sterile saline and tap water for the cleansing of acute traumatic soft tissue wounds. European Journal of Surgery 158(33): 347–350

Ashurst S 1994 Role of nurses in antibiotic therapy. British Journal of Nursing 3(17): 864–865

Bajaja A K, Gupta S C 1986 Contact hypersensitivity to topical antibacterial agents. International Journal of Dermatology 25: 103–105

Bower M, Stein R, Evans T R 1992 The double-blind study of the efficacy of metronidazole gel in the treatment of malodorous, fungating tumours. European Journal of Cancer 28a(45): 888–889

Bryant R 1992 Acute and chronic wounds, nursing management. Mosby Year Book, St Louis

Chisholm C 1992 Wound evaluation and cleansing. Emergency Clinics of North America 10(4): 665–672

Chrinz H, Vibits H, Cordtz T et al 1989 Need for surgical wound dressing. British Journal of Surgery 76(2): 204–205

Cruse P J E, Foord R 1973 A five year prospective study of 23,649 surgical wounds. Archives of Surgery 107: 206–217

Cruse P J E, Foord R 1980 The epidemiology of wound infection. Surgical Clinics of North America 60(1): 27–40

Cullum N 1994 The nursing management of leg ulcers in the community: a critical review of the research. HMSO, London

Duckworth G 1993 Diagnosis and management of methicillin-resistant *Staphylococcus aureus* infection. British Medical Journal 307(23): 1049–1052

Esuvaranathan K, Kaun Y F 1992 A study of 245 infected surgical wounds in Singapore. Journal of Hospital Infection 21: 231–240

Faoagali J, Thong M L 1985 Ten years experience with methicillin-resistant *Staphylococcus aureus* in a large Australian hospital. Journal of Hospital Infection 20: 113–119

Fergason A 1990 A systematic approach to trauma relief. The management of the Accident & Emergency wound. Professional Nurse 6(2): 82–90

Gilcrest B, Reed C 1989 The bacteriology of chronic venous ulcers treated with occlusive hydrocolloid dressings. British Journal of Dermatology 121(3): 337–344

Gould D 1994 The significance of hand drying in the prevention of infection. Nursing Times 90(47): 33–35

Greenwood D 1995 Antimicrobial therapy, 3rd edn. Oxford University Press, Oxford

Hoffman S 1984 Silver sulfadiazine: an antibacterial agent for topical use in burns. Scandinavian Journal of Plastic and Reconstructive Surgery 18: 119–126

Holn D, Pounce B, Burton R 1977 Antimicrobial systems of the surgical wound. American Journal of Surgery 133(5): 597–600

Lawrence C 1994 A novel presentation of saline for wound irrigation. Journal of Wound Care 3(7): 334–337

Lawrence J C, Lilly H A, Kidson A 1992 Wound dressings and the airborne dispersal of bacteria. Lancet 339: 807–809

Linweaver W 1985 Topical antimicrobial toxicity. Archives of Surgery 120: 267–271

Lock P 1979 The effects of temperature on mitotic activity at the edge of experimental wounds. Lock Research Laboratories Paper. Lock Laboratories, Kent

Longfield J N, Townsend T R 1985 Methicillin-resistant *Staphylococcus aureus* (MRSA) risk outcomes of colonised vs infected patients. Infection Control 6(11): 445–450

Lowbury E J 1981 Assessing the effectiveness of antimicrobial agents applied to living tissues. Journal de Pharmacie de Belgique 36: 298–302

Madden J, Edlich R F 1971 Applications of principles of fluid dynamics to surgical wound irrigation. Current Topics in Surgery 1: 85–92

Mishriki S F, Law D J, Jeffery P J 1990 Factors affecting the incidence of post-operative wound infection. Journal of Hospital Infection 16: 223–230

Moore D 1992 Hypochlorites: a review of the evidence. Journal of Wound Care 1(4): 44–53

Morgan D 1993 Is there still a role for antiseptics? Journal of Tissue Viability 3(3): 80–84

Morgan D 1995 Myiasis: the rise and fall of maggot therapy. Journal of Tissue Viability 5(2): 43–51

Morison M, Moffatt C 1994 A colour guide to the assessment and management of leg ulcers, 2nd edn. Mosby, Spain

Myers J A 1982 Modern plastic surgical dressings, Health Society Service Journal 4(18 March): 336–337

Rodeheaver G T 1974 Identification of the wound infection potentiating factors in soil. American Journal of Surgery 128: 8

Rodeheaver G 1988 Topical wound management. Ostomy/Wound Management 4(Fall): 59–68

Rodeheaver G 1995 Conference proceedings. Symposium on Advanced Wound Care & Medical Research Forum on Wound Repair, San Diego, April 30–May 4. Health Management Publications, USA

Russel L 1993 Healing alternatives. Nursing Times 89(42): 88–89

Sedgewick J 1995 Computerised surveillance. Nursing Times 91(10): 59–62

Simpson S 1992 Methicillin-resistant *Staphylococcus aureus* and its implications for nursing practice: a literature review. Nursing Practice 5(2): 2–6

Sleigh J W 1985 Hazards of hydrogen peroxide. British Medical Journal 291: 1706

Sloss J M, Cumberland N, Milner S M 1993 Acetic acid used for the elimination of *Pseudomonas aeruginosa* from burns and soft tissue wounds. Journal of Army Medical Corps 139: 49–51

Surgical Materials Testing Laboratory 1992 The dressing times. Surgical Materials Testing Laboratory Leaflet 5(2). Surgical Materials Testing Laboratory, Bridgend, p 3

Thomas S 1990 Wound management and dressings. The Pharmaceutical Press, London

Thomlinson D 1987 To clean or not to clean? Nursing Times 83(9): 71–74

Willis J 1995 Skin care—principles of hand washing. Nursing Times 91(44): 43–44

Wood R A B 1976 Disintegration of cellulose dressings in open granulating wounds. British Medical Journal 1: 1444–1445

Zamora J 1986 Chemical and microbiological characteristics and toxicity of povidone-iodine solutions. American Journal of Surgery 117: 181–186

4 Wound dressings

Introduction

Wound management research activities over the last 20 years have stimulated increasing interest in this newly developing clinical speciality. This has resulted in much confusion as practitioners struggle to keep up to date with current approaches to wound management. At times, conflicts of opinion have added to this confusion making the selection of appropriate wound treatments into a complex decision requiring a thorough understanding of current philosophies of wound management.

LEARNING OUTCOMES

When you have completed this section you should be able to:

- evaluate the functions of an ideal wound dressing, differentiating between traditional and interactive dressing products
- analyse the range of factors that influence the selection of dressing products
- describe the classification of different types of dressing products
- apply the principle of cost-effectiveness to wound management.

4.1 TECHNOLOGICAL DEVELOPMENTS IN WOUND DRESSINGS

Introduction

Recent advances in the development of wound contact materials has resulted in a rapid proliferation of different types of wound dressings. The speed at which these developments have taken place has left many health professionals feeling out of date and confused as to which dressing to select. Manufacturing technology has resulted in the development of dressing products which have very specific functions such as the ability to absorb exudate, debride devitalised tissue or control odour to name but a few.

Effective wound management relies heavily upon the selection and application of an appropriate wound dressing. But it must be emphasised that although important, the selection of a dressing without holistic wound assessment which takes into consideration the multiplicity of factors known to prolong healing will not ultimately prove successful (see Sect. 2). The management of patients with wounds is a complex activity and as such is much more than merely the selection of an appropriate dressing product.

Activity   5 MINUTES

From your nursing experience, suggest up to six reasons why it may be necessary to dress a patient's wound.

FEEDBACK

There are many reasons why the dressing of wounds can be beneficial. These will always depend on a patient's individual circumstances and wishes. Wound management priorities alter with time; it can therefore prove useful when considering the selection of a particular dressing to define the primary and secondary objectives that will be achieved by dressing a patient's wound. Your answer should have included some of the following:

- to create a warm, non-toxic, moist environment that is conducive to healing
- to promote haemostasis
- to prevent cross-infection
- to treat wound infection
- to reduce pain by excluding air from exposed nerve endings
- to support or immobilise an injured body part
- to control and contain wound exudate and leakage
- to promote autolytic debridement
- to protect exposed tissues from mechanical trauma
- to minimise and contain odour
- to protect the surrounding skin
- to provide psychological support for patient and carers
- to improve quality of life.

New wound dressing technologies

The work of Winter in 1962 on the effects of occlusive dressings and re-epithelialisation rates of superficial wounds stimulated a significant amount of research activity into new dressing materials. The net result of this has been the development of a new generation of dressing products which has transformed and challenged traditionally accepted approaches to wound management and greatly improved the care of patients with compromised tissue viability. As the principle of moist wound healing gained acceptance in clinical practice, researchers began to develop innovative dressing products that were able for the first time to provide conditions at the wound surface that were conducive to healing.

Self-assessment   **5 MINUTES**

How much do you remember about our earlier discussion (Sect. 2.3) which described the provision of a supportive microclimate at the wound surface? Try to recall three conditions known to be important in order to maximise wound healing.

FEEDBACK

One of the fundamental aims of wound management is to provide a controlled set of conditions at the wound site in order to maximise the healing potential of the wound. Your answer should have included three of the following points:

- the maintenance of a moist environment
- the maintenance of a warm environment
- the maintenance of an oxygenated environment
- the maintenance of an acidic environment.

The ideal dressing

Prior to the much publicised work of Winter in the 1960s, Scales (1956) identified several properties considered to be ideal requirements of postoperative surgical dressings. They include:

- high moisture vapour permeability
- non-adherence to the wound surface
- the ability to prevent penetration of capillary loops into the dressing material
- high absorbent capacity
- the provision of a barrier to external contaminants
- good adhesion to the surrounding skin

- composed of hypoallergenic materials
- comfortable to wear
- sterile
- cost effective.

Turner (1985) developed the notion of an ideal dressing even further by refining the minimum criteria for the optimum wound dressing. This classic definition has since become widely accepted by practitioner and dressing manufacturer alike and has provided the framework for the development of many modern wound dressing materials. Turner gives the characteristics of an ideal dressing as:

- maintaining high humidity at the wound/dressing interface
- removing excess exudate and toxic components
- allowing gaseous exchange
- providing thermal insulation
- being impermeable to bacteria
- being free from particulate and toxic contaminants
- allowing removal without causing additional trauma.

Properties of wound dressings

Wound dressings can be broadly categorised as either passive or interactive. A passive dressing is one that simply protects the wound surface by covering it. Some protection against dehydration occurs if moisture is retained at the wound surface; however, this is not always the case. Disadvantages of this type of dressing include their tendency to rapidly become saturated with exudate, dry out and then adhere to the wound surface. Passive dressings are sometimes referred to as traditional dressing products and include products like paraffin gauze and low-adherent dressing pads. Their use should generally be restricted to closed surgical wounds or smaller, lightly exuding superficial wounds.

In contrast, interactive dressings are those that are able to actively interact with the wound surface in order to promote an environment that maximises healing potential. Interactive dressings are sometimes referred to as modern wound contact materials and it is within this area that a rapid expansion of wound dressing products has occurred. Many interactive dressings are also occlusive but the terms should not be used interchangeably. An occlusive dressing is one that totally seals off the wound from the external environment and is either semipermeable or impermeable to moisture. Interactive dressings have been developed from a wide range of different materials, all of which promote the principle of moist wound healing, but their modes of action differ considerably. For the sake of clarity, dressing products are often classified according to their structure and mode of action, although this is becoming more difficult as combination dressings evolve. Current wound dressing research and development activities are exploring methods of actively accelerating the healing process using a variety of innovative approaches including the application of growth factors (Robson et al 1995) and tissue engineering techniques which support the regeneration of new tissue within a matrix substitute.

Self-assessment	10 MINUTES

Use your own words to explain the following terms, giving an example of each:

1. interactive dressing
2. occlusive dressing.

· ·

FEEDBACK

Your answer should have stressed that these two terms are not interchangeable.

- An interactive dressing is one which actively promotes the optimal local environment required to facilitate wound healing. An example would be alginate dressings which on contact with wound exudate form a soft, warm gel. Interactive dressings function in a variety of different ways but their common characteristic is that they do not allow the wound surface to dehydrate and therefore support the philosophy of moist wound healing.
- Occlusive dressings are either impermeable or semipermeable to water and water vapour and effectively seal the wound from the external environment. Hydrocolloids are an example of both occlusive and interactive dressings; alginates, however, are interactive without being occlusive.

· ·

4.2 FACTORS INFLUENCING THE SELECTION OF DRESSINGS

Introduction

The selection of wound dressing products is influenced by a wide range of variables (Flanagan 1992) which are summarised in Box 4.1. Recognition of the significance of all of these factors is important if the most appropriate dressing materials are to be selected. Inappropriate selection of wound dressings may at best be uncomfortable for the patient, or at worst actively delay wound healing.

Box 4.1 Factors influencing nurses' selection of wound dressings

Professional factors

Clinical
1. Wound characteristics—size, appearance, etc.
2. Availability of dressings
3. Properties of dressings
4. Cost-effectiveness of dressings
5. Patient variables—allergies, compliance

Care environment
1. Pressure to conform with established practices
2. Resistance to change
3. Support from colleagues
4. Implementation of research-based practice

Knowledge
1. Lack of knowledge and understanding
2. Reluctance to take responsibility for clinical decisions
3. Lack of experience
4. Conflicting marketing messages from dressing manufacturers
5. Individual bias/preference for particular dressings

Interpersonal factors

Personality
1. Leadership styles
2. Assertiveness
3. Confidence
4. Lack of negotiation skills

Professional relationships
1. Influence of other team members
2. Trust/respect between team members
3. Conflicting opinions/priorities of care
4. Willingness to consult others
5. Team dynamics

Selection of wound dressing products

The first stage when choosing a wound dressing is to perform a comprehensive wound assessment (see Sect. 2 and Fig. 2.7, p. 43) in order to identify the most appropriate treatment objectives and to establish a profile of the patient including any factors that are likely to influence wound healing and selection of dressing materials. The clinical appearance of the wound and its classification (which has been discussed in Sect. 2.7) is an obvious factor influencing choice of dressing materials and will also determine the specific treatment objective required to maximise the healing potential of the wound.

Referring to Section 2.7, define the predominant treatment objective when treating the following types of wound:

- black necrotic wound
- yellow sloughy wound
- red granulating wound
- pink epithelialising wound.

• •

FEEDBACK

You should have said that the predominant treatment objective for a black necrotic wound is debridement and rehydration; for a yellow sloughy wound it is debridement and cleansing; and for both red granulating wounds and pink epithelialising wounds it is protection.

• •

These simple treatment objectives form the basic principles of wound management. Due to advances in the development of wound dressings, all are achievable to some extent by using an appropriate type of interactive dressing material. In some circumstances conservative treatment methods using dressings may actually achieve the intended treatment objective but may do so at a slower rate, e.g. hydrogel dressings can be used to debride necrotic tissue from wounds, but surgical debridement is usually quicker.

Once the general treatment objective of the wound has been determined, then the more specific treatment objectives should be identified taking into consideration a multidisciplinary perspective and the priorities of care identified by the patient. These should then be matched to the predominant functions of each available dressing type (see Table 4.1).

Complete the following boxes by identifying four factors in each box that influence the selection of wound dressings in your clinical setting. An example has been given in each case to start you off.

Wound characteristics
- Position of wound
-
-
-

Wound appearance
- Presence of necrotic tissue
-
-
-

Practical issues
- Dressing availability
-
-
-

Table 4.1 Functions of wound dressings

Major dressing classification	Predominant function of dressing type
Alginates	Absorption
Deodorising dressings	Odour control
Enzymes	Debridement
Foams	Absorption/protection
Hydrocolloids	Absorption/debridement/protection
Hydrofibres	Absorption/protection
Hydrogels	Debridement
Low-adherent primary contact dressings	Protection
Paraffin gauze	Protection
Polysaccharide beads	Absorption/debridement
Polyurethane membranes	Protection
Semipermeable films	Protection
Silicone gel sheets	Remodelling of scars

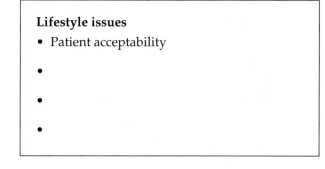

Lifestyle issues
- Patient acceptability

-

-

-

FEEDBACK

In the wound characteristics box you could have listed:

- position of wound
- depth of wound
- size of wound
- shape of wound
- amount of exudate.

In the wound appearance box you could have listed:

- presence of necrotic tissue
- suspected clinical infection
- presence of granulation tissue
- presence of epithelial tissue
- condition of surrounding skin.

In the practical issues box you could have listed:

- dressing availability
- ease of application
- frequency of dressing change
- ability to conform/remain secure
- cost-effectiveness.

In the lifestyle box you could have listed:

- patient's previous experience
- patient's mobility/activity levels
- is the dressing comfortable?
- is the dressing restrictive or bulky?
- patient/carer acceptability.

Professional factors influencing selection of dressing products

In some clinical areas the selection of dressing products continues to cause conflict between colleagues and interprofessional groups. Current philosophies of wound management reflect a major shift from chemical desloughing agents and the use of antiseptics to the promotion of an environment conducive to healing using interactive dressing products. This corresponds with the recognition and emergence of nursing's unique contribution to the management of patients with chronic wounds. Such differences in perspective are often responsible for triggering role conflict and deterioration of communication within the multidisciplinary team. Nurses within such teams may experience difficulty when trying to make wound management decisions based upon research-based practice as decisions relating to what type of dressing to use may be linked with issues relating to power, status and leadership (Flanagan 1992). The influence that medical staff exert on the selection of dressings is variable and tends to be more prescriptive within the acute hospital setting in comparison with the community. Traditionally community nursing staff have more autonomy than their hospital colleagues, but may experience frustration when effective dressing regimes are altered when patients either attend outpatient appointments or are admitted to hospital. As cost-effectiveness of treatment assumes an ever greater importance, the use of many wound dressings is being restricted in the mistaken belief that overall cost savings are being made. Issues of power and control also relate to the professional relationships that nurses have with each other. At some time in their career, most practitioners have experienced disappointment when colleagues have changed a patient's dressing regime without prior consultation and often without any supportive rationale.

The influence of these professional issues on dressing selection can be quite profound but is often difficult to identify. In relation to wound management, emphasis is often placed upon the acquisition of clinical knowledge which is often achieved at the expense of the development of advanced interpersonal skills such as assertiveness and clinical decision making. Selection of appropriate wound dressings depends on a combination of all of these skills and the application of theory to practice. In many settings nurses are coordinating the management of patients with compromised tissue viability. Taking responsibility for clinical decision making is a fundamental characteristic of professional accountability (see Sect. 7.1).

4.3 CLASSIFICATION OF PRIMARY CONTACT WOUND DRESSINGS

Introduction

Advances in the development of primary wound contact layers over the last 20 years have meant that a wide range of different dressing materials has become available to practitioners. The development of the more recent dressing products are all based upon the fundamental principle of promoting moist wound healing. There is a wide variety of dressing products currently available on the market with new products being constantly developed. As a consequence, selection of dressing materials has become increasingly more complex as the range of dressing products gets larger. In an attempt to simplify the selection of wound management products, dressings are usually classified according to generic name. However, classification of wound dressings is becoming increasingly more complex since not all products sharing the same classification work in exactly the same way and manufacturers are beginning to develop dressing products that are a combination of one or more of the generic groups.

Activity   30 MINUTES

The following pages provide a full classification, according to generic group, of the wound dressing products currently available.

1. Read carefully the information in Tables 4.2 to 4.18 on properties, clinical indications and practice guidelines given for each type of dressing.

2. Put a tick against those products which you have recently used or are currently using and, at the same time, consider whether they are the best choice available for the particular types of wounds that you commonly see.

3. Against each product a space has been left for the current price and its availability in your clinical setting. During the next week or so gather the information needed to complete the blanks.

Information regarding product prices may be obtained from the following sources:

- the dressings budget holder
- local wound management interest group
- local specialist nurses—tissue viability, infection control
- pharmacy/supplies department
- direct from manufacturers or company representatives.

As prices and availability of dressing products frequently change, it may be useful to record these details in pencil.

Alginate dressings

Generic description

Calcium alginate dressings are derived from seaweed. They produce a moist gel in the presence of exudate. Alginates rich in mannuronic acids (Sorbsan) form soft gels; alginates rich in glucuronic acids (Kaltostat) form firmer gels. An alternative classification is as type 1 or 2 dressings: type 1 contain calcium alginate fibres (Sorbsan); type 2 contain calcium-sodium alginate fibres (Kaltostat).

Table 4.2 Alginate dressings

Product name	Manufacturer	Presentation	Current cost	Availability Y/N
Comfeel Plus	Coloplast	Sheet dressing		
Comfeel SeaSorb	Coloplast	Cavity filler		
Sorbsan*	Maersk	Sheet and packing		
Sorbsan Plus*	Maersk	Sheet dressing		
Sorbsan SA*	Maersk	Adhesive island		
Kaltostat	Convatec	Sheet and packing		
Kaltostat Fortex	Convatec	Sheet dressing		
Kaltogel*	Convatec	Sheet dressing		
Tegagen	3M Healthcare	Sheet dressing		
Nu-gel	Johnson & Johnson	Amorphous gel		
Kaltocarb	See Deodorising dressings			
Dermasorb Spiral	ConvaTec	Cavity filler		

*See text headed 'Properties'

Properties

- Provides many characteristics of the optimum environment for healing.
- Highly absorbent dressing, capable of absorbing moderate to high levels of exudate.
- On contact with exudate, the alginate fibres form a hydrophilic gel (through an ion exchange mechanism) which conforms to the wound surface.
- Once gel has formed, it facilitates autolytic debridement of moist slough and necrotic tissue.
- Acts as an haemostat.
- Some alginate dressings are soluble in normal saline.*
- Reduces pain by keeping nerve endings moist.

Clinical indications

- Moderate to heavily exuding wounds —pressure sores, leg ulcers, donor sites.
- Can be used on infected wounds.
- Useful for filling irregularly shaped wounds such as cavities, abscesses and sinuses.
- Useful for debriding moist devitalised tissue.
- These characteristics make it suitable for use on malignant and fungating wounds.

Practice guidelines

- Only use on exuding wounds, as dressing is inactive in a dry environment.
- Patients may report a transient 'burning' sensation if the dressing is applied to wounds with little or no exudate.
- Dressings sometimes adhere to wound; loosen by irrigating with normal saline.
- Any residual alginate fibres should be irrigated with normal saline.
- When filling cavities, care should be taken to ensure that the alginate is not tightly packed into the wound. Over-tight packing may impede free drainage of exudate and lead to wound deterioration.

- At dressing change, all alginate fibres in direct contact with the wound should have formed a gel. If the alginate fibres remain dry, it is likely that the wound is not producing sufficient exudate; either the time between dressing changes requires extending or the dressing should be discontinued.

Deodorising dressings

Generic description

A range of low-adherent dressings that are combined with either activated charcoal cloth or activated carbon in order to reduce wound odour. The deodorising agent is combined with various other materials including alginates, foams or low-adherent wound contact layers.

Properties

- Absorbent dressing—low to moderate level of exudate.
- Contains deodorising agents, capable of controlling/reducing offensive wound odours.
- Contains 0.15% silver, absorbs bacteria and inhibits bacterial growth within the dressing.*
- Some activated charcoal layers are in direct contact with the wound and are able to absorb bacteria and wound toxins.*

Clinical indications

- Use for exuding, malodorous wounds —malignant and fungating wounds.
- Can be used on infected wounds.

Practice guidelines

- Can be used in conjunction with other dressings.
- Can be combined with metronidazole gel to control anaerobic bacteria associated with malignant wounds. Topical metronidazole may induce antibiotic resistance; therefore use should be restricted.

Table 4.3 Deodorising dressings

Product name	Manufacturer	Presentation	Current cost	Availability Y/N
Actisorb Plus*	Johnson & Johnson	Sheet dressing		
Carbonet	Smith & Nephew	Sheet dressing		
Kaltocarb	Convatec	Sheet dressing		
Lyofoam C	Seton	Sheet dressing		
Lyofoam E C	Seton	Sheet dressing		
*See text headed 'Properties'				

- Dressing changes should be frequent so that exudate build-up is avoided.
- Avoid cutting Actisorb Plus as carbon fibres could leak into the wound.

Enzymatic debriding agents

Generic description

A mixture of proteolytic enzymes—streptokinase and streptodornase presented as a sterile dry powder in a vial.

Properties

- Contains a mixture of streptokinase and streptodornase which are proteolytic enzymes that are able to break down fibrin and fibrinogen and facilitate wound debridement. Technically, enzymatic debriding agents should be classified as biological cleansers rather than wound dressings.

Clinical indications

- Wounds containing necrotic or sloughy tissue.
- Contraindicated for use with wounds which have exposed structures—muscle, nerve endings, blood vessels, e.g. fungating wounds.
- Can be used on infected wounds.

Practice guidelines

- Needs to be reconstituted with sterile normal saline prior to application.
- Avoid shaking the vial vigorously when reconstituting as denaturing of the enzymes may occur.
- Remains stable for 24 hours if stored in a refrigerator.
- The enzymes need to penetrate hard eschar to be effective, which necessitates either the cross-hatching of dry scabs or injecting underneath the surface.
- Alternative application methods include gentle mixing with amorphous hydrogels prior to use.
- Requires the use of a secondary dressing.

Foam dressings

Generic description

Polyurethane foam dressings with a hydrophilic action providing a low-adherent wound contact layer. Some of these dressings have moisture-vapour-permeable backings which are hydrophobic, preventing vertical strike-through. Exudate is absorbed horizontally; once the dressing is saturated, exudate becomes visible at the dressing edges as lateral strike-through.

Properties

- Provides many characteristics of the optimum environment for healing.
- Absorbent dressings—low to high levels of exudate (see individual manufacturer's instructions).
- Foams have good thermal insulating properties.
- Permeable to water vapour which prevents the wound bed from drying out.

Clinical indications

- Low to heavily exuding wounds—pressure sores, leg ulcers, burns, donor sites.
- Useful for filling larger cavity wounds such as dehisced surgical incisions, pilonidal sinuses, pressure sores.*
- Shaped dressings are available for dressing tracheostomies and drain sites.†
- Foam dressings release easily from fragile skin, making them useful for patients with delicate or sensitive skin.

Practice guidelines

- Can be used on a range of wounds —low to heavily exuding.
- Retains absorbent capacity under compression bandaging.
- Foam cavity fillers require a secondary dressing.
- Self-adhesive foams are also waterproof which allows bathing and showering.

Table 4.4 Enzymatic debriding agents				
Product name	Manufacturer	Presentation	Current cost	Availability Y/N
Varidase	Lederle	Dry powder		

Table 4.5 Foam dressings

Product name	Manufacturer	Presentation	Current cost	Availability Y/N
Allevyn	Smith & Nephew	Sheet dressing		
Allevyn adhesive	Smith & Nephew	Adhesive island dressing		
Allevyn Cavity Wound Dressing*	Smith & Nephew	Cavity dressing		
Allevyn Tracheostomy†	Smith & Nephew	Sheet dressing		
Cavi-care*	Smith & Nephew	Cavity dressing		
Cutinova cavity*	Beiersdorf	Sheet dressing		
Cutinova foam	Beiersdorf	Sheet dressing		
Cutinova thin	Beiersdorf	Adhesive sheet dressing		
Lyofoam	Seton	Sheet dressing		
Lyofoam A	Seton	Adhesive island dressing		
Lyofoam Extra	Seton	Sheet dressing		
Lyofoam T†	Seton	Sheet dressing		
Tielle	Johnson & Johnson	Adhesive island dressing		
Lyofoam C	See Deodorising dressings			

* and † see text headed 'Clinical indications'

Hydrocolloid dressings

Generic description

Dressings consist of a hydrocolloid base containing a variety of constituents including gelatine, pectin and sodium carboxymethylcellulose in an adhesive polymer matrix. The hydrocolloid base is hydrophilic in contrast to the adhesive matrix which is hydrophobic.

The outer layer of these dressings is a combination of waterproof polyurethane foams and films which prevents vertical strike-through.

Properties

• Dressings which provide many characteristics of the optimum environment for healing.

Table 4.6 Hydrocolloid dressings

Product name	Manufacturer	Presentation	Current cost	Availability Y/N
Comfeel Ulcer Dressing*	Coloplast	Sheet, paste, powder		
Comfeel Plus Ulcer Dressing†	Coloplast	Sheet dressing		
Comfeel Transparent Dressing‡	Coloplast	Sheet dressing		
Comfeel Pressure Relieving Dressing§	Coloplast	Sheet dressing		
Dermasorb†	Convatec	Cavity filler		
Granuflex E*¶	Convatec	Sheet dressing		
Granuflex	Convatec	Paste		
Granuflex Extra Thin‡	Convatec	Sheet dressing		
Tegasorb	3M	Sheet dressing		
Tegasorb Thin‡	3M	Sheet dressing		

* and † see text headed 'Properties'
‡, § and ¶ see text headed 'Clinical indications'

- Absorbent dressings—low to high levels of exudate.
- On contact with exudate the hydrocolloid slowly absorbs fluid, forming a soft, viscous gel.
- Some hydrocolloids have a cross-linked adhesive matrix which forms a cohesive mass as it absorbs exudate making dressing removal easier.*
- Facilitates autolytic debridement of slough and necrotic tissue.
- Rehydrates dry wounds promoting a moist wound environment.
- Promotes pain relief by keeping exposed nerve endings moist.
- Some hydrocolloids are combined with calcium alginate to improve exudate absorption.†

Clinical indications

- Sheet hydrocolloids—low‡ to moderate¶ exudate levels—shallow wounds.
- Paste hydrocolloids—increased absorption. Useful for filling cavities or sinuses.
- Powder hydrocolloids—highest absorptive capacity—moderate to high exudate levels.
- Indicated for local pressure relief.§
- Useful for debridement of both dry and moist devitalised tissue.
- Can be used at all stages of healing from debridement to protection of epithelial tissue.

Practice guidelines

- Debridement action can cause an initial apparent increase in wound size, of which patients and carers should be aware.
- Hydrocolloids produce a characteristic odour at dressing change, of which patients and carers should be aware.
- Many hydrocolloid sheets have low-profile edges that increase wearing times.
- Hydrocolloids are self-adhesive and waterproof, facilitating bathing or showering.
- Hydrocolloid residue should be irrigated from the wound surface; they can occasionally be difficult to remove from the surrounding skin.

Hydrofibre dressings

Generic description

Non-woven absorbent, fibrous dressings manufactured from Hydrofibre (sodium carboxymethylcellulose).

Properties

- Provides many characteristics of the optimum environment for healing.
- Absorbent dressing—low to heavily exuding wounds.
- On contact with exudate the dressing fibres swell and rapidly form a gel which remains an integral part of the dressing.
- The integrity of the dressing is maintained in both dry and wet states when it is gelled.
- Conforms well to cavity wounds.
- Facilitates autolytic debridement of slough and necrotic tissue.
- Promotes pain relief by keeping exposed nerve endings moist.

Clinical indications

- Low to heavily exuding wounds—pressure sores, leg ulcers.
- Can be used on infected wounds.
- Can be used at all stages of healing from debridement to protection of granulation tissue.

Practice guidelines

- Releases easily from drier wounds, but if necessary release can be facilitated by moistening with normal saline.
- The presence of normal saline or exudate causes the dressing fibres to gel rapidly.
- Requires a secondary dressing.

Hydrogel dressings

Generic description

Hydrogel dressings have a high water content and contain insoluble polymers. Constituents vary

Table 4.7 Hydrofibre dressings				
Product name	Manufacturer	Presentation	Current cost	Availability Y/N
Aquacel	Convatec	Sheet dressing		
		Cavity filler		

Table 4.8 Hydrogel dressings

Product name	Manufacturer	Presentation	Current cost	Availability Y/N
AquaForm	Robert Bailey & Sons	Amorphous gel		
Clearsite	NDM	Sheet dressing		
Clearsite Island dressing	NDM	Adhesive island dressing		
Geliperm	Geistlich	Sheet dressing Amorphous gel		
Intrasite Gel	Smith & Nephew	Amorphous gel		
Spenco 2nd Skin	Spenco Medical UK	Sheet dressing		
Sterigel	Seton	Amorphous gel		
Granugel	Convatec	Amorphous gel		

depending on the manufacturer but include modified carboxymethylcellulose, hemicellulose, agar, glycerol, pectin. Hydrogels have marked fluid-handling properties; fluid absorption is usually at the expense of fluid-donating properties.

Properties

- Provides many characteristics of the optimum environment for healing.
- Varying amounts of fluid-absorbing capacity —low to moderate levels of exudate.
- Fluid-donating properties facilitate autolytic debridement of dry and moist slough and necrotic tissue.
- Rehydrates dry wounds providing a moist wound environment.
- Promotes pain relief by keeping exposed nerve endings moist.
- Sheet hydrogels swell slightly as they absorb exudate.
- Amorphous hydrogels progressively lose viscosity as they absorb exudate.

Clinical indications

- Sheet hydrogels—low to moderately exuding *flat* wounds—pressure sores, leg ulcers, minor burns, traumatic wounds.
- Amorphous hydrogels—low to moderately exuding wounds, necrotic or sloughy wounds —pressure sores, sinuses, cavity wounds, extravasation injuries.
- Useful for rapid debridement of both dry and moist devitalised tissue.
- Amorphous hydrogels are useful for filling irregularly shaped cavities, abscesses, sinuses.

- Can be used at all stages of healing from debridement to protection of granulation tissue.

Practice guidelines

- Amorphous hydrogels should be removed from the wound by irrigation with normal saline.
- Sheet dressings and amorphous gels can act as a carrier for medicaments such as metronidazole gel.
- Rapid debridement action can initially appear to increase the size of the wound, of which patients and carers should be aware.
- Amorphous hydrogels require direct contact with the wound. Effectiveness is compromised if subjected to direct local pressure such as compression bandaging.
- Sheet hydrogels allow inspection of the wound through the dressing and do not require a secondary dressing.
- Use of hydrogels is sometimes associated with increased skin maceration at the wound edges especially if applied to highly exuding wounds.

Low-adherent primary contact dressings (non-medicated)

Generic description

Dressings made from a variety of materials including cotton/acrylic fibres and knitted viscose. Many are coated with low-adherent materials, e.g. aluminium or perforated films. Some are combined with an absorbent layer, others are not. Newer generation low-adherent dressings are composed of non-adherent materials such as silicone and polyamide net which cause minimal disturbance to the tissues.

Table 4.9 Low-adherent primary contact dressings (non-medicated)

Product name	Manufacturer	Presentation	Current cost	Availability Y/N
Cutilin	Beiersdorf	Sheet dressing		
Interface V-C	Vernon Carus	Sheet dressing		
Metalline	Lohmann	Sheet dressing		
Melolin	Smith & Nephew	Sheet dressing		
Mepital*	Molnlycke	Sheet dressing		
NA Dressing	Johnson & Johnson	Sheet dressing		
Release	Johnson & Johnson	Sheet dressing		
N-A Ultra*	Johnson & Johnson	Sheet dressing		
Tegapore*	3M	Sheet dressing		
Tricotex	Smith & Nephew	Sheet dressing		
Telfa	Kendall	Sheet dressing		

* See text headed 'Properties' and 'Clinical indications'

Properties

- Many are low-adherent rather than non-adherent.
- These dressings are not highly absorbent; some contain an absorbent layer, others require backing with an absorbent secondary dressing.
- Dressings allow strike-through when saturated with exudate and require frequent changing.
- The new generation of low-adherent dressings* has been developed to release easily from the wound surface and some can be left in situ for extended periods of time.

Clinical indications

- Dry to medium exuding wounds—surgical wounds healing by primary intention, superficial wounds.
- Homeostasis should be achieved before using Tegapore or Mepital on donor sites.
- Can be used to protect surgical incisions and recently healed wounds.
- Newer low-adherent interface layers* can be used for larger, exuding wounds, burns, or for patients who have extremely fragile skin.

Practice guidelines

- Strike-through will occur when used to cover exuding wounds, necessitating dressing change.
- Remove with care. If adherent, loosen with normal saline.
- Skin maceration may be associated with the use of some of these dressings.
- Require securing with a secondary dressing, tape or bandages.

Low-adherent primary contact dressings (medicated)

Generic description

Knitted viscose dressing impregnated with 10% povidone-iodine in a water-soluble polyethylene glycol base.

Properties

- Has low absorbency properties.
- Contains 10% povidone-iodine, reduces bacterial growth.

Table 4.10 Low-adherent primary contact dressings (medicated)

Product name	Manufacturer	Presentation	Current cost	Availability Y/N
Inadine	Johnson & Johnson	Sheet dressing		

- The polyethylene glycol base is water soluble and is therefore easily removed from the skin or wound surface.

Clinical indications

- Dry or low-contaminated exuding wounds —traumatic wounds, superficial burns and skin-loss injuries
- Prophylaxis and treatment of a wide range of microorganisms including bacterial and fungal infections.
- This dressing should be used with caution for pregnant or lactating women owing to the possible side-effect of elevated serum iodine levels.

Practice guidelines

- Change dressing when orange-brown colour changes to white indicating the release of the povidone-iodine.
- Free iodine content is low, but sensitivity to povidone-iodine has been reported.
- Remove with care, as it may adhere to dryer wound surfaces; if so, it can be effectively loosened using normal saline.
- Requires a secondary dressing.
- Dressing requires changing frequently if levels of antibacterial activity are to be maintained.
- A maximum of four dressings should be applied at any one time.

Polysaccharide bead dressings (non-medicated)

Generic description

Hydrophilic, sterile beads of dextranomer (carbohydrate polymer) mixed with glycol and water to form a paste which is contained within a low-adherent nylon bag or is available as a foil-wrapped paste.

Properties

- The dextranomer beads absorb exudate. The process of capillary action removes slough and bacteria from the wound surface.

- Materials with low molecular weight are absorbed into the structure of the beads.
- Once the dextranomer is fully saturated it will fail to absorb further fluid and requires replacement.
- Dextranomer is able to debride moist necrotic tissue effectively.

Clinical indications

- Should only be used on exuding sloughy or necrotic wounds—leg ulcers, pressure sores, surgical wounds.
- Can be used on infected wounds.
- The paste should not be used in narrow sinuses, as removal can be difficult.

Practice guidelines

- Discontinue dressing once the wound bed has been fully debrided, as dextranomer can cause discomfort when applied to clean, granulating wounds.
- The dextranomer beads are not effective if allowed to dry out.
- The dextranomer pads should be held in place using a semi-occlusive dressing.
- These dressings should be moistened with saline to ease removal.
- Once the wound has been cleansed, new dressings should be applied while the wound surface is still moist.
- Occasionally transient stinging pain is associated with the use of these dressings. This can be minimised by ensuring that the wound is moistened with saline before application of a fresh dressing.

Polysaccharide bead dressings (medicated)

Generic description

Hydrophilic beads of cadexomer impregnated with iodine (0.9%); cadexomer is a modified starch hydrogel.

Table 4.11 Polysaccharide bead dressings (non-medicated)				
Product name	Manufacturer	Presentation	Current cost	Availability Y/N
Debrisan Absorbent Pads	Kabi Pharmacia	Absorbent pads		
Debrisan Beads	Kabi Pharmacia	Paste dressing		

Table 4.12 Polysaccharide bead dressings (medicated)

Product name	Manufacturer	Presentation	Current cost	Availability Y/N
Iodosorb Powder	Perstop Pharma	Powder		
Iodosorb Ointment	Perstop Pharma	Ointment		

Properties

- Absorbent dressing; on contact with exudate a moist gel is formed.
- Iodine is not released until the dressing is moistened by wound exudate and the beads begin to swell.
- The iodine exerts an antimicrobial effect; in addition bacteria are removed from the wound surface by the process of capillary action.

Clinical indications

- Low to heavily exuding sloughy wounds —traumatic lacerations, abrasions.
- Can be used on infected wounds.
- This dressing must not be used during pregnancy or with patients with thyroid disease or suspected iodine sensitivities, owing to the risk of systemic absorption.

Practice guidelines

- The powder is indicated for moderate to heavily exuding wounds that contain slough or pus.
- The paste is indicated for moderate to heavily exuding wounds.
- The ointment is indicated for lightly to moderately exuding wounds.
- These dressings change colour from orange-brown to white when the iodine has been absorbed, indicating the need for dressing change.
- If the dressing dries out it can be removed from the wound bed by gentle irrigation with normal saline.
- Some patients report slight discomfort when the dressing is first applied; the ointment or paste preparations are less likely to have this effect.

- Over 1 week, applications should not exceed 50 g of paste and 150 g of Iodoflex.
- All require the use of a secondary dressing.

Polyurethane membrane dressings

Generic description

Absorbent polyurethane membrane covered by a semipermeable polyurethane film. The wound contact layer is covered with a pressure-sensitive hydrophilic adhesive.

Properties

- Absorbent dressing that responds to varying levels of exudate production by altering the moisture vapour permeability of its outer layer.
- Provides a moist environment at the wound surface without overdrying.
- Remains impermeable to bacteria and water.

Clinical indications

- Lightly to moderately exuding wounds —pressure sores, leg ulcers, abrasions, lacerations.
- Not recommended for use on infected wounds.

Practice guidelines

- Can be used on a range of wounds —low to moderately exuding.
- The dressing is self-adhesive and waterproof, facilitating bathing and showering.
- Exudate travels laterally through the dressing.
- The dressing can be cut to fit awkward areas and overlapped if necessary.

Table 4.13 Polyurethane membrane dressings

Product name	Manufacturer	Presentation	Current cost	Availability Y/N
Spyrosorb	Convatec	Sheet dressing		

Semipermeable film dressings (non-medicated)

Generic description

Transparent, adhesive-coated, polyurethane, semipermeable films.

Properties

- Provides many of the characteristics of the optimum environment for healing.
- Has no absorbency properties.
- Different semipermeable films exhibit varying degrees of water vapour permeability.
- Semipermeable films are impermeable to water and microorganisms.
- These dressings trap exudate at the wound surface providing a moist environment.

Clinical indications

- Wounds producing low amounts of exudate —superficial pressure sores or leg ulcers, surgical wounds, scalds, abrasions, minor lacerations.
- Can be used prophylactically to prevent pressure sores by reducing friction forces acting on the skin.
- Some semipermeable films have higher water vapour permeability making them suitable for intravenous fixation.*
- Often used as a secondary dressing, e.g. to hold hydrogels in place.

Practice guidelines

- Only use on lightly exuding wounds; copious exudate production will cause dressing leakage and skin maceration.
- Use with care on fragile or blistered skin; careful removal is essential to minimise trauma.
- These dressings are not designed to be removed daily. The acrylic adhesive becomes less adherent with time, making removal easier.
- These dressings are transparent and therefore facilitate wound inspection.
- Their use is not recommended on clinically infected wounds.

Semipermeable film dressings (medicated)

Generic description

Semipermeable, adhesive, polyurethane films, containing a controlled release antimicrobial agent.

Properties

- This dressing has the same properties as non-medicated films, but is combined with antimicrobial agents such as silver.
- The antimicrobial agents dissolve in water or water vapour leaving no solid residue and deliver a continuous antibacterial effect.

Table 4.14 Semipermeable film dressings (non-medicated)

Product name	Manufacturer	Presentation	Current cost	Availability Y/N
Bioclusive	Johnson & Johnson	Sheet dressing		
Cutifilm	Beiersdorf	Sheet dressing		
Opsite	Smith & Nephew	Sheet dressing		
Opsite I.V. 3000*	Smith & Nephew	Sheet dressing		
Tegaderm	3M	Sheet dressing		
Tegaderm IV*	3M	Sheet dressing		
*See text headed 'Clinical indications'				

Table 4.15 Semipermeable film dressings (medicated)

Product name	Manufacturer	Presentation	Current cost	Availability Y/N
Arglaes Controlled Release Dressing	Pharmaplast	Sheet dressing		

Clinical indications

- Wounds producing low amounts of exudate —superficial pressure sores, leg ulcers or burns, surgical wounds, abrasions, intravenous cannula sites.
- Suitable for infected wounds that are not producing high levels of exudate.

Practice guidelines

- Only use on lightly exuding wounds; copious exudate production will cause dressing leakage.
- These films will darken gradually following application to the wound.
- Other topical agents, i.e. antiseptics and antibiotics, should not be used in conjunction with medicated films as different antimicrobial agents may induce sensitivity reactions.

Silicone gel dressings

Generic description

A soft, conformable, transparent dressing consisting of silicone gel which is 3–4 mm thick.

Properties

- Chemically inert, conformable.
- Softens and flattens scar tissue; the precise mode of action is unknown.
- Conforms well to body contours without leaving adhesive residues on the surface of the skin.

Clinical indications

- For use on recently healed wounds with raised or hypertrophic scars—burns, skin grafts, surgical scars.
- Used to minimise scar formation and to reduce scar contracture.
- Not recommended for patients with a known allergy to silicone.
- Not recommended for use on open wounds.

Practice guidelines

- Comfortable and simple for the patient to self-manage.
- Can be worn underneath pressure garments or bandages.
- Wear time should be gradually increased in order to acclimatise the skin surface.
- The scarred area should be gently washed daily with warm water.
- Suitable for multiple re-use; should be washed daily in mild, non-detergent soap.

Paraffin gauze dressings (non-medicated)

Generic description

Open mesh, cotton, rayon, viscose or gauze impregnated with white or yellow soft paraffin (tulle gras literally means 'greased net').

Properties

- Low-adherent wound contact material. Paraffin reduces the adherence of the dressing.

Table 4.16 Silicone gel dressings

Product name	Manufacturer	Presentation	Current cost	Availability Y/N
Cica-care	Smith & Nephew	Sheet dressing		
Silicone Gel Sheets	Spenco Medical	Sheet dressing		

Table 4.17 Paraffin gauze dressings (non-medicated)

Product name	Manufacturer	Presentation	Current cost	Availability Y/N
Cutinet	Beiersdorf	Sheet dressing		
Jelonet	Smith & Nephew	Sheet dressing		
Paranet	Vernon-Carus	Sheet dressing		
Paratulle	Seton	Sheet dressing		

- These dressings are not highly absorbent.
- Dressings allow strike-through especially in the presence of exudate.

Clinical indications

- Low to medium exuding wounds—clean, superficial wounds, split thickness skin grafts, minor burns.

Practice guidelines

- Should only be used on lightly exuding wounds.
- Remove with care as this type of dressing has a tendency to dry out and adhere to the wound bed. Irrigation with saline is of limited value as paraffin has hydrophobic properties.
- Can shed fibres into the wound.
- Paraffin gauze dressings should be multilayered to minimise the risk of adherence and cut to shape to avoid risk of surrounding skin maceration.
- Requires frequent dressing changes to avoid drying out and damage to granulation tissue.
- Use of these dressings has been associated with reports of patient discomfort, especially if left in situ for any length of time.
- Requires the use of a secondary dressing.

Paraffin gauze dressings (medicated)

Generic description

Open mesh, cotton, rayon or gauze impregnated with white or yellow soft paraffin. The paraffin base is combined with a variety of antimicrobial agents.

Properties

- Low-adherent wound contact material. Paraffin reduces the adherence of the dressing.
- Contains various antimicrobials depending on the manufacturer. Bactigras (chlorhexidine acetate 0.5%), Sofra-Tulle (framycetin and 10% lanolin), Serotulle (chlorhexidine acetate BP 0.5%).

- Systemic absorption may occur in wounds covering 30% or more of the body surface (Carville 1995).

Clinical indications

- Low- to medium-contaminated exuding wounds—superficial traumatic wounds.
- Prophylaxis and topical treatment of wound infections.
- Ineffective release of antimicrobials from the paraffin base has been reported (Thomas 1983).

Practice guidelines

- Should only be used on lightly exuding minor wounds.
- Remove with care as has tendency to dry out and adhere to the wound bed.
- Can shed fibres into the wound.
- Irrigation with saline is of limited value as paraffin has hydrophobic properties.
- Requires multilayering and cutting to shape as indicated previously.
- Hypersensitivity reactions and acquired resistance have been reported in medicated tulles that do not contain chlorhexidine.

Dressing infected wounds

Colonisation of chronic wounds is common and is not usually a contraindication to the use of most dressing products. Where systemic or local wound infection is suspected or develops during treatment, appropriate adjunctive therapy should be given and the progress of the wound monitored daily (see Sect. 3.3). This may mean changing a dressing for the purposes of inspection more frequently than would otherwise be necessary. Infected wounds usually produce high levels of exudate, making those dressings with low absorbency unsuitable for the management of infected wounds. If exudate is allowed to leak from dressings, the bacterial barrier property of the dressing will be compromised and the dressing should be replaced. For current information regarding the suitability of a particular dressing product

Table 4.18 Paraffin gauze dressings (medicated)				
Product name	Manufacturer	Presentation	Current cost	Availability Y/N
Bactigras	Smith & Nephew	Sheet dressing		
Sofra-Tulle	Roussel	Sheet dressing		
Serotulle	Seton	Sheet dressing		

for use on infected wounds, advice should be sought from the manufacturers and their instructions followed at all times.

To test your understanding of wound dressing products, complete the following questions by ticking the correct statements.

1. Cadexomer iodine is a:

   a. monosaccharide
   b. disaccharide
   c. trisaccharide
   d. polysaccharide.

2. Which of the following are suitable uses of semipermeable film dressings?

   a. Low-exuding superficial wounds
   b. Highly exuding superficial wounds
   c. Low-exuding cavity wounds
   d. Highly exuding cavity wounds.

3. Which of the following are suitable for dressing large cavity wounds?

   a. Alginate dressings
   b. Amorphous hydrogels
   c. Foam cavity dressings
   d. Hydrocolloid paste dressings.

4. The following is a description of which type of dressing?

   These dressings are available in a variety of forms which contain a high water content combined with insoluble polymers. They have advanced fluid-handling properties and are capable of both absorbing fluid from and donating fluid to the wound site.

   a. Hydrocolloid
   b. Hydrogel
   c. Hydrofibre
   d. Alginates.

5. Which of the following are suitable for debriding dry necrotic tissue?

   a. Alginates
   b. Hydrogels
   c. Hydrocolloids
   d. Polysaccharide bead dressings.

6. Which of the following dressings are useful for patients who have fragile, delicate skin?

   a. Foam dressings
   b. Semipermeable film dressings

   c. Silicone gel dressings
   d. Paraffin gauze dressings.

7. Complete the following boxes by inserting the generic names of appropriate types of dressing. It may be useful to list only those dressings that are currently available in your clinical practice environment.

Dressings suitable for cavity wounds

   •

   •

   •

Dressings suitable for debriding dry necrotic wounds

   •

   •

   •

Dressings suitable for debriding moist necrotic wounds

   •

   •

   •

Dressings suitable for lightly exuding wounds

   •

   •

   •

Dressings suitable for moderately exuding wounds

-
-
-

Dressings suitable for highly exuding wounds

-
-
-

FEEDBACK

Your answers should have been as follows.

1. The right answer is (d). Cadexomer iodine is a polysaccharide.

2. The right answer is (a). Semipermeable film membranes are only suitable for use on low-exuding flat wounds. Large amounts of exudate will collect under the dressing eventually causing leakage and in some instances may increase the likelihood of maceration of the surrounding skin. Semipermeable films are only suitable as a secondary dressing for cavity wounds when used in conjunction with an absorbent cavity wound filler.

3. The right answer is that all could be used, depending on the amount of exudate produced by the wound. Amorphous hydrogels and hydrocolloid pastes have a tendency to seep out of the wound as they absorb exudate. This tendency is exacerbated by the effects of local pressure especially if the wound is in the sacral area.

4. The right answer is (b). All of these dressings contain a high water content except alginates. All have advanced fluid-handling properties, but only hydrogels are manufactured from insoluble polymers.

5. The right answers are (b) and (c). Both hydrocolloids and hydrogels facilitate autolytic debridement of wounds by rehydrating dry eschar as a result of their high water content. Alginates and polysaccharide beads, however, are both inactive in a dry wound environment.

6. The right answers are (a) and (c). Foam dressings and silicone gel dressings both release easily from both the wound surface and the surrounding skin. The use of silicone gel dressings should be reserved for the management of scar tissue following healing; silicone helps remodelling of scar tissue and protects the surrounding skin, which can remain delicate for some time.

7. Your answers should be similar to those given in Box 4.2. Whenever possible, the generic dressing type has been listed. Individual product names have only been used to differentiate a product from the rest of its generic group, if the rest of that product category is not suitable.

The information given above indicates broad practice guidelines for the selection and choice of dressing products. More comprehensive product information is available in the form of manufacturers' written instructions which should always be referred to before using a new product for the first time.

Decision-making framework for the selection of dressings

The selection of dressing products is a complex clinical decision-making skill that depends on many variables. The framework presented in Box 4.3 summarises the main steps of selecting a suitable dressing product, whilst an overview of the whole process can be seen in Figure 4.1.

The selection of wound dressings is likely to remain a complex decision as more and more products become available as technological advances increase. Figure 4.2 summarises the clinical indications for the selection of wound dressing by generic group and is intended as a framework only. Unfortunately for those wound problems that are relatively uncommon such as management of fungating wounds, the choice of suitable dressing products is likely to remain restricted. In contrast, choice of dressings suitable for the management of simpler wounds has proliferated in recent years and for many practitioners has increased levels of confusion. Good quality research in the form of controlled randomised trials in order to evaluate the efficacy of dressing products is urgently required in order to clarify this confusing situation.

Box 4.2 Types of wounds and suitable dressings

Dressings suitable for cavity wounds
- Alginate dressings
- Allevyn Cavity Wound Dressing
- Cavi-care dressing
- Cutinova cavity dressing
- Hydrocolloid pastes
- Dermasorb
- Hydrofibre cavity filler
- Amorphous hydrogel dressings
- Polysaccharide bead dressings

Dressings suitable for debriding dry necrotic wounds
- Hydrocolloid dressings
- Hydrofibre dressings
- Hydrogel dressings

Dressings suitable for debriding moist necrotic wounds
- Alginate dressings
- Hydrocolloid dressings
- Hydrofibre dressings
- Hydrogel dressings
- Polysaccharide bead dressings

Dressings suitable for lightly exuding wounds
- Adhesive Island dressings
- Foam dressings
- Hydrocolloid sheet dressings
- Hydrofibre dressings
- Hydrogel dressings
- Low-adherent primary contact dressings
- Polyurethane membrane dressings
- Semipermeable film dressings
- Paraffin gauze dressings

Dressings suitable for moderately exuding wounds
- Alginate dressings
- Foam dressings
- Hydrocolloid paste and sheets
- Hydrofibre dressings
- Hydrogel dressings
- Low-adherent primary contact dressings
- Polyurethane membrane dressings
- Polysaccharide bead dressings

Dressings suitable for highly exuding wounds
- Alginate dressings
- Foam dressings
- Hydrocolloid powder and sheets
- Hydrofibre dressings
- Polysaccharide bead dressings

Box 4.3 Decision-making framework for the selection of dressings

1. Assess the wound taking into consideration previous treatments and patient priorities.
2. Define and prioritise the specific treatment objectives required to effectively manage the wound.
3. Define what should be the primary and secondary functions of the wound dressing.
4. Define what the specific performance criteria of the dressing should be.
5. Identify any contraindications to the use of the wound dressing.
6. Consider the advantages of using various types of dressing products.
7. Consider the constraints of using various types of dressing products.
8. If considering using a combination of dressing types for the management of a wound, identify what advantages this will have over the use of a single dressing type.
9. Always follow the manufacturers' instructions.
10. Establish whether the dressing is currently available in your clinical setting.
11. Consider all other available alternative options.
12. Consider the cost-effectiveness of your chosen dressing regime.
13. At dressing change, review the effectiveness of the dressing's ability to meet the defined performance criteria.
14. Review patient satisfaction with the current dressing regime.

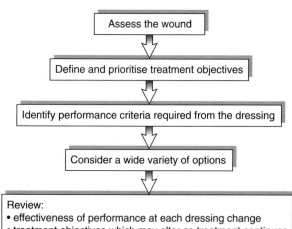

Fig. 4.1 Summary of the clinical decision-making process when selecting wound dressings.

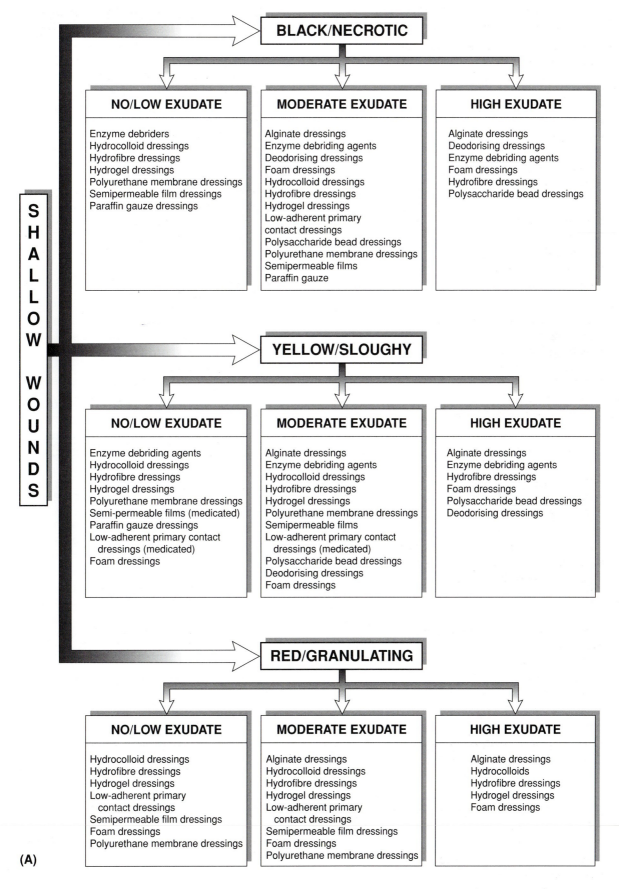

Fig. 4.2 (A) Selection of wound dressings. The dressings included are not exhaustive and are intended as a user guide only. For further details of each generic dressing group, refer to pages 72–83.

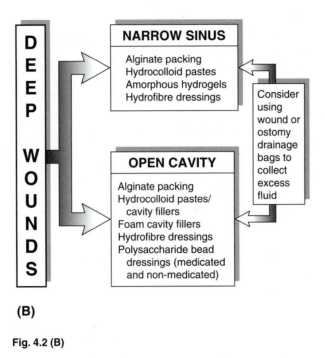

(B)

Fig. 4.2 (B)

4.4 COST-EFFECTIVENESS OF TREATMENTS

Introduction

Over the last decade, scarcity of health service resources has increased awareness of the need to ensure delivery of cost-effective health care. Expenditure on wound care continues to be a significant drain on resources which can be difficult to quantify. Estimates vary, but many authors agree that the management of patients with wounds or compromised tissue viability accounts for in excess of £1000 million per annum in the UK alone (Bennett & Moody 1995). At the same time there is mounting evidence that significant cost savings can be achieved in wound management without compromising quality of care (Thomas 1995).

Basic principles of health economics

Health economics is based upon the principle that health care resources will always be scarce relative to need, which inevitably means that decisions will have to be made concerning the allocation of available resources to priority services. Scarcity of resources means that any decision to allocate funds will always be at the expense of other health care needs elsewhere. Budget holders are therefore required to justify decisions related to resource management and need to demonstrate that allocation decisions are supported by explicit criteria. A fundamental criterion used for economic evaluation is that of 'efficiency' which specifically relates to the need to maximise benefits from all available resources.

Cost-benefit analysis in wound healing

Cost-benefit analysis is a method of economic evaluation which attempts to identify all gains (benefits) associated with implementing a particular intervention against all losses (costs); these are usually expressed in monetary terms. Economic principles state that the only interventions that are valid are those where the benefits exceed the value of the costs. When considered in relation to the provision of health services such as wound management, economic principles can be difficult to apply as many aspects of health care prove difficult to quantify in economic terms. Indeed, results from a recent cost-benefit analysis exercise commissioned by the DoH in 1993 into the cost of pressure sores proved to be highly controversial. The report (Touche Ross 1993) concluded that the cost of pressure sore prevention was substantially higher than the cost of pressure sore treatment if the significant costs of staff time required to implement preventive interventions were taken into consideration (see Table 4.19). Staff costs are significant as pressure sore preventive strategies will always need to be applied to a larger number of 'at-risk' patients than those who actually go on to develop pressure sores. If costs associated with staff time are excluded from this analysis, then the costs of pressure sore treatment far exceed preventive costs (see Table 4.20). This report excluded quality of life costs to the patient and potential litigation costs to health authorities and therefore failed to represent the complexity of this issue. This example highlights the inherent difficulties of costing health care services, especially when trying to quantify concepts such as quality of life. Clearly there are ethical dilemmas associated with the delivery of health services which prevent the rigid application of economic principles alone. The question is not whether to treat patients with existing wounds, but whether the higher cost of a particular treatment can be justified in terms of extra benefits gained, such as increased healing rates and earlier discharge from care. This concept is of particular relevance when considering either prophylaxis or preventive interventions which may prove to be an inefficient use of resources.

Self-assessment — 15 MINUTES

Try to list the potential costs (losses) and benefits (gains) associated with the use of a modern interactive dressing such as a hydrocolloid for management of a patient with a chronic pressure sore when compared with the use of a 'cheaper' alternative traditional dressing such as paraffin gauze.

FEEDBACK

Your answer should have included the majority of the following points.

Costs

1. Treatment costs:
   - consumables—dressings, bandages, dressing packs, tapes, gloves, etc.
   - wound-cleansing agents
   - medications—antibiotics, analgesics, etc.
   - diagnostic procedures—swabs, X-rays
   - surgery
   - therapy sessions—physiotherapy, etc.
2. Staff time
3. Specialist nursing/medical services
4. Staff education
5. Overheads
   - utilities
   - equipment replacement
6. Opportunity costs—extended length of hospital stay.

Benefits

1. Alleviation of pain and suffering
2. Increased patient satisfaction
3. Increased patient compliance
4. Decrease in wound size/healing of wound
5. Reduced nursing time (staff costs)
6. Reduced hospital stay/length of treatment time.

Table 4.19 Estimated comparison of overall hospital costs* for pressure sore prevention and treatment per annum in England (Touche Ross 1993)

Annual hospital costs	Lowest cost (including staff time)	Highest cost (including staff time)
Treatment costs	£180 million	£321 million
Prevention costs	£180 million	£755 million

* Figures based upon estimated costs of a typical general hospital of 600 beds which were then extrapolated to give an estimated total cost of pressure sore prevention and treatment for the whole of England.

Table 4.20 Estimated comparison of pressure sore prevention and treatment costs per annum for a typical general hospital (England) (Touche Ross 1993)

Single hospital costs	Lowest cost/year (excluding staff time)	Highest cost/year (excluding staff time)
Treatment costs	£459 476	£710 663
Prevention costs	£135 293	£310 185

Allowances need to be made for 'overhead' items such as utilities (heating, power, water) even if care is carried out in the patient's own home. In this case, utility costs relate to the costs associated with running support services such as the health clinic and community nurse travelling costs as well as care that is provided in unsocial hours as this incurs higher labour charges. Calculating costs which serve as averages of the typical labour and consumables required to provide a particular type of service is referred to as 'standard costing'. Today, computerised information systems provide the necessary support for resource allocation within the health services as data is collected about the patients and the 'episodes' of care that they receive. An 'episode' of care is defined as a course of treatment and care prescribed for one main diagnosis or set of symptoms, usually by a single consultant or GP. An 'episode' of care may consist of an inpatient stay, a series of outpatient attendances or support provided by community nursing services.

Self-assessment   **10 MINUTES**

Identify three factors that will inevitably increase the 'standard costing' of providing an 'episode' of care for a patient with a chronic venous leg ulcer.

FEEDBACK

Anything which lengthens the patient's episode of care will inevitably increase costs, which is why it is notoriously difficult to build in these average costs for those patients with chronic or complex wounds. The most commonly occurring incidents that increase the cost of providing wound care that you should have included in your answer are:

1. the onset of wound complications such as wound infection or wound breakdown which increase costs not only by prolonging healing times but by increasing the need for diagnostic procedures and medications, etc.

2. lack of available resources such as access to specialist advice in the form of a leg ulcer clinic or specialist nurses, or lack of availability of compression bandages.

3. uncompliant patients, who may not for various reasons follow the advice and treatments suggested by nursing and medical staff (see Sect. 6).

4. failure to implement research-based practice which reduces treatment costs by improving healing rates.

Cost-effectiveness analysis in wound care

Cost-effectiveness analysis (CEA) is a simpler method of economic evaluation with many more published studies relating to wound management than cost–benefit analysis. CEA should be used when the efficacy of alternative treatments is being compared to determine if a single benefit is affected, e.g. wound healing rates. Consideration must be given to all the costs that vary between the alternative dressing and treatment regimes. Many dressing evaluations in the literature claiming to be CEAs, only estimate the costs of consumables such as dressings and bandages without taking into consideration the hidden but significant costs of nursing time, staff education and overheads. Many clinical trials are designed to demonstrate such benefits by attempting to compare the efficacy and cost-effectiveness of different types of dressing products but often fail owing to the difficulty of expressing all of the associated costs and benefits in monetary terms. Ohlson et al (1994) evaluated the use of hydrocolloid versus saline-soaked gauze dressings and identified a reduction in ulcer area as the benefit measure. Costs of nursing time including frequency and length of visit and travelling time were included in addition to the costs of the dressing materials in order to effectively demonstrate cost-effective treatment.

Economic evaluation is undertaken to assist resource allocation decision making and normally requires more data than are usually provided by clinical trials and product evaluations. The difficulty of quantifying broader outcome measures such as quality of life inevitably increases the complexity of these studies. With the increasing scarcity of health care resources, nurses in collaboration with multidisciplinary colleagues should be seeking to evaluate wound care interventions, focusing not only on clinical effectiveness but also on whether interventions represent good value for money. The ultimate aim is to provide high quality wound care whilst achieving significant cost savings.

SUMMARY

This section has reviewed recent advances in the development of wound dressing materials. In it you have learnt that:

- An increasingly wide range of wound dressings are becoming available, many of which are wound specific and therefore capable of performing a defined function.

- Selection of wound dressings has become more complex as choice increases and more products become available.

- Holistic wound assessment is an essential prerequisite to the selection of wound dressings and should always involve the identification of specific treatment objectives.

- The new generation of wound dressings are technologically advanced and are designed to promote the principle of moist wound healing and provide the optimal local environment for healing.

- The selection of the correct dressing product is an important factor in wound management, but is only one part of the overall process which should always be supported by accurate and objective wound assessment that utilises contributions from the multidisciplinary team.

- Scarcity of health care resources means that cost-effectiveness of wound management will have to be determined in order to provide high quality care as well as value for money.

REFERENCES

Bennett G, Moody M 1995 Wound care for health professionals. Chapman Hall, London

Carville K 1995 Wound care manual. Silver Chain Foundation, Western Australia

Flanagan M 1992 Variables influencing nurses' selection of wound dressings. Journal of Wound Care 1(1): 33–43

Ohlson P, Larsson K, Lindholm C, Moller M 1994 A cost-effectiveness study of leg ulcer treatment in primary care. Scandinavian Journal of Primary Health Care 12: 295–299

Robson M C, Phillips L G, Lawrence W T 1995 The safety and effect of transforming growth factor-beta for the treatment of venous stasis ulcers. Wound Repair and Regeneration 3: 157–167

Scales J T 1956 Development and evaluation of a porous surgical dressing. British Medical Journal 2(Oct): 962–981

Thomas S 1983 Improvements in medicated tulle dressings. Journal of Hospital Infection 4: 391–398

Thomas S 1995 The cost of wound care in the community. Journal of Wound Care 4(8): 350–354

Touche Ross 1993 The cost of pressure sores. Touche Ross, London

Turner T 1985 Which dressing and why? In: Westerby S 1985 Wound care. Heinemann Medical Books, London

Winter G 1962 Formation of the scab and the rate of epithelialisation of superficial wounds in the skin of the domestic pig. Nature 193: 293–294

5 Management of complex wounds

Introduction

Complex wounds present problems which are many and varied and often cause difficulties for the patients, their carers and health professionals alike. The majority of wounds, irrespective of aetiology, heal relatively quickly and without complication. Problem wounds may be of either an acute or chronic nature, but will all have a significant impact on the patient's quality of life. Those unfortunate to have complicated wounds often express frustration at the relatively slow rate at which their wound appears to improve and for many this can be a lonely and frightening experience.

This section is aimed to help you identify the management principles required to care for patients with a variety of commonly occurring wound problems and to facilitate the development of problem-solving skills relevant to the complexities of clinical practice.

LEARNING OUTCOMES

When you have completed this section, you should be able to:

- identify a range of wound management problems frequently reported by patients and carers
- review the management principles of caring for patients with malignant wounds
- review the management principles of caring for patients with non-healing leg ulcers
- review the management principles of caring for patients with fistulae and sinuses
- review the management principles of caring for a patient with neuropathic foot ulcers.

5.1 COMMON WOUND MANAGEMENT PROBLEMS

Problem wounds, whether they are chronic or acute, need careful management if they are to heal effectively. However, normal healing can be compromised by the presence locally at the wound surface of the following conditions:

- local infection
- excessive slough production
- excessive exudate/haematoma production
- presence of necrotic tissue
- inadequate drainage
- dehydration/desiccation.

These problems have been described from a health professional's perspective. Common wound management problems experienced by patients are often different. The following problems relating to wound management commonly cause considerable distress to patients, their carers and their families:

- wound leakage
- pain/discomfort
- lack of sleep
- offensive odour
- increased dependence on carers
- altered body image
- reduced quality of life
- loss of confidence/self-esteem.

All of these problems have the potential to reduce patient compliance and therefore need to be approached sensitively, involving both the patient and carers as much as possible with planned care. These difficulties are multidisciplinary in nature and as such require collaboration from the whole team in order to utilise a variety of different skills and perspectives and to make effective clinical decisions based upon informed practice.

Activity 5 MINUTES

Think of one patient for whose wound management you are responsible.

1. What local conditions exist which might compromise the healing of the wound?
2. In your own experience, which of the above problems experienced by patients do you think causes them the most distress?

FEEDBACK

This exercise will help you to appreciate the differences in the way that problems are perceived by you and the patient and make you more aware of the wide variety of problems which must be considered in overall management of the situation.

5.2 MANAGEMENT OF MALIGNANT WOUNDS

Introduction

Patients with malignant wounds have many complex and difficult obstacles to overcome. Wounds usually present as ulcerating or fungating. Thankfully, fungating wounds are uncommon, but have a profound psychological impact on patients and their families and present many challenges to those responsible for managing a patient's care.

Fungating wounds can be defined as lesions that are products of cancerous infiltration of the epithelium, resulting in a protruding, nodular growth which is prone to infection, bleeding and malodorous exudate (Foltz 1980, Fitzgerald & Sims 1987).

Patient assessment

Thorough assessment will help to identify the specific problems affecting the patient, family and friends and will allow them to be prioritised from the patient's perspective. The following criteria should be considered when planning care:

* clinical and social history
* cause and stage of disease
* treatment and prognosis
* the patient's and family's knowledge of the diagnosis
* nutritional assessment
* psychological impact of the wound for the patient and carers
* impact of the wound on quality of life
* availability of resources and social support network.

The principles of managing patients with malignant wounds

The management principles when caring for a patient with a malignant wound should aim to maximise healing whilst taking into account the specific problems related to wound aetiology.

General management principles

These would include:

* the identification of realistic treatment objectives that promote the patient's quality of life
* effective pain management and symptom control to promote patient comfort
* the prevention of any further wound deterioration or complications
* the provision of an aesthetically acceptable dressing
* the need for psychological and spiritual support to promote self-esteem and patient acceptance.

Specific management principles

These will vary depending on the cause and stage of disease and the location and severity of the wound, but would include some or all of the following:

* control of wound odour
* management of excessive exudate production
* prevention and control of haemorrhage
* care of the skin surrounding the wound
* care of irradiated skin
* prevention and control of wound infection.

Control of wound odour

Malodorous wounds often cause psychological distress for patients and will often lead to feelings of loneliness, depression, repulsion and social isolation. These psychological problems will certainly affect the patient's quality of life and may well actually delay the process of wound healing although further studies in this area need to be carried out (Van Toller 1994). The most common causes of odour associated with malignant wounds are the presence of necrotic tissue, fistula formation into the bowel and anaerobic wound infection. The main source of malodour associated with this type of wound derives from the compounds putrescine and cadavarine which are extremely offensive and difficult to disguise (Van Toller 1994). Odour may be controlled using a variety of different approaches, including wound debridement and topical agents.

Wound debridement. Wound debridement may be a quick method of reducing odour, but needs to be carefully evaluated as the potential risk of haemorrhage is great. Often the presence of a hard, dry eschar on the surface of the wound may actually be a useful way of controlling smell. Large areas of liquefied slough or necrotic tissue have a tendency to be extremely offensive and may be gently debrided using a dressing with a high water content such as a hydrogel or hydrocolloid.

Topical agents. Dressings may in some instances help to control smell. The use of carbon impregnated dressing products can be particularly important. Carbon can be combined with a variety of dressing materials including alginates, foams and dry dressings (see Sect. 4.3). Self-adhesive dressings such as foams, hydrocolloids and semipermeable films mask odour by effectively sealing the wound, whilst the use of wound drainage or ostomy bags can effectively drain wound exudate and isolate offensive odours. The use of topical metronidazole gel can in many instances reduce odour commonly associated with fungating wounds and can help to eradicate the anaerobic bacteria responsible for the offensive odour (Thomas & Hay 1991). However, continuous therapy is required as the anaerobes quickly multiply once treatment is discontinued. Metronidazole can also be given systemically to achieve similar results but can cause nausea for some patients. Room deodorants, adequate ventilation and appropriate disposal of soiled dressings and linen are also effective measures that can help to reduce this distressing problem.

Management of excessive exudate and skin protection

Many malignant wounds produce large amounts of exudate, which cause dressings to leak leading to skin maceration, excoriation, discomfort and lack of confidence. Wound dressings need to be capable of absorbing large amounts of exudate and should have the ability to hold fluid away from the surface of the surrounding skin. Foam or alginate dressings are particularly suited to this purpose and should be firmly held in place to lessen the risk of leakage. Patients with breast wounds should be encouraged to wear a well-fitting bra to help facilitate this process and to give a reasonable aesthetic appearance. If dressings are unable to contain exudate adequately, wound drainage or ostomy bags can be used and are available in a variety of different sizes. Specialised advice may be sought from ostomy nurses who also have a great deal of experience of protecting delicate or damaged skin.

Minimisation of trauma and haemorrhage

The surface of fungating wounds in particular is extremely vulnerable to the effects of trauma. Any adhesive product requires careful use as the increased vascularity of these wounds leads to an increased risk of bleeding. For this reason, extreme care is required when surgically debriding malignant wounds, which should always be done under medical supervision. Spontaneous haemorrhage can occur as the tumour infiltrates surrounding blood vessels and can be extremely frightening for the patient and carers. Haemostasis can be achieved by simple compression or by using topical haemostats such as alginate dressings, stomahesive powders or, in severe bleeds, adrenaline, which must always be prescribed by medical staff. The use of low-adherent dressings is vital and care should be taken when irrigating the wound surface in order to minimise tissue disturbance.

Self-assessment   5 MINUTES

List four types of dressings that may be helpful when managing fungating wounds.

FEEDBACK

You may have mentioned a variety of dressings that offer advantages in dealing with the problems associated with the management of fungating wounds. The most frequently used include:

1. alginate dressings as these absorb exudate, conform easily to the wound surface and can help to control haemorrhage
2. foam dressings as these absorb high levels of exudate and release easily from the wound surface
3. hydrogel dressings as they can promote gentle wound debridement and help to control odour associated with necrotic, sloughy wounds
4. hydrocolloid dressings which absorb exudate and help to debride smaller areas of slough or necrotic tissue again reducing wound odour
5. low-adherent wound contact dressings combined with activated charcoal which absorb some exudate and help to reduce wound odour.

Care of irradiated skin

Radiotherapy is a commonly used treatment which aims to destroy malignant cells. Unfortunately any healthy skin within the treatment area will also inevitably be damaged in the process. Skin reactions range in severity but will get progressively worse as treatment progresses. There are three types of skin reaction associated with the use of radiotherapy.

• Erythema—usually appears after the first few weeks of treatment and is characterised by warm, red, skin which feels tight.

- Dry desquamation—characterised by red, dry, itchy, sensitive skin.
- Moist desquamation—characterised by red, sore, blistered and excoriated skin which produces exudate. Areas commonly affected include the chest wall, groin and skin folds.

The main aims of treatment include:

- minimising patient discomfort and further skin reactions
- reducing the physiological effects of radiotherapy.

The treatment area should be kept clean and dry; it should be gently washed daily, avoiding the use of soaps, and then be carefully patted dry. Talcum powder and skin creams should be avoided as they may contain metallic substances which may potentiate radiotherapy reactions. Mechanical trauma should be avoided and is often caused by shaving, constrictive clothing and adhesive dressings or tapes. Extremes of temperature should also be avoided and the patient encouraged to wear loose-fitting cotton clothing. Exposure of the affected area to sunshine will also exacerbate skin damage and should be avoided, skin should be protected with a sunscreen (SPF 15 +). Dry desquamation should be moisturised using a bland, non-metallic, prescribed cream. Damaged irradiated skin can be made more comfortable by the application of a soothing dressing which can also help to minimise further trauma if left undisturbed in between treatments. Advice should be sought from individual radiotherapy departments but the following dressing types can be useful: simple low-adherent products, silicone low-adherent sheets, hydrogels in sheet or amorphous presentations, foam dressings or hydrocolloids (see Sect. 4.3). Some centres have had considerable success with the use of fixation sheets which are applied directly to damaged skin and left intact for 5–7 days. The covered areas are carefully washed and dried daily; the dressing is finally removed after soaking with a vegetable oil which loosens it without causing any further skin damage (Carville 1995). Improvements in adhesive technology have resulted in the increased use of adhesive dressings for the management of patients suffering from these skin problems. A wise precaution is to ensure that the adhesive borders of such dressings come into contact with non-damaged skin only.

Prevention and control of wound infection

Moist areas and the presence of necrotic and sloughy tissue in malignant wounds mean that the risk of wound infection by both anaerobic and aerobic bacteria is unfortunately high. For the general management principles of infection refer to Section 3.3.

The effective management of patients with malignant wounds is dependent on the utilisation of many skills and therefore should always involve a patient-led approach to care which makes the best use of the multidisciplinary team.

Activity   10 MINUTES

Take a few minutes to study Plate 5 (between pp. 22 and 23) and the brief patient details in Box 5.1 and then answer the questions below:

Box 5.1 Mrs Williams

Mrs Williams is a 77-year-old woman, who lives with her husband. She has recently presented at her GP's surgery with a large fungating breast wound which she has been managing for the last 4 years on her own. She has sought help because the wound has become particularly offensive, has recently started to bleed quite profusely at times and she has generally found it increasingly more difficult to effectively contain the high exudate levels being produced by the wound. She is obviously a very independent woman who would prefer where possible to manage this wound herself.

1. Before discussing the management of this wound with Mrs Williams, what information would be beneficial in order to help plan the appropriate care and management of this complex wound?
2. Suggest three needs that this patient might have in relation to controlling her symptoms.
3. What criteria do you think that Mrs Williams will want to be fulfilled by a wound dressing? Try to think of at least five.

FEEDBACK

Your answers should have included the following points.

1. Various issues would need to be sensitively explored with Mrs Williams prior to specifically focusing attention on the practical management of the wound itself. If at all possible these discussions should involve her husband, although it is not unusual in such circumstances for other close family members to be unaware that such problems exist. The following points would, if possible, need to be explored further:

- What is the patient's and family's knowledge and acceptance of the diagnosis and prognosis of her condition?
- Have all treatment options been discussed, e.g. radiotherapy, surgery?
- What effect has this wound had on her quality of life?
- What particular aspects of managing her wound cause her the biggest difficulties?
- What is her ability to continue self-caring for her own wound?
- What formal or informal support systems is she likely to accept?
- What resources and support from the multidisciplinary team are available?
- How has she managed her wound in the past, which approaches have been helpful and which have not?

2. Assessment of the difficulties being faced by Mrs Williams should take into account her priorities for wound care. Advice given should be as practical as possible and treatment options should allow her to continue to take an active role in the management of her wound for as long as she wishes to do so. Her previous experience of managing this wound should also be acknowledged.

   At this point in time, her specific symptom control needs are likely to include:

   - absorption and control of wound exudate levels
   - control of bacterial and/or fungal wound infections
   - control of associated wound odour
   - pain control
   - reduction of wound and skin trauma at dressing change.

3. Mrs Williams is going to want a dressing that fulfils most, if not all, of the following criteria:

   - easy to use and quick to change
   - conformable to the breast area.
   - comfortable to wear and cosmetically acceptable
   - highly absorbent, yet not bulky
   - capable of containing offensive odours
   - will not cause additional tissue trauma or bleeding on removal
   - can be left in place for a few days at a time without leaking
   - available for use in the community.

The successful management of this patient's fungating lesion will primarily depend on the relationships that are fostered between the multidisciplinary team and herself. Facilities available within her own home environment will also greatly influence the suggested treatment options.

5.3 MANAGEMENT OF NON-HEALING LEG ULCERS

Introduction

Without a doubt the main cause of delayed healing of ulcers of the lower limb is failure to identify and treat the underlying cause (Morison & Moffatt 1994). There are, however, many other factors that cause delayed wound healing. Those widely recognised as being of importance are:

- psychosocial problems
- restricted mobility
- dependent limb oedema
- malnutrition
- poor compliance.

Patient assessment

Accurate patient assessment is required when a patient presents for the first time with a leg ulcer, in order to determine:

- the underlying aetiology of the ulcer
- which previous treatments have been used
- any associated factors that may prolong healing
- the patient's attitude to the ulcer
- the patient's social environment and support network.

A detailed nursing history combined with some simple investigations will in most cases help to determine the underlying pathology of the patient's leg ulcer. The aetiology of the majority of leg ulcers is approximately as indicated in Figure 5.1.

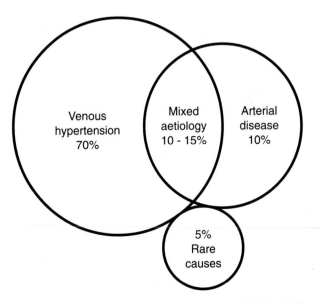

Fig. 5.1 Aetiology of leg ulceration (based on data in Callum 1992).

Before deciding on the treatment of any patient with a leg ulcer, the underlying aetiology must be determined. In addition to a thorough patient history, the ulcer and the limb should be carefully assessed. Some of the general differences between the appearance of arterial and venous ulcers have already been described in Section 2.9. Clinical observation should always be confirmed by an assessment of the arterial status of the limb using Doppler ultrasound (see Sect. 2.9). Whatever the cause of the ulcer appears to be, it is also important to exclude the rarer causes of ulceration, especially if the ulcer has been slow to heal, or has an atypical appearance.

Patients should always be referred to medical staff for a more detailed vascular assessment if the following conditions apply:

- patients who are younger and mobile as they may benefit from vein surgery
- patients who have ulcers that are not responding to treatment within 3 months
- patients with an ankle brachial index of 0.7 and below should be referred to the vascular surgeon
- patients with suspected rarer causes of ulceration
- any patient where the aetiology of ulceration is uncertain.

If there is any uncertainty regarding the underlying pathology of an ulcer, the patient must be referred to medical staff as soon as possible. Specialist advice is important for those patients with arterial disease including those with diabetes mellitus and rheumatoid arthritis as a more comprehensive vascular assessment is required to determine the extent of the disease and the appropriate management.

Principles of managing patients with leg ulcers

The most important objective when managing patients with leg ulcers is to determine the underlying aetiology so that appropriate treatment can be implemented.

General management principles for patients with venous leg ulcers

The main principles to be aware of are:

- accurate assessment of the underlying aetiology of the ulcer
- correction of the underlying cause of the ulcer
- identification and improvement of any associated factors that may prolong ulcer healing
- provision of the optimal local environment at the wound surface to maximise healing
- maintenance of patient compliance with treatment
- prevention of complications associated with ulcer pathology.

Once the aetiology of the ulcer has been determined, the treatment objectives should reflect the specific management principles appropriate to the cause of the leg ulcer.

Specific management principles for patients with venous ulcers

Chronic venous hypertension is the most common cause of venous ulcers. Therefore the primary aim of venous leg ulcer management should focus on the reversal of venous and capillary hypertension by:

- reducing the high pressure exerted on the superficial venous system
- encouraging venous return to the heart
- increasing calf muscle pump function by improving patient mobility or foot and ankle exercises
- discouraging oedema by reducing the pressure difference between the capillaries and surrounding tissue.

It is widely accepted that sustained graduated compression from the toes to the knee provides the optimum conditions for improvement of venous hypertension. Compression therapy can be provided using a variety of different methods. Choice of method will depend upon:

- resources available, including availability of equipment and training
- locally determined treatment protocols/clinical practice guidelines
- patient mobility
- the size and shape of the patient's leg
- patient preference.

Activity   10 MINUTES

Read Article 7 in the Reader (p. 180) and answer the following question:

Describe three factors that will influence the amount of pressure exerted by a compression bandage.

● ●

FEEDBACK

Three variables that will affect the amount of pressure exerted by a compression bandage are:

- *Bandage tension:* which primarily depends on the amount of extension or stretch applied by the person putting the bandage on to the patient's leg.

- *Layers of bandage:* two layers of bandage will exert twice as much pressure on the tissues as a single layer. There needs to be a consistent number of bandage layers applied to the leg. In the majority of application techniques this will be two layers, as each turn of the bandage usually overlaps the previous one by 50%.
- *Limb radius:* as long as bandage tension and number of layers applied to the limb remain constant, a bandage will exert a higher pressure on the diameter of a smaller leg than on a larger one. This ensures that in a normally shaped leg, at constant tension, a compression bandage is capable of producing a higher pressure at the ankle than at the calf. Therefore the natural shape of the lower limb helps to achieve graduated pressure which will facilitate the reduction of venous hypertension and the control of oedema.

Another variable affecting the amount of tension applied by a compression bandage relates to the amount of elastomeric fibres within it. The tensile force generated by these fibres when extended exerts pressure on the limb. It is therefore important to read the instructions supplied by individual bandage manufacturers, as an indication is given of how much pressure on average can be exerted by the bandage when applied at a given tension.

Specific management principles for patients with arterial ulcers

Management of these patients is usually conservative and is concerned with the maintenance of the limb. If arterial insufficiency is due to a local problem such as an atherosclerotic arterial occlusion, surgical intervention may be appropriate. In instances where there is more widespread arterial involvement such as in diabetes mellitus or rheumatoid arthritis, any treatment will be closely monitored by medical staff. Nursing responsibilities include symptom relief, local wound management, patient education and psychological support.

Under no circumstances should any type of compression therapy be applied to a limb with an ankle pressure index of 0.8 or below without medical supervision.

The conservative management principles of caring for patients with arterial ulcers are:

- management of underlying disease
- avoidance of mechanical trauma and prevention of any further deterioration in limb condition
- daily examination of the legs and feet
- maintenance of skin hygiene
- avoidance of sudden changes of temperature, which can cause thermal trauma

- maximisation of arterial blood flow to the feet, avoiding constrictive clothing or shoes
- elevating the head of the bed, always resting legs in a dependent position
- regular assessment and review by chiropodist/podiatrist
- effective pain control.

Specific management principles for patients with ulcers of mixed aetiology

Patients with ulcers of mixed vascular origin will exhibit the characteristics of both arterial and venous ulcers which can make assessment and treatment difficult. The use of Doppler ultrasound is vital to accurately determine the ratio of venous arterial mix. It must also be remembered that the vascular status of a limb is dynamic and can change quickly; therefore regular reassessment using the doppler is recommended. Some authors suggest that this procedure is repeated at 3-monthly intervals (Simon et al 1994). Treatment objectives vary, depending on whether venous or arterial disease is the predominant factor. The primary aim of management of this type of ulcer is to:

- determine the degree of arterial insufficiency, which will influence the decision to apply modified compression or not
- regularly reassess the vascular status of the limb
- follow the principles for managing venous/arterial ulcers depending on which is the predominant aetiology.

Leg ulcers cause considerable distress and discomfort for patients. There are many causes of leg ulceration making accurate assessment a fundamental priority in the care and management of this group of patients. Appropriate management based upon objective assessment can do much to alleviate the suffering associated with this chronic condition.

Activity   20 MINUTES

Read the case history in Box 5.2 and then answer the following questions.

1. Study Plate 6 (between pp. 22 and 23). Briefly assess Mrs White's wound, listing at least six problems that this type of wound may cause from her perspective.
2. Now describe from your own perspective any additional problems that may arise from caring for a patient with this type of wound.
3. What five investigations would you wish to perform in order to identify which factors may be responsible for the delayed healing of this wound?

Box 5.2 Mrs White

Mrs White is an 82-year-old widower who lives alone. She has had a leg ulcer intermittently for the past 11 years. This episode of ulceration has lasted for 3 years and the wound is becoming progressively worse. The ulcer is particularly troublesome at night, when it has a tendency to leak and is more painful. Despite some support from the community nursing services, the ulcer is gradually enlarging and getting deeper. Mrs White is very disheartened by this lack of progress and feels that there is nothing more that can be done to help her.

4. In your experience, what additional factors could be responsible for the delayed healing rate of this type of wound? Think of at least four common problems and two less common problems.

FEEDBACK

1. Difficulties commonly reported by patients with leg ulcers include:

   - excess wound exudate and dressing leakage
   - heavy and oedematous legs
   - maceration of the skin surrounding the ulcer
   - dry, itchy, sensitive skin surrounding the ulcer
   - wound pain and/or discomfort
   - lack of mobility
   - social isolation
   - lack of sleep.

2. From a nursing perspective you may have noted the following additional problems:

   - excessively sloughy wound that may impair the growth of granulation tissue
   - potential risk of wound infection that may prolong the inflammatory response
   - risk of skin sensitivities/allergies that may cause further skin deterioration and limit the choice of dressing
   - risk of low patient compliance
   - uncertain ulcer aetiology so that commencement of appropriate treatment is delayed.

   Remember, if there is any uncertainty about the underlying ulcer pathology, the patient should be referred as quickly as possible to medical staff for a detailed assessment.

3. The following tests should be routinely performed on all patients presenting with ulceration of the lower leg:

   - Doppler ultrasound to determine the vascularity of the limb. The absence or

presence of palpable foot pulse is not sufficient as they may be masked by oedema, or be congenitally absent (Barnhorst & Braner 1968). Studies have also indicated that lack of pedal pulses has a positive predictive value for significant arterial disease in only 35% of cases (Moffatt 1995).

   - wound swab—only if clinical signs of infection are present (see Sect. 2.6).
   - patch testing to determine the presence of skin sensitivities or allergies.
   - urine test to exclude undiagnosed diabetes.
   - full blood count—haemoglobin levels may be low and are relatively easily corrected. A raised erythrocyte sedimentation rate (ESR) may indicate infection and vasculitis associated with rheumatoid arthritis or systemic lupus erythematosus.

4. Although the majority of leg ulcers are relatively easily identified as either venous or ischaemic in origin, a significant proportion will either be of mixed aetiology, result from rare causes or be complicated by the following problems:

   - Common problems
     —lack of mobility/fixed ankle joint
     —wound infection
     —skin sensitivities/allergies
     —scratching leading to repeated local trauma
     —inadequate treatment—aetiology not established
     —underlying ischaemia and/or diabetic neuropathy
     —poor social conditions
     —lack of patient motivation/compliance
     —patient application of home remedies and treatments.
   - Less common problems
     —vasculitis (most often associated with rheumatoid disease)
     —malignancy (confirmed by tissue biopsy)
     —osteomyelitis (confirmed by X-ray) which could be due to rare infections, e.g. leprosy, syphilis, tuberculosis
     —lymphoedema, which causes characteristic thickening of the dermis.

5.4 MANAGEMENT OF SINUSES AND FISTULAE

Introduction

The presence of sinuses or fistulae in a wound will always delay healing and inevitably makes patient management more complex. Fistulae may develop spontaneously and are often associated with inflammatory diseases or are a postoperative complication following surgery. Patients with large wounds complicated by fistulae are faced with many distressing problems such as a large disfiguring wound which may expose internal organs and produce copious amounts of offensive discharge. A major difficulty for these patients is coping with altered body image and loss of self-esteem.

External fistulae are usually a result of trauma, infection, malignancy, obstruction, surgery or radiation damage. They may also be associated with large cavity wounds and sinus formation following wound dehiscence and represent a major challenge to the multidisciplinary team.

Self-assessment 2 MINUTES

Define briefly what is meant by the term fistula.

● ●

FEEDBACK

A fistula is an abnormal track connecting two or more structures or spaces. This can involve a communicating tract from one body cavity or hollow organ to another hollow organ or to the skin (Bryant 1992). Fistulae may be internal or external and are described as internal when connecting two internal organs, e.g. enterocolonic, where the intestine and the colon are connected. External fistulae join an internal organ to the skin, e.g. vesicocutaneous where the bladder connects with the skin.

● ●

Self-assessment 2 MINUTES

Define briefly what is meant by the term sinus.

● ●

FEEDBACK

A sinus is a blind-ending tract which opens on to an epithelial surface; it may indicate the presence of a chronic abscess or foreign body deep within the tissues.

The differences in structure between a sinus and a fistula can be seen in Figure 5.2.

● ●

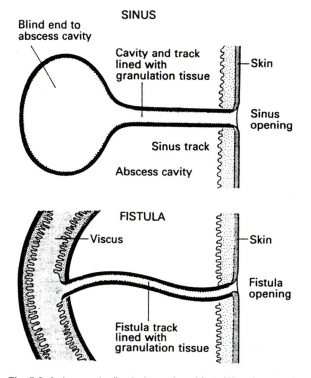

Fig. 5.2 A sinus and a fistula (reproduced from Westaby 1985 by kind permission).

Many of the principles of caring for patients with sinuses and fistulae are similar; where possible management of these types of patients will be described together, but for the sake of clarity the principles of caring for these patients have been listed separately.

Principles of caring for patients with a sinus

The presence of a sinus within a wound indicates that there is a foreign body or abscess deep within the tissues causing a focal point for infection and a marked inflammatory response.

General management principles

Without appropriate treatment sinuses have a tendency to heal, only to recur again at a later date. This is because only superficial bridging of epithelial tissue has occurred at the sinus opening, which prevents free drainage of fluid and removal of the causative foreign body. Therefore the most appropriate treatment for sinuses is surgical intervention where the sinus is either completely excised or is laid open to facilitate growth of healthy granulation tissue from the wound base.

General management principles therefore include:

• providing optimal conditions for closure of the sinus

- effective symptom control to promote patient comfort
- promotion of patient independence and mobility.

Specific management principles

These principles focus specifically on the provision of those conditions known to promote closure of sinuses, which are:

- to establish the size and extent of the sinus
- to remove any foreign bodies from the sinus tract
- to encourage free drainage of exudate
- to promote growth of granulation tissue from the base of the sinus
- to absorb excess exudate and protect the surrounding skin.

Principles of caring for patients with fistulae

Conservative treatment is the commonest approach to the management of patients with fistulae and includes creating the optimal conditions for spontaneous closure of a fistula or preparation of the patient for surgical intervention.

General management principles

Many patients with fistulae are severely debilitated and immunocompromised. Fistula development may prove to be a life-threatening complication requiring a high level of medical and nursing intervention. General management principles include:

- the identification of realistic treatment objectives that promote the patient's quality of life
- providing optimal conditions for closure of the fistula
- effective symptom control to promote patient comfort
- the promotion of patient independence and mobility
- the need for psychological support to promote self-esteem and acceptance.

Specific management principles

These will vary depending on the origin and location of the fistula and the type and amount of fluid drainage, but would include some or all of the following:

- accurate assessment of fistula output
- the maintenance of fluid and electrolyte balance
- the maintenance of nutritional support
- care of the skin surrounding the fistula
- effective management of fistula effluent and odour.

We will look at each of these in more detail.

Accurate assessment of fistula output

It is essential to determine the cause, type and amount of exudate for any patient with a complex draining wound in order to manage and evaluate healing potential and to plan appropriate treatment objectives. Excessive wound drainage may lead to a variety of complications including abscess formation, wound infection, septicaemia, skin excoriation, sinus or fistula formation and wound dehiscence. It is therefore important to assess the likely origin of wound drainage by observing colour, consistency, odour, type and amount of exudate produced. If possible, samples of drainage fluid should be collected for laboratory analysis. This is especially important when managing high output fistulae which drain in excess of 500 ml of fluid in 24 hours, as analysis of effluent may be helpful in determining the patient's electrolyte and fluid balance. A low output fistula is defined as one that produces less than 500 ml of fluid in 24 hours (Doughty & Broadwell Jackson 1993). Fluid replacement and electrolyte balance are dependent on the origin of the fistula and the amount of fluid drained, making a thorough patient history necessary including details of the nature and type of any previous surgical procedures.

Maintenance of fluid and electrolyte balance

Accurate monitoring of fluid intake and output together with laboratory analysis of blood form the basis of fluid and electrolyte replacement therapy. The loss of electrolytes that are secreted from the gastrointestinal tract by high output fistulae, if uncorrected, will result in circulatory collapse. Fluids may be replaced orally, enterally or parenterally depending on the patient's physical condition, the type of fistula and the amount of fluids required.

Maintenance of nutritional support

Malnutrition is a common complication that many patients with complex wounds and fistulae will experience. Nutritional support not only increases the likelihood of spontaneous closure of fistulae (Rombeau & Rolandelli 1987) but maximises healing potential of other associated wounds. A negative nitrogen balance resulting from excessive loss of protein-rich fluids, increased metabolic needs and a reduced protein intake contribute to malnutrition and will further compromise tissue viability. The calorific requirements of patients with severe tissue damage is dependent on the size of the wound and the patient's pre-existing physical condition. In particular, patients with fistulae require additional calories owing to the large amounts of protein-rich fluid that are lost daily from the fistula. Detailed nutritional assessment will be required on an ongoing basis by the nutritional support team to confirm that the patient's nutritional requirements are met.

An undesirable consequence of enteral feeding and oral intake may be increased fistula output which may further compromise electrolyte and fluid balance and may prolong the closure of the fistula tract. Total parenteral nutrition is the method of choice for those patients with high output fistulae. Many fistulae will spontaneously close within 4–8 weeks; after this time if fistula drainage is persistent and the patient is free from infection surgical intervention may be indicated.

Care of the skin surrounding the fistula or sinus

The primary consideration when caring for the skin surrounding a fistula or sinus is to protect it from coming into contact with drainage fluid. For the management of smaller sinuses the use of highly absorbent dressing materials should be sufficient to adequately contain discharging wound exudate. The objective of using a dressing in this situation should be to encourage absorption and free drainage of exudate whilst protecting the surrounding skin from maceration. There are several types of dressing materials that are particularly suited to the management of sinuses which are described in greater detail in Section 4.3.

The skin surrounding a fistula is extremely vulnerable owing to the digestive enzymes found in the discharging effluent. There are various methods of protecting the skin surrounding fistulae and larger sinuses which are briefly described in Table 5.1.

Self-assessment   4 MINUTES

1. Which of the following is used to absorb moisture from excoriated skin?
   a. Filler pastes
   b. Adhesive barriers
   c. Protective powders
   d. Protective films.

2. Protective films may be used for all of the following except:
   a. protection of the skin from the effect of adhesives
   b. prevention of skin maceration
   c. prevention of skin erosion from irritant effluent
   d. provision of a secure seal between skin and appliance.

FEEDBACK

1. The most suitable products for absorbing excess moisture at the skin's surface are the protective powders and the adhesive barriers; these are usually made from pectin, gelatine, carboxymethylcellulose, karaya and sterculia gums, which are all highly absorbent. As well as absorbing fluid they also have a protective function which helps to provide favourable conditions for re-epithelialisation.

2. Protective films have a variety of uses but will not adequately prevent skin excoriation from irritants such as digestive enzymes. They have a particularly useful role in skin protection when combined with other products such as adhesive barriers, filler pastes and protective powders.

Table 5.1 Skin care products

Product	Action and application
Protective films	These create a waterproof barrier when used on intact skin and should be used as a preventive measure. Available as skin wipes or sprays that dissolve to leave a film coating on the skin which also increases the adhesiveness of appliances
Protective powders	Absorb exudate and protect the surrounding skin. Any excess should be removed from the skin's surface before application of appliances
Filler pastes	These contain various constituents including gelling and film-forming agents and thickeners. Pastes should be thinly applied to the skin for protection and used to fill cracks and uneven surfaces in order to prevent leakage of effluent
Adhesive barriers	These flat wafers are composed of various compounds that are able to absorb water, adhere to damp skin and soothe excoriated areas. Wafers can be cut to size or may be an integral part of an appliance or presented as a ring shape

Effective management of fluid output and odour

Ostomy and wound drainage appliances vary in type and design. Selection depends on the following factors:

- type of wound/stoma
- location of wound/stoma
- amount of fluid produced in 24 hours
- individual patient needs and preferences.

Appliances are available as one or two pieces; two-piece appliances allow access to the wound without the need to remove the protective adhesive wafer. Some one-piece appliances contain access ports to facilitate wound management. This allows the appliance to remain in situ for a few days without compromising the need to irrigate or pack the wound. If output is excessive an additional drainage bag will need to be attached to the original one. Appliances are available that have suitable connecting points which minimise the risk of leakage. Wide bore tubing and wide-ended drainage bags are necessary for patients with fistulae that produce output containing undigested food if blockages are to be avoided. If the wound is in a difficult area such as the groin, a flexible one-piece appliance capable of moulding to the skin's contours will be most practical and comfortable for the patient. Urostomy appliances usually have non-return valves making them useful for managing fistulae that drain large amounts of digestive enzymes so that backflow is prevented from damaging the skin surrounding the fistula.

Suction can be used to facilitate drainage of high output fistulae. Care must be taken to ensure that suction is gentle in order to avoid unnecessary trauma to the surrounding tissues. Suction drains are usually used in combination with ostomy or wound drainage appliances where the drain is inserted into the fistula through an access port in the appliance. Drainage should be recorded if appropriate.

Much of the odour associated with fistulae can be minimised by effective containment of effluent by ensuring that the appropriate fillers, wafers and appliances are used in order to prevent embarrassing leakage for the patient. Systemic antibiotics may be required to control pathogens responsible for creating odour in infected wounds and should be prescribed as indicated. Proper disposal of effluent is essential, whilst the use of air fresheners, deodorants, incense or aromatherapy oils may be helpful for some patients. Many may find the use of air fresheners more unpleasant than the original odour and individual wishes should be respected at all times.

Self-assessment — 10 MINUTES

1. Define what is meant by a low output and a high output fistula.
2. List three methods of maintaining fluid replacement for a patient with a high output fistula.
3. List three life-threatening complications that may affect patients with fistulae.
4. Taking into consideration your answers to the question above, define five goals for the nursing management of the patient with a fistula.

FEEDBACK

Your answers should have included the following points.

1. A low output fistula is one which drains less than 500 ml of fluid in a 24-hour period, whilst a high output fistula will drain in excess of 500 ml within 24 hours.

2. Maintenance of fluid and electrolyte balance for patients with high output fistulae can be achieved by the following methods:

- orally
- enterally
- parenterally.

3. The most commonly occurring life-threatening complications that may affect patients with fistulae are:

- fluid and electrolyte imbalance
- malnutrition
- sepsis.

4. In order to prevent these complications careful patient assessment and monitoring is required. Nursing intervention should therefore focus on:

- accurate assessment of patient's fluid balance
- correction and maintenance of fluid and electrolyte imbalance
- monitoring of patient's nutritional status
- correction and maintenance of nutritional support
- assessment for signs and symptoms of local or systemic infection.

Activity — 10 MINUTES

Read the case history presented in Box 5.3 and refer to Plate 7 (between pp. 22 and 23).

Box 5.3 Mrs Edwards

Mrs Edwards is a 52-year-old woman who has a long history of Crohn's disease. Following major abdominal surgery 3 weeks ago, she is making a slow recovery which has been complicated by the breakdown of her suture line and the formation of several small fistulae.

1. When planning the management of Mrs Edwards what factors would you take into consideration when assessing her suitability for an appropriate drainage system?
2. Describe the advantages from Mrs Edwards' perspective of having an adhesive drainable appliance for the management of her fistulae.

· ·

FEEDBACK

1. Preplanning and careful assessment will help to ensure that the most effective ostomy or wound drainage system is selected to meet Mrs Edwards' needs. There is a wide variety of appliances and drainage bags available today; many are specifically designed to deal with particular patient problems. Your answer should have included the points listed below.

   • Location of the fistulae; are they close to other wounds, scars or skin folds that may complicate the application of a drainable appliance? Will the patient if necessary be able to empty and care for the drainable appliance?
   • Determine the size and location of the fistula openings within the wound. Are they small and easily identified or large and irregular in shape? Do the fistulae open up deep within the wound or at more superficial sites?
   • Determine exactly how many fistula openings are present. Are they all together so that they could be contained using one appliance? Are there any signs of tracking or fistula openings at different sites?
   • Assess the amount and type of drainage. Are there likely to be any digestive enzymes or bile present in the effluent that could cause severe skin irritation? Does the effluent contain undigested food that may cause the drainage system to block? Are the fistulae producing low or high output over 24 hours?
   • Assess the surrounding skin condition looking for signs of irritation, excoriation, blistering or inflammation. Does the patient have any known allergies to adhesives or dressing tapes?

   • Discuss with Mrs Edwards her posture and mobility. Determine in what positions she likes to lie in bed in order to determine the optimal positioning of the drainage bag, so that it is not affected by skin folds or pulled or kinked whilst sleeping. Checking the location of skin folds when sitting is also important for the same reason.

2. The likely advantages of an adhesive drainable appliance for Mrs Edwards would be the following.

   • It contains the effluent and minimises odour associated with fistulae.
   • The skin surrounding the fistulae is protected and kept dry, which enhances patient comfort.
   • Use of the drainage system encourages mobility and only minimally restricts activities of living.
   • The drainage system can be effectively disguised under clothing, which increases patient confidence and morale.
   • The appliance can be left in situ for a few days at a time, which minimises disruption and lessens time spent managing the fistulae and reapplying wound dressings.
   • The system allows free drainage of effluent which creates the best conditions for spontaneous closure of the fistulae.

· ·

5.5 MANAGEMENT OF NEUROPATHIC FOOT ULCERS

Introduction

Diabetic foot problems cause significant pain, disability and mortality world-wide. It is estimated that up to 50% of non-traumatic amputations of the lower limb occur in people with diabetes (Levin et al 1993). The World Health Organization through the St Vincent Declaration, to which the UK is a signatory, aims to reduce major amputations in people with diabetes by 50% (WHO 1990). A greater understanding of the aetiology of this commonly occurring problem is essential for nurses who may be the only members of the multidisciplinary team to have regular contact with this particular group of patients.

Patient assessment

Peripheral sensory neuropathy is probably the most common single cause of foot ulceration in diabetic patients (Young & Boulton 1991) with as many as one-fifth of foot ulcers being due to peripheral vascular disease alone. However, foot ulcers have a tendency to occur as a result of a combination of factors, commonly:

- peripheral vascular disease
- peripheral neuropathy
- wound infection.

Careful assessment of the foot and skin condition is of paramount importance in the prevention of these ulcers. Patients identified as being at risk should be encouraged to inspect their feet daily and carry out meticulous foot hygiene. Any patient who has suffered from foot ulceration in the past should always be considered as being at risk because recurrence is extremely common. Once skin damage occurs, deterioration can be extremely rapid and may quickly lead to serious complications such as infection. Elderly patients living alone are at particular risk, especially if vision is impaired and their mobility restricted.

Peripheral neuropathy affects the peripheral sensory, motor and autonomic nerves of the lower limb. This has several main effects, the reduction or loss of sensation, the absence of sweating, and foot deformities due to alterations in the biomechanics of the foot. Foot deformities develop as small muscles in the foot atrophy; this causes clawing of the toes and results in the metatarsal heads becoming more prominent. These changes cause alterations in gait, and the resultant build-up of repeated and prolonged local pressure causes callus formation and the eventual ulceration of the skin (see Fig. 5.3).

Neuropathic ulcers usually develop from deep within the tissues. A collection of fluid develops underneath the callus which leads to abscess formation and eventual ulceration. Usually the ulcerated area is initially very small and to the uninitiated looks insignificant. By the time the ulcer enlarges and starts to discharge fluid a great deal of tissue damage has often occurred and the wound is often infected and tracks deep within the tissues involving tendon and bone. Patient and carer education is therefore of primary importance if these ulcers are to be detected early and treated before lasting damage occurs.

Causes of leg ulcers

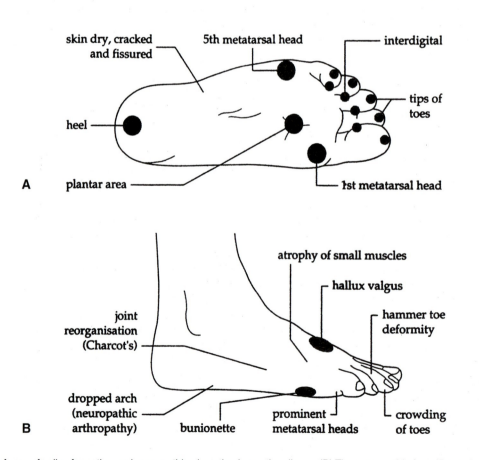

Fig. 5.3 (A) Areas of callus formation and neuropathic ulceration beneath calluses. (B) The neuropathic foot. (Reproduced from Morison & Moffatt 1994 by kind permission.)

Name the three types of peripheral neuropathy, briefly describing the effects that each has upon the foot.

FEEDBACK

The three types of peripheral neuropathy, which can occur in isolation or together, are:

- *Sensory neuropathy*. Loss of sensation increases the risk of mechanical, thermal and chemical trauma. Pain serves an important protective function; without this, the patient is either unaware that damage has occurred or believes that tissue damage is of no consequence.
- *Motor neuropathy*. This causes atrophy of the small muscles in the foot which eventually causes deformities such as hammer toes and gait changes. Disruptions in gait cause localised and repetitive stresses to develop, which eventually will result in callus formation and lead to ulceration.
- *Autonomic neuropathy*. This causes an inability to sweat which results in dry, cracked skin which is more prone to bacterial or fungal growth. These microorganisms are able to penetrate into the soft tissues quickly and combined with repetitive gait stresses may cause abscess formation, gangrene and amputation.

Principles of caring for patients with neuropathic ulcers

Because of the serious complications of neuropathic ulceration, preventive foot care is of fundamental importance. Detailed assessment is necessary in order to determine if the patient is suffering from ischaemia, neuropathy or both.

General management principles

- Accurate identification of those patients at risk of developing foot ulcers.
- Adequate monitoring and control of diabetes.
- Appropriate referral to specialist services, i.e. chiropody and vascular consultation.
- Targeting of specialised educational programmes at those patients considered to be at risk of developing foot ulcers.
- Continued support and follow-up of those patients with or at risk of developing foot ulcers.

Specific management principles

Patients with foot ulcers do not fight sepsis well and often present late with complicated wounds that are often slow to heal. In order to maximise healing of these wounds it is necessary:

- to assess the full extent of tissue damage
- to undertake radical local debridement of callus, eschar and necrotic tissue
- to control and eradicate infection
- to relieve localised pressure from the ulcer bed
- to absorb ulcer exudate levels whilst encouraging free drainage of the lesion
- to facilitate patient compliance.

Assessment of full extent of tissue damage

It is important when assessing the patient with an ulcerated foot to try to determine the predominant aetiology of the lesion. Collection of a detailed patient history may reveal many clues as to the origin of the ulcer's pathology. Deformities of gait are usually associated with neuropathy, while a history of pain more often than not will indicate the presence of peripheral vascular disease and ischaemia. Careful assessment of the feet and lower limbs will provide further evidence of either ischaemia, neuropathy or both. Unfortunately, a mixed aetiology is found in as many as 40% of patients attending foot hospitals in the UK (Young & Boulton 1991).

It can therefore be difficult in practice to differentiate between neuropathic and ischaemic foot ulcers; Table 5.2 summarises the main differences between these ulcer types.

Assessment of the depth, extent and type of tissue involvement of any patient with a foot ulcer is of primary importance if the wound is to be appropriately managed and further complications minimised. This necessitates rapid debridement of any callus or necrotic tissue so that the full extent of the wound can be determined. Radiological investigations can help to determine the extent of any bony involvement, the presence of osteomyelitis or any foreign bodies that may be deeply embedded within the tissues.

The term 'diabetic ulcer' is commonly used by health professionals to describe foot ulcers that may be frequently associated with patients who are diabetic. This term is incorrect and misleading as it suggests that the aetiology of all foot ulcers is linked to the pathophysiological changes seen in the microcirculation and nerve supply of the diabetic foot. The aetiology of a foot ulcer in a diabetic patient is one or other, or a combination, of two underlying pathologies, namely ischaemia and neuropathy.

Table 5.2 Differentiating between ischaemic and neuropathic foot ulceration

Signs and symptoms	Ischaemic ulcer	Neuropathic ulcer
Callus formation	Not present	Present commonly on planter surface under metatarsal heads
Foot deformity	Not present	Present—claw toes, hallux valgus, hammer toes
Ulcer onset	Rapid	Gradual
Ulcer position	Usually on or between toes	Associated with areas of local pressure and callus formation
Pain/discomfort	Severe rest pain, often worse at night	None, nerve function tests reveal an insensate foot
Surrounding skin condition	Atrophic, shiny skin. Dusky pink turning pale on elevation	Dry, fissured skin, absence of sweating
Foot temperature	Cool	Normal
Pedal pulses	Absent or diminished	Normal

Radical local debridement

These wounds are prone to infection, especially if the patient is diabetic. Surgical local debridement of all nonviable tissue is recommended (Levin 1988) in order to prevent the accumulation of slough and debris at the ulcer's surface and to remove callus, all of which provide an ideal medium for bacterial growth. Debridement is often undertaken in theatre so that a wide excision can be made, the wound can be fully explored and any abscesses be drained. The reason for such an 'aggressive' approach should be discussed with patients and their relatives beforehand. Smaller foot ulcers should be referred to the chiropodist for effective debridement of callus and advice sought regarding which types of dressings to use. Although the use of high water content dressings (hydrogels and hydrocolloids) has been successful in the conservative management of these lesions, some of the properties of these types of dressing may be unsuitable for neuropathic foot ulcers.

Control and eradication of infection

Systemic antibiotic therapy is the mainstay of treatment of foot ulceration and should follow antibiotic sensitivity testing. There is no place for the use of topical antibiotics or medicated dressings (Thomas 1990). Patients with infected foot ulcers should be admitted to hospital without delay. The diabetic foot does not tolerate the existence of pus under pressure and this will inevitably lead to rapid deterioration of tissue damage and cause fluctuations in blood sugar levels. Antibiotics may be given intravenously for 5–7 days followed by a further period of oral antibiotic therapy. Surgical debridement will also allow deep tissue biopsies to be sent for microscopy and culture so that antibiotic therapy can be targeted more accurately.

Self-assessment | 5 MINUTES

Which of the following may indicate osteomyelitis?

1. A non-healing foot ulcer.
2. Abnormal X-ray film findings.
3. A deep tissue biopsy.
4. All of the above.

FEEDBACK

All of the above are likely to confirm the diagnosis of osteomyelitis. Early referral is of utmost importance. If infection is left untreated the chances of eventual amputation of the limb are significantly increased.

Reduction of localised pressure

Patients should be referred to a chiropodist so that the need for specially adapted footwear which reduces the pressure normally exerted over the bony prominences can be identified. Padding of the foot or toes with foams or wools should only be attempted under the close supervision of a chiropodist. Padding incorrectly inserted into a shoe can lead to an increase in pressure points and may increase the risk of tissue breakdown. Special insoles of polyethylene foam have energy-absorbing properties; they can be heated and individually moulded to the foot in order to cushion and redistribute weight more evenly. Total contact casting where the foot is encased within a plaster of Paris or lighter-weight walking cast may be indicated for the effective management of neuropathic ulcers and have the added advantage of promoting patient mobility, while distributing the pressures exerted when walking across the whole sole of the foot. Whenever possible the patient should be encouraged to elevate the leg, unless ischaemic pain makes this impractical, as this will help to improve oedema and relieve the local pressure points that result from weight-bearing. Bed-rest is perhaps the most effective method of pressure relief, but is probably the most difficult to enforce.

Absorption of ulcer exudate

Appropriate dressing selection is important, but is not the mainstay of the treatment or management of this group of patients. Excessive tissue maceration should be avoided especially between the toes as this increases the likelihood of infection, and dressings need to be changed at frequent intervals. Any cavities should be gently filled using absorptive dressing materials that are able to encourage free drainage of exudate; foam and alginate dressings have been used with considerable success (Foster et al 1994).

Self-assessment   15 MINUTES

Briefly describe five essential characteristics that a dressing for patients with foot ulceration must have.

• •

FEEDBACK

Your answer should have included most of the following points:
    A dressing for patients with foot ulcers should:

• perform well within the enclosed environment of the shoe and not be too bulky
• withstand the constant local pressures and shear stresses exerted when walking, without slipping or bottoming out
• provide optimal conditions for healing by maintenance of the ulcer in a moist but not macerated condition
• absorb the large amounts of exudate that these wounds produce when under pressure
• avoid plugging the wound—diabetic lesions in particular will deteriorate rapidly if free drainage is prevented
• be capable of easy, non-traumatic removal, as most wounds of this type will require inspection and assessment every 24–48 hours owing to the rapid rates of deterioration commonly seen.

• •

Patient compliance

Patient education and compliance is fundamental in preventing and minimising the complications of foot ulceration. Unfortunately, experience suggests that although many diabetic patients understand the aetiology of foot ulceration, many do not consider themselves to be personally at risk; an even greater number of patients are totally unaware of their increased 'at-risk' status (Masson et al 1989). There is still an obvious need for improvement in the provision of educational programmes for this susceptible group of patients and their carers.

    Once healed, the patient is in the highest risk category for the development of subsequent ulcers. Foot care, continued education and careful follow-up are all necessary to try to prevent recurrence.

Activity   15 MINUTES

Take a few minutes to examine Plate 8 (between pp. 22 and 23) and the brief patient details supplied in Box 5.4 and then answer the questions below.

Box 5.4 Mrs Patel

Mrs Patel is 48 and has reluctantly sought the advice of her general practitioner as a small, but deep wound on the sole of her left foot under the first metatarsal head has failed to heal since she injured it 4 months ago. She is a shy person who speaks very little English and relies heavily on her eldest son who is 13 to translate for her. On examination she has a lot of hard skin and callus formation on her feet which may be due to the fact that she spends much of her time walking either barefoot or in open-toed sandals. She does not share the GP's concern about her wound because it is relatively dry and does not cause her any pain.

1. List any factors that you consider may have contributed to the formation of the ulcer on Mrs Patel's foot.
2. What is the most likely aetiology of this wound? Give a brief rationale to support your decision.
3. What advice concerning the care of her feet would you give to Mrs Patel?

• •

FEEDBACK

1. There would be a number of factors contributing to the formation of this patient's

foot ulcer. All of the following should have been identified:

- delayed healing following minor trauma several months ago
- the increased risk of trauma resultant from the wearing of open-toed sandals or walking barefoot
- reluctance to seek help and advice from health care professionals
- lack of understanding of the potential seriousness of lesions of this type
- limited ability to speak English
- prolonged delay between initial injury and presentation at GP surgery.

2. Your answer should have identified that this wound is most likely to have been caused by either ischaemia, neuropathy or a combination of the two. In this particular case, the wound appears to be neuropathic in origin, with the possibility of some ischaemic involvement. It would be of particular importance to exclude the possibility that Mrs Patel has undiagnosed diabetes as this would greatly increase her risk of sepsis and localised wound infection. In practice it is difficult to differentiate between neuropathic and ischaemic ulceration. Mrs Patel's history and examination of her foot suggest a neuropathic ulcer as these:

- tend to occur over weight-bearing areas of the foot
- are usually well defined but initially dry and covered with a scab
- are often surrounded by thick callus formation
- are present on a foot with good colour but dry, cracked skin
- are usually painless and cause the patient little or no concern
- have usually been present for some time.

3. Any advice given to Mrs Patel will have to be simple as she has a limited understanding of English. In many areas, specialised foot care advice is available in written form in a variety of languages and dialects. Much of the following information could be discussed in the presence of her son so that he can translate for her, giving her the opportunity to ask questions.

The role of the community nurse in the context of patient advice and prevention of these problems cannot be overemphasised. All patients should be given the following advice, much of which is unpopular.

- Wash feet daily using soap and warm water. The skin should be dried well, paying particular attention to areas between the toes.

- If feet are very dry, they should be lightly moisturised.
- Patients should be warned of the dangers of walking barefoot and should take particular care to avoid any trauma to their feet and toes.
- Any injury, however small, should be carefully monitored and should preferably be assessed by a health professional.
- Feet should be inspected daily for signs of trauma and ischaemia.
- The chiropodist should cut toenails and treat any callus formation as well as other localised foot problems.
- Home remedies and topical applications should always be avoided.
- Avoid extremes of temperature; hot water, hot-water bottles and sitting close to fires may cause tissue damage, especially in the insensate foot.
- All footwear should be fitted properly to avoid constriction of the feet and toes as well as undue friction which can occur if shoes are too big.
- In particular, sandals with thongs between the toes should not be worn, as this increases risk of unnecessary trauma.
- Shoes should not be worn without socks or stockings.
- Specialist footwear, which is tailored to specific patient requirements, should be measured and fitted by appropriately qualified members of the team.
- Patients should be encouraged wherever possible to reduce smoking and comply if diabetic with dietary advice.

Management of patients with foot ulcers represents a challenge to the multidisciplinary team. Many of these ulcers continue to fail to heal, owing to problems of maintaining patient compliance and because many patients receive inadequate or inappropriate care. A basic understanding of the underlying principles of managing this type of wound will do much to prevent the serious complications that so frequently occur. Early detection and appropriate referral to those members of the team with specialist skills will ultimately lessen the risk of amputation and increase the likelihood of successful rehabilitation.

Your role in caring for patients with complex wounds

Nurses are in a unique position within the multidisciplinary team to make an important contribution to the patient's progress and as such are usually primarily responsible for assessing wounds. Accurate, objective and holistic assessment can make early detection of wound complications possible. Whilst effective clinical decision making based upon research-based practice increases the likelihood of solving the patient's wound-related problems, health professionals are not yet in a position to heal all wounds. They can, however, make a significant contribution to the alleviation of patient distress and discomfort caused by complex wounds.

Activity   **20 MINUTES**

You may find it useful to note down any details of local members of the multidisciplinary team who may be of use to you when caring for patients with complex wounds. Extra space has been provided so that you can update your records or add additional information as required.

Resources available locally to me for the support of patients with tissue viability problems include:

Title	Name	Telephone number	Address/other details
Tissue viability nurse specialist			
Diabetic nurse specialist			
Dermatologist			
Chiropodist/podiatrist			
Stoma nurse specialist			
Orthotist			
Vascular surgeon			
Social worker			
Palliative care team			

SUMMARY

This section has focused on specific types of complex wounds and has emphasised the need for:

• comprehensive patient assessment taking into consideration the psychosocial, environmental and educational needs of patients with complicated wounds

• detailed planning of care, involving the identification of both general and specific treatment objectives

• involvement of collaborative practice involving a multidisciplinary team approach

• regular objective evaluation and reassessment of the patient's problems which actively involves both patient and carers

• problem solving using a flexible and creative approach.

USEFUL ADDRESSES

The Wound Care Society
PO Box 170
Huntingdon PE18 7PL

Tissue Viability Society
Wessex Rehabilitation Association
Salisbury District Hospital
Wiltshire SP2 8BJ

REFERENCES

Barnhorst D A, Braner H B 1968 Prevalence of congenitally absent pedal pulses. New England Journal of Medicine 278: 264–265
Bryant R 1992 Acute and chronic wounds, nursing management. Mosby Year Book, St Louis
Callum M 1992 Prevalence of chronic leg ulceration and severe chronic venous disease in western countries. Phlebology 7(suppl): 6–12
Carville K 1995 Wound care manual. Silver Chain Foundation, Western Australia

Doughty D, Broadwell Jackson D 1993 Gastrointestinal disorders. Mosby, St Louis

Fitzgerald V, Sims R 1987 A positive approach. Community Outlook (Nov): 18–21

Foltz A 1980 Fungating and ulcerating malignant lesions: a review of the literature. Journal of Advanced Nursing 7(2): 8–13

Foster A, Greenhill M, Edmonds M 1994 Five case studies illustrating the use of hydrocellular cavity dressings in the management of large post-surgical wounds in infected diabetic feet. Proceedings: 4th European Conference on Advances in Wound Management. Macmillan, London

Levin M E 1988 The diabetic foot: pathophysiology, evaluation, and treatment. In: Levin M, O'Neal L W, Bowker J H (eds) The diabetic foot, 4th edn. C V Mosby, St Louis, pp 1–50

Levin M, O'Neal L W, Bowker J H 1993 The diabetic foot. Mosby Year Book, London

Masson E A, Angle S, Roseman P 1989 Diabetic ulcers—do patients know how to protect themselves? Practical Diabetes 6(1): 22–23

Moffatt C 1995 Ankle pulses are not sufficient to detect impaired arterial circulation in patients with leg ulcers. Journal of Wound Care 4(3): 134–138

Morison M, Moffatt C 1994 A colour guide to the assessment and management of leg ulcers, 2nd edn. Mosby, Spain

Rombeau J, Rolandelli R 1987 Enteral and parenteral nutrition in patients with enteric fistula and short bowel syndrome. Surgical Clinics of North America 67(3): 551–568

Simon D A, Frank L, Williams I M 1994 Progression of arterial disease in patients with healed venous ulcers. Journal of Wound Care 3(4): 179–180

Thomas S 1990 Wound management and dressings. The Pharmaceutical Press, London

Thomas S, Hay N P 1991 The antimicrobial properties of two metronidazole medicated dressings used to treat malodorous wounds. Pharmaceutical Journal 3(2): 264-266

Van Toller 1994 Invisible wounds: the effects of skin ulcer malodour. Journal of Wound Care 3(2): 103–105

Westaby S (ed) 1985 Wound care. Heinemann Medical Books, London

World Health Organization (Europe) 1990 Diabetes care and research in Europe: the St Vincent Declaration. Diabetic Medicine 7: 360

Young M J, Boulton A J M 1991 Guidelines for identifying the at-risk foot. Practical Diabetes 8(3): 103–105

FURTHER READING

Boulton A M J, Conner H, Cavanagh P R 1993 The foot in diabetes. John Wiley, Chichester

Morison M, Moffatt C 1994 A colour guide to the assessment and management of leg ulcers, 2nd edn. Mosby, Spain

The impact of wounds on the quality of life

Introduction

Current philosophies of nursing reflect a holistic approach to care which is becoming more evident in the management of patients with wounds, as nurses and nursing assume greater responsibility in this emerging speciality. Provision of health services has traditionally concentrated on meeting the physical needs of wounded patients, whilst the influence of an individual's psychosocial and spiritual needs has been either underestimated or neglected. Holistic wound management must give equal importance to all dimensions of health if it is to facilitate a smooth transition to either complete healing or acceptance of palliative care.

LEARNING OUTCOMES

When you have completed this section you should be able to:

- discuss the impact that wounds may have on the lifestyle of individuals and their families
- explore the psychological and social needs of patients with wounds and their families
- explore significant factors that may have an effect on patient motivation and compliance
- discuss current philosophies of effective health education approaches.

6.1 LIVING WITH WOUNDS: THE PATIENT'S PERSPECTIVE

Introduction

There is a growing body of research interest in the relationship between psychological factors and the healing of wounds; indeed many studies have been able to demonstrate an important correlation between rates of wound healing and psychological factors, although the exact mechanism of these influences is not fully understood (Ryan 1989, Hyland et al 1994).

Quality of life

The majority of wounds will heal without complication and with a good cosmetic result; advances in surgical techniques and the development of wound dressings have greatly contributed to this effect. Members of the general public and many health professionals therefore often assume that wound healing is non-problematic and simple to achieve and may fail to consider the wider implications that non-healing wounds have for the individuals concerned and their families. It is, however, generally recognised that certain types of wounds, such as malignant wounds or wounds causing facial disfigurement, are more likely to cause psychological distress which may affect compliance with treatment and patient acceptance. What is often not acknowledged is the fact that any type of wound whether visible or concealed, acute or chronic, large or small may have profound psychological effects on the individual concerned.

Activity   5 MINUTES

Drawing on your own experience, list as many characteristics of wounds as you can identify which may cause psychological distress for patients and their families.

FEEDBACK

Characteristics that you are likely to have included in your answer are listed in Box 6.1.

Box 6.1 Factors commonly associated with wounds that cause psychological distress

- Visible wounds of the face, neck and hands
- Wounds affecting body image—surgery to the breast, reproductive organs
- Surgery affecting body function—formation of ostomies, amputation of limbs
- Wounds associated with life-threatening diseases—malignancies
- Malodorous wounds—faecal fistulae, fungating wounds
- Large wounds with extensive tissue loss—burns
- Wounds that interfere with quality of life—pain, high levels of exudate
- Accidental wounds caused by trauma

For particular types of wound there may be more than one of these factors exerting an effect on an individual at any one time, e.g. the presence of a malignant tumour of the head and neck is likely to cause distress due to the cumulative effects of the majority of influences listed in Box 6.1.

• •

'Quality of life' is a term that first emerged in the USA in the 1950s and has become increasingly referred to by health professionals in relation to the process of patient rehabilitation over the last decade. It remains a very difficult concept to define and although many health professionals feel that they have an intuitive understanding of the term there are those who believe that lip-service is paid to the concept of holistic care, with particular reference to quality of life measures (Price & Harding 1993). Psychologists argue that quality of life is a complex phenomenon and should be considered as being composed of separate core domains (Fallowfield 1990) as shown in Table 6.1.

Although definitions of quality of life vary, most authors agree that this concept must reflect a broad range of interrelated dimensions all of which have particular relevance to the support and management of patients with wounds.

Table 6.1 Defining quality of life (adapted from Fallowfield 1990 and Todd 1992)

Core domains	Typical items
Psychological	Adjustment to illness Emotional state—depression, anxiety Cognitive and intellectual ability Self-esteem and self-concept
Social	Engagement in social/leisure activities Personal and sexual relationships Social support networks Social roles associated with illness Social isolation
Occupational	Ability to perform paid employment Ability to carry out activities of living
Physical	Pain Mobility Sleep Appetite and nausea Sexual functioning

Increasingly, quality of life measures are being used to evaluate the efficacy of wound management interventions with the emphasis being placed on the patient's experience and perceptions of qualitative aspects such as psychological well-being. This type of assessment is becoming more common as a method of identifying patient-centred outcome measures of health care and as a method of establishing priorities by health care managers. There is a variety of existing scales that can be used to measure quality of life from a general perspective (Bowling 1991) but growing interest in this area has resulted in the development of specific quality of life measures for patients suffering from leg ulcers (Hyland et al 1994) and surgical cavity wounds (Price et al 1994). Such tools could easily be adapted for use with other patients suffering from different types of chronic wounds and help to identify from the patient's perspective the consequences of having a wound that is slow to heal. Patients included in the quality of life study by Price et al (1994) all had either pilonidal sinuses or abdominal cavity wounds which were granulating and without clinical complications and would usually be classified by health professionals as being 'routine'. In contrast, patients reported that their mobility had been severely restricted by the presence of their surgical wounds and that most had been confined to their homes during the period that it took for the wound to heal, which on average was 2–3 months. As a direct consequence of this, the majority of patients stated that their social activities had been significantly limited, which also affected other members of the household. This study demonstrates that the presence of surgical wounds has a substantial impact on the lives of patients, including disturbed sleep patterns, decreased appetite, increased discomfort and feelings of unhappiness. The significance of the effects of less complex wounds on a patient's quality of life are often not recognised by health professionals, which has direct implications for both health education on discharge and the provision of support by the community nursing services.

The experience of pain

The level of pain or discomfort experienced by patients with wounds is directly correlated with the amount of sleep loss and restriction in activities that they report (Hyland et al 1994). Pain appears to be a major determinant of patients' experiences associated with their wounds and has a tendency to negatively affect all other quality of life indicators such as feelings of well-being, depression and loss of

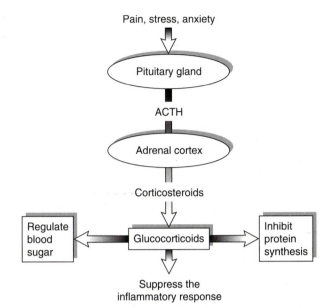

Pain, stress, anxiety

Pituitary gland

ACTH

Adrenal cortex

Corticosteroids

Regulate blood sugar ← Glucocorticoids → Inhibit protein synthesis

Suppress the inflammatory response

Fig. 6.1 Psychological and physiological responses to pain, stress and anxiety.

confidence. Wound pain is often underestimated by health professionals and can lead to muscle tension, fatigue and anxiety which if inadequately managed can delay healing by depressing the action of the immune system. Pain and psychological stress are inextricably linked and have many physical consequences including the stimulation of the pituitary gland which secretes adrenocorticotrophic hormone (ACTH) which in turn stimulates cortisol release from the adrenal cortex (see Fig. 6.1). These corticosteroids regulate the production of glucocorticoids which cause the breakdown of the body's store of glucose, raising blood sugar levels. Glucocorticoids suppress the immune system by reducing the mobility of macrophages which in turn reduces the normal inflammatory response. In addition, glucocorticoids also increase the rate of protein breakdown which directly inhibits collagen synthesis. Patients who are anxious and in pain have an increased risk of wound infection, so it is of paramount importance that pain and anxiety levels are adequately assessed and that appropriate interventions are administered and evaluated. Pain assessment tools have been demonstrated to be effective in clinical practice (Ballie 1993), but unfortunately are not widely used, perhaps due to lack of knowledge, or an underestimation of the severity of pain that the patient is experiencing.

Make a list of causes of wound pain that a patient may experience. Try to think of at least five.

FEEDBACK

Your answer should have included some of the common causes of painful wounds:

- wound site—thoracic wounds, fingertip injuries
- depth of wound—shallow wounds with exposed nerve endings are more painful than deeper wounds where nerve endings have been destroyed
- localised pressure—due to fluid or haematoma accumulation
- localised tension—due to tight suture materials
- presence of foreign bodies—grit, drains, etc.
- wound infection
- ischaemia
- excessive handling of tissues during surgery
- hypertrophic scar tissue/contractures
- skin sensitivities/allergies
- patient anxiety
- inappropriate wound management.

Innovations in reducing wound pain include the administration of analgesia prior to surgery, the infiltration of local anaesthetic into the affected area (Wall 1988) and the use of patient-controlled analgesia (Thomas 1993).

Improvement in pain assessment techniques and recognition of the severe and debilitating effects that painful wounds have, not only on patients but on their families, will do much to relieve distress. As practitioners, we must remember that providing appropriate wound management is just one of our responsibilities and must be combined with the appropriate psychological support of the patient and family unit if we are to fulfil our aim of providing holistic care.

Define the four core domains that psychologists believe are representative of the concept of 'quality of life'.

FEEDBACK

Your answer should have covered the following points.

- Although various models attempting to encapsulate the meaning of quality of life exist, all agree that this concept must represent a broad range of interrelated health behaviours. The dimensions most frequently cited are: psychological, social, occupational, physical.

. . . .

6.2 PSYCHOLOGICAL ASPECTS OF WOUNDING

Introduction

People who are disfigured through the effects of surgery, disease or trauma and their families have to learn to cope with the long-term effects of mutilation, the results of which may be visible or concealed. The process of healing has previously been discussed in detail from a physiological perspective, but it also involves complex psychological and social consequences that have a substantial impact on the wounded person's quality of life. Changes in body image produced by wounds and the stress associated with the effects of trauma often have a profound and disturbing psychological effect which often passes unrecognised by health professionals who may be ill-equipped and unprepared to deal with this situation.

Body image

Some wounds will severely alter a person's body image. Coming to terms with disfigurement and alterations in appearance can take many months and often years to achieve and unfortunately for some individuals is never successfully accomplished. This process is largely dependent on the reactions of those who surround the injured person; the attitude of others towards him or her will greatly influence that person's acceptance and self-esteem (Partridge 1993). The relationships that are developed early in the recovery process between patient and carers are of paramount importance and the comforting of patient, family and friends calls for highly developed interpersonal skills. Many health professionals feel totally inadequate when faced with the role of counsellor and comforter of those affected by injury. Disfigured patients are extremely sensitive to non-verbal cues and are often able to sense if health professionals are uncomfortable in their presence, all of which serves to heighten feelings of fear, frustration and isolation (Topping 1992).

The experiences of those who have suffered from traumatic injuries, surgery and wounds are all individual but always represent a major life crisis. However, there are reported broad similarities in the psychological reactions that those affected experience. Based upon his own personal experience and from supporting many disfigured people, Partridge (1993) describes the transitional process following injury as a series of stages (Fig. 6.2) and describes the movement from one stage to another as slow and erratic. The following factors are felt to influence an individual's capacity for adaptation:

- personality
- intelligence
- age
- social support system
- socioeconomic status
- level of self-esteem prior to injury.

Recovery following disfigurement is difficult owing to a number of factors. A person's self-image is the picture that the person has of him/herself in his/her own mind and has become particularly important in today's society, where a great deal of emphasis is placed on attractiveness. This message is constantly reinforced by cultural and media images which have a tendency to link disfigurement and scars with negative traits.

Activity   5 MINUTES

Take some time to consider how the media and fairy stories tend to portray images of the proverbial 'baddy'. List any common visual characteristics that you can and then try to identify the feelings that these images may be associated with.

. . . .

FEEDBACK

You may have listed some of the following characteristics:

- scars
- hunchbacks
- walking with a limp
- close-set eyes
- warts
- thin lips
- thick-set necks
- patches over eyes
- hooked noses
- ugliness

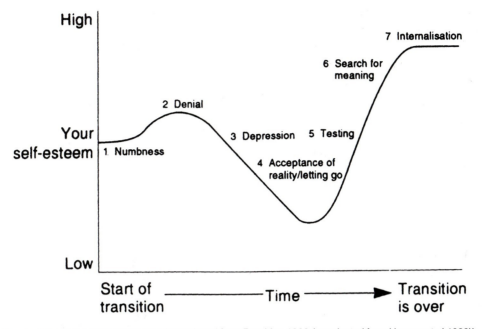

Fig. 6.2 Changes in self-esteem during transition (reproduced from Partridge 1993 (as adapted from Hopson et al 1988)).

- missing limbs, hands or digits
- having a prosthesis—hooks, false limbs.

These images traditionally tend to evoke negative feelings from a very early age and reinforce the powerful message that disfigurement is not comfortably accepted in our society.

Those suffering from facial disfigurement are particularly hard hit as the face is extremely important in defining public identity and is involved in every social interaction, however small. The ultimate effect of these experiences can be self-consciousness, lack of confidence and self-imposed social isolation. Partridge (1996) defines the 'scared syndrome' (Table 6.2) as a useful way of summarising the reactions of both disfigured people and those that they encounter and emphasises the damage that these negative reactions will have if allowed to persist.

Positive approaches to care

During hospitalisation, injured people require the unconditional support of those around them and the

Table 6.2 The SCARED syndrome (reproduced from Partridge 1990 by kind permission)

You			They	
Feel	Behave		Behave	Feel
Self-conscious		S		Sympathy
	Submissive		Staring	
Conspicuous		C		Caution
	Clumsy		Curiosity	
Angry		A		Anguished
	Apathy		Awkwardness	
Resentful		R		Reluctant
	Regressive		Rudeness	
Empty		E		Embarrassed
	Excluded		Evasiveness	
Different		D		Dread
	Defenceless		Distance	

use of highly developed interpersonal skills. Empathy should seek to console without pretending that no difficulties exist and both the families and the injured person should be given as much information as they appear to want and need, remembering that emotions may well be volatile and that psychological defence mechanisms such as denial will often be present. Feelings of hostility, anger and guilt are commonly expressed and may well be directed at staff who often experience feelings of inadequacy and self-doubt. Support groups for patients and staff alike may be useful in some instances.

Honest and realistic advice needs to be given to patients and their families in order that informed decisions can be made concerning future treatments, although expectations about surgery and medical treatments tends to remain high. Figure 6.3 illustrates the extended support network that is available for injured people and their families.

When planning the care of patients with complex wounds, consideration must be given to the psychological, spiritual and social needs of the patients, their families and friends. The effect of altered body image is an individual and extremely complex phenomenon that can take many years to resolve. The skill of nursing is based upon the concept of nurturing and comforting (Table 6.3). The development of a sensitive nurse–patient/family relationship combined with practical nursing care will do much to facilitate the healing of body and mind.

Activity   5 MINUTES

Referring to Partridge's description of the scared syndrome, list and compare the feelings experienced by disfigured people and those around them.

● ●

FEEDBACK

The work of Partridge describes what he believes to be the typical type and sequence of reactions experienced by facially disfigured people and the people around them.

Disfigured person's feelings:

- Self-conscious
- Conspicuous
- Angry
- Resentful
- Empty
- Different.

Other people's reactions:

- Staring
- Curiosity

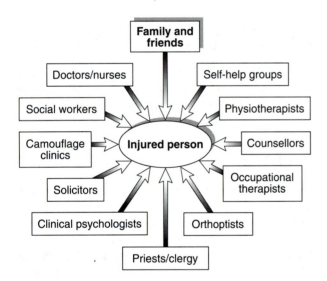

Fig. 6.3 Extended support network.

Table 6.3 The healing partnership (adapted from Carville 1995)		
	Nurse interventions	*Patient/family responses*
Psychological nurturing	Provides advice and information Counselling skills Suggests alternative therapeutic approaches to healing	Feels supported and involved Verbalises fears and needs Visualises positive outcomes
Spiritual nurturing	Fosters the development of: faith, hope, love, prayer and peace	If desired is able to respond to faith, hope, love, prayer and peace
Social nurturing	Fosters the development of: • relationships • caring • trust • confidence • carer/family support	Has positive interaction with: • family • friends • carers

- Awkwardness
- Rudeness
- Evasiveness
- Distance.

Partridge describes this combination of feelings as two sets of negatives which repel each other, creating a chasm which increases social isolation and frustration.

6.3 PATIENT COMPLIANCE AND MOTIVATION

Introduction

Patient motivation to comply with wound management treatments and therapies is of paramount importance if the eventual goal of healing is to be achieved. There has been in recent years a growing interest in the exploration of those factors affecting compliance in longer-term wound treatments such as the management of patients with chronic leg ulcers (Moffatt & Franks 1995). The phenomenon of patient non-compliance is poorly understood, yet has significant implications for both the patient and those responsible for providing health services.

Factors influencing compliance

Although patient compliance is recognised as a factor contributing to the recurrence or non-healing of chronic wounds such as leg ulcers (Muir Gray 1983), it is also an important influence in the management of acute wounds such as traumatic or surgical wounds. Early patient discharge and the increased provision of day-surgery units, means that many patients with acute wounds are discharged home within hours of surgery with the expectation that they will be either self-caring or receive limited support from community nursing services. These factors potentiate the tendency for non-compliance with treatment, especially as the general public often do not understand the principles of caring for wounds and the opportunity to fully explain treatment rationales may not always be available.

The stereotypical image of the non-compliant patient is of an elderly person with a long-standing leg ulcer who is socially isolated and is resistant to healing. This assumption is not substantiated by research and appears to be based upon anecdotal evidence (Moffatt 1995). Indeed, studies examining issues relating to the quality of life of this group of patients suggests the opposite to be true (see Sect. 6.1). Work in this area is beginning to document the profound debilitating effects that leg ulcers have from the patients' perspective. Recurrence rates of venous leg ulceration are well documented although estimates vary considerably (Moffatt 1995) (see Table 6.4).

Rates are difficult to compare, as ulcer recurrence can be measured at different time intervals and various methods of applying graduated compression are invariably used but not always documented. Details concerning compliance in other areas of wound management are not readily available and require further research if the factors influencing patient compliance are to be fully understood.

Table 6.4 Comparison of ulcer recurrence rates for patients with chronic venous leg ulcers

Author	Year	Ulcer recurrence at 1 year
Monk & Sarkany	1983	69%
Cornwall	1990	53%
Wright et al	1991	22%

Activity   **20 MINUTES**

Using your own experience, list as many as possible of the variables that may affect a patient's ability to comply with wound management interventions.

FEEDBACK

Depending on the type of patients that you regularly care for, you will have identified various variables that influence a patient's ability or desire to comply with treatment. It is important to recognise that in many instances, adherence to wound management regimes is extremely difficult owing to a combination of unrealistic professional advice and limitations in the patient's home environment.

For the sake of clarity, factors relating to patient compliance have been summarised into three broad categories, which are not intended to be mutually exclusive.

1. *Patient factors:*
   - Lack of knowledge
   - Lack of motivation
   - Lack of self-esteem
   - Beliefs/attitudes—concerning illness and effectiveness of treatment.

2. *Treatment factors:*
   - The impact of treatment upon patient lifestyle
   - Length of proposed treatment
   - Complexity of treatment
   - Ability to comply with treatment
   - Comfort associated with treatment regime.

3. *Lifestyle factors:*
   - Environmental limitations—inadequate housing
   - Resource limitations—financial, transport facilities
   - Occupational limitations—need to work/resume household duties.

· ·

There are ethical implications that require exploration when considering the dynamics of patient compliance (Burkhardt 1986). Compliance implies the use of a coercive, authoritarian approach in which the patient is expected to follow the suggested treatment regime. Current philosophies of nursing support the notion of equal partnership between patient and carer in the negotiation process, but in practice, an attempt is often made by health professionals to influence and change the patient's behaviour.

Factitious wounds

An extreme form of non-compliance is the management of a patient with a factitious wound. As health professionals we tend to make the assumption that all patients wish their wounds to heal; unfortunately, this is not always the case. Occasionally, some patients either inflict their own wounds or contribute to non-healing. Wounds produced in this way are defined as 'factitious' (Lyell 1972). The underlying problems are extremely complex and are psychological in nature rather than physical. Treatment strategies therefore need to be aimed at resolving the psychological difficulties that the patient is experiencing, and the patient may benefit from referral to the psychiatric team. This type of extreme non-compliance is not common, but may affect people of all ages with a variety of different wound types, which can make classification of this type of wound extremely difficult. Typically, patients presenting with factitious wounds are young women who are psychologically immature and who use the wound as a method of avoiding social contacts and relationships; a characteristic of these patients is that they have been unsuccessfully managed by a number of different treatment centres. It is interesting that this type of behaviour is sometimes exhibited by older patients with chronic wounds, who may be interfering with their ulcers in order to prolong social contact with community nursing services. Early identification of patients with factitious wounds is important if resources are not to be wasted and the patient is to receive specialist support (Baragwanath et al 1994). However, it has been estimated that over 30% of this type of wound will remain unhealed even at long-term follow-up (Sneddon & Sneddon 1975).

Activity   5 MINUTES

Briefly describe the principles of care that could prove helpful when supporting a patient with a suspected factitious wound.

· ·

FEEDBACK

Management of this type of situation can be difficult and frustrating for all those involved and requires a great deal of sensitivity. The circumstances of individual patients are obviously very different, but generally accepted principles include the following.

1. Comprehensive wound assessment together with a detailed medical and social history is fundamentally important to establish this difficult diagnosis.
2. It may be helpful to admit the patient to hospital for a short period of close observation. At the same time, investigations can be completed to exclude the presence of any other underlying pathology.
3. Referral to the psychiatric team so that follow-up and support can be initiated and opportunity is given to explore the psychological nature of the problem without confrontation. Psychotherapy can be of help for some patients.
4. Primary wound dressings need to be carefully selected in order that they promote the principle of moist wound healing, are comfortable and do not cause additional trauma on removal. However, consideration must be given to the long-term economic implications of supplying 'high'-cost dressing materials at a time when the patient's goal is to prolong healing.

· ·

Studies have shown that even with nursing support, supervision and availability of appropriate treatments, significant numbers of patients do not comply with the management of chronic wounds (Ruckley 1992). This has many implications for the delivery of tissue viability services, especially as changes in the provision of health services mean that increasing numbers of patients with chronic wounds will be cared for within their own homes. In some instances, assistance offered by health professionals may not be welcome in an individual's own home, for a variety of reasons including a lack of understanding of the benefits of treatment or an unwillingness to receive help from others.

6.4 HEALTH EDUCATION

Introduction

People require knowledge and information before they can make the decision to comply with treatment. As previously discussed, it is important for patients to have an understanding about the aetiology of their wounds, factors that influence healing and the rationale for treatment. This is of particular significance if there is a variety of alternative treatment choices available or treatment is likely to be time consuming or uncomfortable.

Strategies for effective health promotion

From the 1970s onwards there has been a shifting emphasis from medical domination to lay participation in care which has been reflected in health education trends; most would agree that the nurse's health education role is an integral part of nurse–patient interaction. Yet the majority of nurses persist with the simplistic behavioural change approach to health education, which assumes that if individuals are given information they will subsequently follow the advice of health professionals (Mackintosh 1995).

Evidence continues to suggest that when patients have received detailed information and the opportunity to ask questions about chronic wounds, then they are more likely to comply with treatment regimes (Cameron & Gregor 1987). In this study, patients who understood the basics of the pathophysiology of leg ulcer formation demonstrated greater commitment to the use of compression bandaging and calf-muscle pump exercises. However, it must be remembered that not all patients will welcome this type of information or interpret that it is their responsibility to act upon it.

Highly developed interpersonal and teaching skills are integral to the implementation of effective patient education. The skilled nurse needs to be able to identify gaps in the patients' knowledge, sense how much information they want, judge whether timing is right and focus language and information to the appropriate level. Effective patient education is extremely difficult to evaluate, but owing to the economic implications of non-healing wounds, has become an increasingly important strategy used to facilitate patient compliance.

Activity   5 MINUTES

Look at Reader Article 8 (p. 186) and evaluate the effectiveness of this patient education guide for people living with leg ulcers. Briefly summarise why this teaching aid is likely to enhance the health promotion messages that the author is trying to convey.

FEEDBACK

This patient information sheet effectively puts into practice the principles of health education which include the following.

- The topic has direct relevance to the patient.
- Written information is reinforced by large, clear diagrams.
- Written information has been kept to a minimum and is jargon free.
- Common patient difficulties have been anticipated and presented in the form of simple questions and answers.
- The most important messages are reinforced in large, bold print.

Therapeutic communication

Two major types of behaviour have been identified in relation to nurse–patient interaction. Nurses are described as adopting either a position-centred or person-centred approach to care (Kasch & Knutson 1985). The position-centred approach traditionally assumes that the role of the health professional confers authority to give advice and issue instructions without considering the beliefs or expectations of the patient. Alternatively, the person-centred approach is based upon joint commitment and takes into consideration the patients' and families' beliefs, needs and attitudes. The development of a collaborative relationship between nurse and patient appears to be a major factor influencing compliance. To effectively facilitate any lasting changes in behaviour, both nurse and patient need to be actively involved in any decision-making process. It is well recognised that a team approach that fosters a therapeutic relationship, where the nurse provides knowledge, expertise and support and the patients share their thoughts, feelings and beliefs, is much more likely to succeed (Di Matteo & Di Nicola 1982).

The recent shift to counselling techniques in health education is an attempt to address the balance of professional power and control over the patient and also emphasises that patient education should focus on the social context of health rather than solely on the individual as a determinant of behaviour (Caraher 1995). Therapeutic communication in nursing is not new and has been described as a three-phase cycle of facilitation, transition and action (Gazda et al 1975). The essential features of the facilitation phase are listening and talking in a manner which is empathetic, non-directive and non-judgemental, where it is important to allow patients to express their thoughts, feelings and attitudes. It is during the transition phase that the patient's problems are defined and explored. The action phase is where the problem solving begins; the focus is on patient participation whilst the nurse provides support and helps to plan mutually acceptable strategies. Two current approaches to health education that have relevance to wound management are illustrated in Table 6.5. Both focus on self-empowerment which encourages individuals or groups to take responsibility and have greater control over the health choices that they make. Both of these contemporary approaches to health promotion aim to increase the individual's self-esteem and develop social skills. The goal of the humanistic approach for health education is to facilitate health-related decision making by modifying the individual's self-concept and enhancing self-esteem, so that people are in a better position to identify their own health needs and take action to meet them. On the other hand, the aim of the community development approach to health education focuses on groups so that they identify common interests, are motivated by each other and work together for the benefit of each other.

Activity 2 MINUTES

Complete Table 6.5 by giving an example of both the humanistic and the community development approaches to health education.

FEEDBACK

There are many examples of types of patients with wounds or compromised tissue viability that could benefit from these approaches to health education.

- *Humanistic approach*—e.g. paraplegic patients who need to prevent pressure sore formation and protect their skin from the effects of trauma, or the development of self-care skills for a patient with a newly formed colostomy.
- *Community development approach* —e.g. establishment of a local self-help group such as the National Eczema Society, or the establishment of a healed ulcer clinic to provide support and follow-up services for those patients whose leg ulcer treatment has been successful.

In the past, health promotion and health education activities have concentrated on the individual, in an attempt to influence and change behaviour, but this has resulted in some instances in the phenomenon of victim blaming (Crawford 1980). Where non-compliance is seen as the sole responsibility of the individual concerned and the wider implications of the social and political influences on health are ignored, patients with non-healing wounds are often categorised as non-compliant. Further work is required to explore the effects on chronic wound healing of limited health resources and inadequacy of patients' living conditions.

Table 6.5 Strategies for health education (adapted from Mackintosh 1995)		
	Self-empowerment humanistic approach	*Community development approach*
Focus	The individual	A group
Goal	To facilitate decision-making, improve self-confidence enhance motivation	To work together in a supportive environment, learn from each other and enhance motivation
Rationale	Enhanced self-esteem encourages identification of individual health needs and action to meet them	Realistic advice can be shared, individuals can appreciate that others experience similar problems. Helps to avoid social isolation
Example		

SUMMARY

This section has begun to explore the psychological and socioeconomic needs of patients, families and carers. In it you have learnt that:

- An important correlation exists between wound healing and psychological needs, although the exact relationship between the two is not fully understood.

- Quality of life is a complex phenomenon that is difficult to define but is increasingly being used as a method of evaluating patient-centred outcome measures of health.

- Wound pain is often underestimated by health professionals and if left unresolved will increase psychological stress and anxiety, which are known to delay healing.

- Psychological reactions to injury or disfigurement follow characteristic patterns, identification of which can greatly influence the patient's capacity for eventual acceptance.

- Patient compliance is dependent on a multitude of factors which do not only relate to the individual and his or her lifestyle.

- The traditional focus of health education has altered from one of behavioural change to a move towards a self-empowerment, humanistic approach.

- Nurses have an important role as providers of information rather than as indoctrinators.

REFERENCES

Ballie L 1993 A review of pain assessment tools. Nursing Standard 7: 23, 25–29

Baragwanath P, Shutler S, Harding K G 1994 The management of a patient with a factitious wound. Journal of Wound Care 3(6): 286–287

Bowling A 1991 Measuring health: a review of quality of life measurement scales. Oxford University Press, Oxford

Burkhardt C 1986 Ethical issues in compliance. Topics in Clinical Nursing 7: 4, 9–16

Cameron K, Gregor F 1987 Chronic illness and compliance. Journal of Advanced Nursing 12: 671–676

Caraher 1995 Nursing and health education: victim blaming. British Journal of Nursing 4(20): 1190–1213

Carville K 1995 Wound care manual. Silver Chain Foundation, Western Australia

Cornwall J 1990 Update on leg ulcer survey. Journal of District Nursing 8(11): 9–10

Crawford R 1980 Healthism and the medicalisation of everyday life. International Journal of Health Services 10(3): 365–367

Di Matteo M R, Di Nicola D D 1982 Achieving patient compliance. Pergamon Press, New York

Fallowfield L 1990 The quality of life: the missing dimension in health care. Souvenir, London

Gazda G M, Walters R P, Childers W C 1975 Human relations development: a manual for health sciences. Allyn & Bacon, London

Hopson B, Scully M, Stafford K 1988 Transitions. Mercury, London

Hyland M E, Ley A, Thomson B 1994 Quality of life of leg ulcer patients: questionnaire and preliminary findings. Journal of Wound Care 3(6): 294–298

Kasch C, Knutson K 1985 Patient compliance and interpersonal style: implications for practice and research. Nurse Practitioner 10(3): 52–64

Lyell A 1972 Dermatitis artifacta and self-inflicted disease. Scottish Medical Journal 17: 187–196

Mackintosh N 1995 Self-empowerment in health promotion: a realistic target? British Journal of Nursing 4(21): 1273–1278

Moffatt C J 1995 Recurrence of leg ulcers within a community ulcer service. Journal of Wound Care 4(2): 57–61

Moffatt C J, Franks P 1995 The problem of recurrence in patients with leg ulceration. Journal of Tissue Viability 5(2): 64–66

Monk B E, Sarkany I 1983 Outcome of treatment of venous stasis ulcers. Clinical Dermatology 7(4): 397–400

Muir Gray J A 1983 Social aspects of peripheral vascular disease in the elderly. Churchill Livingstone, London, pp 191–199

Partridge J 1990 Changing faces: the challenge of facial disfigurement. Penguin, Harmondsworth (Reprinted 1990 by Changing Faces, London)

Partridge J 1993 The psychological effects of facial disfigurement. Journal of Wound Care 2(3): 168–171

Partridge J 1996 Facial disfigurement: the full picture. Changing Faces, London

Price P, Harding K G 1993 Defining quality of life. Journal of Wound Care 2(5): 304–306

Price P, Butterworth R J, Bale S 1994 Measuring quality of life in patients with granulating wounds. Journal of Wound Care 3(1): 49–50

Ruckley C 1992 Treatment of venous ulceration. Phlebology 7(suppl 1): 22–26

Ryan T J 1989 Pressure sores: prevention, management and future research—a medical perspective. Palliative Medicine 3: 249–255

Sneddon I, Sneddon J 975 Self-inflicted injury: a follow up study of 43 patients. British Medical Journal 3: 527–530

Thomas N 1993 Patient and staff perceptions of PCA. Nursing Standard 7(28): 37–39

Todd C 1992 Quality of life and diabetes audit. Health Psychology Update 11: 9–14

Topping A 1992 The trauma of burns. Wound Management 2(3): 8–9

Wall P D 1988 The prevention of postoperative pain. Pain 33: 289–290

Wright D D I, Franks P J, Blair S D 1991 Oxerutins in the prevention of reoccurence in chronic venous ulceration: randomised controlled trial. British Journal of Surgery 78: 1269–1270

FURTHER READING

Partridge J 1994 Changing faces: the challenge of facial disfigurement, 2nd edn. Available from Changing Faces, a registered charity, 1–2 Junction Mews, London, W2 1PN

7 Provision of a comprehensive wound management service

Introduction

This final section aims to briefly explore the combination of influences that are responsible for shaping the future development of services for patients with compromised tissue viability as research findings begin to challenge traditional approaches to the delivery of wound care services.

LEARNING OUTCOMES

At the end of this section, you should be able to:

- explore issues relating to professional and legal accountability in relation to the development of wound management services
- analyse the contribution of the clinical nurse specialist to the provision of wound management services
- identify likely trends in the development of services for patients with poor tissue viability.

7.1 LEGAL AND PROFESSIONAL ISSUES

Introduction

Nursing's quest for professional status has inevitably led to the establishment of clearer lines of responsibility and accountability. Increased accountability has meant that nurses have had to examine their own practice, develop a discrete body of knowledge that is research based and justify their own actions. One of the major characteristics of professional status is the freedom that practitioners have to make judgements on an individual basis and act accordingly in the light of their professional knowledge. Accountability creates many professional dilemmas and raises many questions. This section aims to introduce the principles of accountability without discussing in detail any specific legislation or professional codes of practice which are necessarily dependent upon the country you are currently practising in.

The need for accountable practice

The principles of accountable practice are based upon the public's need for trust and confidence in the professional; nowhere is this more apparent than within the health services. Accountability can be defined as a combination of legal, moral and professional obligations which are based upon professional codes of conduct. These codes of conduct reflect society's expectations that each nurse will maintain professional standards and support the primacy of patient interest (Ralph 1990).

Self-assessment   5 MINUTES

Identify at least four groups to whom nurses are accountable.

• •

FEEDBACK

The main groups that nurses are accountable to include: the patient; family and friends; the general public; their employer; their professional body and themselves.

Many contemporary influences affect nursing accountability (see Fig. 7.1).

The application of accountability to clinical practice is becoming increasingly more complex as levels of nursing responsibility and scope of professional practice expand to represent the multitude of different clinical settings in which nurses work.

• •

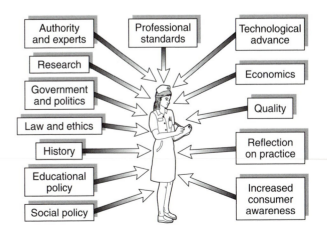

Fig. 7.1 Current influences on professional accountability.

Consider your own professional practice, identifying three ways in which you are able to demonstrate professional accountability. For example, you might be able to say that you always base your nursing practice on proven research, or you always maintain up-to-date and accurate information.

FEEDBACK

The examples that you may have listed will probably be specific to the practice area in which you work. However, your answer should relate to the following principles of accountable practice:

- maintaining and improving professional knowledge and competence
- basing practice on research
- defining acceptable standards of care
- accurate documentation
- practising patient advocacy by representing the patient's interests
- risk management—monitoring of complaints/adverse incident reports
- examination of high-risk areas of care
- evaluation of standards of practice.

The implementation of these principles enhances the ability of practitioners to justify clinical decision making in greater detail and therefore rationalise their current practice.

One means of protecting the general public from unsafe practice is the requirement for qualified nurses to be recorded on a central professional register. The nursing profession is also governed by codes of professional conduct which will vary slightly from country to country but are based upon a common set of principles. Such professional codes of conduct represent a statement of the profession's values and act as a sound philosophical framework upon which professional practice can be based. Professional codes of conduct help to define standards of practice and are intended to protect both the general public and the professional nurse against unsafe or outdated practice. Themes commonly represented by nursing's professional codes of conduct include:

- an emphasis on nursing as a collaborative profession
- the importance of continued professional education
- the maintenance of standards of care so that patients receive skilled professional nursing.

Litigation and the concept of negligence

Codes of professional conduct are also a means of determining the standards against which allegations of professional misconduct are judged. Litigation claims are unfortunately becoming increasingly more common within nursing practice, with the total number of malpractice cases rising on an annual basis in some countries (Tingle 1991). In the UK, it is alleged that litigation claims are threatening some health authorities with near bankruptcy (Sims 1991). Since 1991 in the UK, the costs of clinical negligence claims have been borne by health trusts and directly managed units, increasing the similarities between the UK and the provision of health services in other countries. The impact of these changes has many implications for the speciality of tissue viability, where significant claims have successfully been made for patients suffering from pressure sores and the frequency of such claims is increasing all the time as the general public become more litigious.

In order to successfully establish negligence, the patient (the plaintiff) or the patient's representative must be able to demonstrate that the investigation, diagnosis and/or treatment fell below the standard of reasonably competent practitioners (Dimond 1990). This does not refer to the highest professional standard that a nurse might attain, but the standard of care which could be reasonably expected of an average practitioner.

In cases of negligence it is the responsibility of the plaintiff to demonstrate on the 'balance of probabilities' (more likely than not) that the practitioner and/or his or her employer was under a duty of care and that there was a breach of the appropriate standard of care and that the plaintiff suffered harm as a result of that breach (Dimond 1990).

Try to identify at least three circumstances specifically relevant to wound management where a patient could make a claim of negligence.

FEEDBACK

- The development of pressure sores in a patient who previously had intact skin.
- The application of compression bandaging to the limb of a patient with established peripheral vascular disease.
- The development of haemorrhage or nerve damage following a nurse's decision to surgically

debride a necrotic wound using a scalpel or other sharp instrument.

- The failure to nurse a patient on a suitable support surface following the identification of the patient as being at 'high risk' of developing pressure sores.

The common factor in all of these examples is the plaintiff's ability to demonstrate that harm or damage has occurred. Negligence can also be proven due to a failure to act such as in the final example, where the nurse has a responsibility to identify any situation which may prove harmful to the patient. Nurses are well placed within the multidisciplinary team to act as patient advocates, which is a fundamental component of exercising professional accountability. Advocacy has been defined as: 'doing what is morally and ethically right on behalf of the patient not the institution' (Wiseman 1990). Several facets of advocacy can be identified all of which have direct relevance to tissue viability. They include:

- monitoring informed consent
- providing patients with information on alternative therapies
- mediating on the patient's behalf
- acting as a coordinator of care.

There are no easy answers to some of the professional dilemmas that nurses face. However, it is fundamentally important that nurses continue to explore the issues related to accountability and responsibility. Today nurses are expected to be assertive and ask questions as part of the process of challenging the views of other members of the multidisciplinary team. However, nurses must resist the urge to practise defensively and need to respond to the professional challenges that increased accountability brings. Accountability must be seen as an integral part of every nurse's practice and not just associated with the justification of crisis situations.

7.2 DEVELOPMENT OF TISSUE VIABILITY NURSE SPECIALISTS

Introduction

It is well recognised that improvements in quality of care can be achieved by the development of nurse specialism (Storr 1988, Wright 1991). The introduction of clinical nurse specialists is a significant development in nursing and has become increasingly more common within the 'purchaser–provider' system of health care as quality of care and cost-effectiveness assume greater importance.

The role of the clinical nurse specialist

Numbers of tissue viability nurse specialists have dramatically risen in the last decade in the UK as both purchasers and providers of health care recognise that mismanagement of patients with wounds is both costly and unnecessary. An essential function of a clinical nurse specialist is to act as a positive role-model at a time when the professional role of the nurse is challenged by economic constraints and limited health care resources. A number of factors make it difficult for nurses to be aware of contemporary developments within each specialist area of clinical practice.

Activity   2 MINUTES

Identify two reasons why you are unable to keep up to date with all of the specialist areas of nursing which your role encompasses.

FEEDBACK

For most nurses the sheer time element involved in keeping abreast of new developments within nursing is a major difficulty. Other reasons include: rapid technological advances in each specialist field; the lack of consensus among specialists resulting in conflicting messages; and the increased responsibilities of qualified nurses, resulting in increased role diversification.

A tissue viability specialist nurse can assist all members of the multidisciplinary team to overcome these problems by providing expertise and acting as a resource to facilitate clinical decision making.

The primary focus of the clinical nurse specialist should be clinical: theoretical and clinical expertise should be used to promote professional nursing practice and quality care (Caruso & Payne 1990). The clinical nurse specialist role is complex and much debated (Hamric & Spross 1983, Storr 1988)—the most commonly cited sub-roles include those of:

- practitioner
- educator
- consultant
- researcher
- change agent
- staff and patient advocate.

A clinical nurse specialist does not practise nursing in the traditional manner; experience and education, together with the freedom from daily patient care, allow the specialist to make an objective assessment of wound management problems and offer innovative solutions (Fenton 1985). Education is an integral component of the clinical nurse specialist's role; examples include the identification of staff training needs, the formulation of wound management guidelines and protocols and the development of patient education materials.

The concept that nurses should consult other nurses outside their immediate area of work is relatively new (Barrown 1983). One benefit of the consultative process is that not only can clinical nurse specialists assist practitioners with the assessment of complex tissue viability problems, but they can also facilitate a holistic approach to the management of wounds. The clinical nurse specialist can significantly improve communication between all members of the multidisciplinary team, removing what can often be a significant obstacle to effective wound management. Another important role of the clinical nurse specialist which is of particular relevance to tissue viability has been identified by Fenton (1985) as that of making bureaucracy respond to patient needs. This is referred to as 'massaging the system' and links closely with the concept of patient advocacy.

Tissue viability nurse specialists are in an ideal position to generate research which will range from communication of research findings and facilitation of research awareness to implementation and involvement in research activities. Inherent within the role of nurse specialist is the expectation that he or she will act as a change agent. A key issue here is that the specialist nurse must have the support of both peers and managers in order to effectively influence practice; the development of good professional relationships is fundamental when trying to implement change. Indeed many health service managers introduce the role of tissue viability nurse with the specific objective that they will advise budget holders of the most cost-effective preventive care and treatment options available.

There are many problems inherent within the role of the clinical nurse specialist, including:

- role ambiguity
- unrealistic expectations
- professional isolation
- lack of managerial support
- limited career development.

The role of the tissue viability specialist nurse appears to have additional difficulties in that one of its focal points is promoting cost-effective practice. This is a particularly stressful activity as the majority of tissue viability nurse specialists in the UK do not control their own budget (James 1994) and spend a great deal of their time attempting to influence budget holders to release funds that are increasingly in short supply. Many specialist nurses experience considerable pressure when faced with this responsibility, especially when recommending that significant sums of money are spent on preventive care and treatments, the effectiveness of which are not always quantifiable (Hill 1995). This will remain a difficult task until there are methodologically sound clinical trials to support the various claims of product manufacturers, in particular those of pressure-reducing equipment.

Activity · 10 MINUTES

List what you consider to be the core skills required of a clinical nurse specialist.

FEEDBACK

Your answer should have included some of the following points:

- advanced interpersonal skills—assertiveness, listening skills, negotiation skills
- leadership skills—acts as a positive role model
- teaching skills—colleagues, patients and carers
- presentation skills—meetings, conferences
- general management skills—time management, organisational skills
- research skills—research awareness, conducts and participates in research
- professional networking skills—collaborative practice
- political awareness—local and national
- change-management skills—ability to plan, initiate and support changes in practice.

The role of the clinical nurse specialist is paramount in maintaining quality of service and the identification of important areas for quality improvements and can facilitate a more structured approach to patient care through the implementation of clinical practice guidelines and research-based care. The tissue viability specialist nurse should be in the forefront of establishing and auditing clinical standards in order to improve the care and management of all patients with compromised tissue viability.

Activity · 10 MINUTES

Find out if your trust or unit employs a tissue viability nurse specialist. If so record his or her details below.

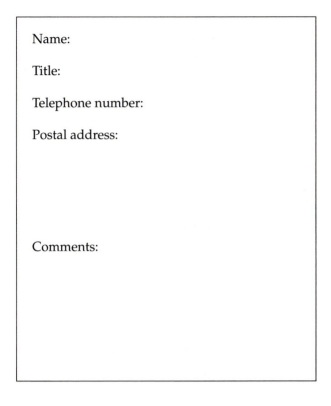

Name:

Title:

Telephone number:

Postal address:

Comments:

7.3 THE FUTURE OF TISSUE VIABILITY SERVICES

Introduction

Tissue viability services have developed considerably over the last decade, which has resulted in substantial improvements in care for those patients with wounds. Specialist wound care units are now beginning to emerge offering patients a comprehensive range of support services and the combined expertise of a wide range of health professionals. As governments become increasingly aware of the economic implications of chronic wounds, it is hoped that specialist services for patients with wound problems will become more commonplace resulting in the establishment of more wound care units and the appointment of tissue viability nurse specialists.

Community care

Radical changes in the provision of health care and the advancing age of the general population, inevitably mean that the management of chronic wounds is poised to rise higher on the political agenda as the costs of providing tissue viability services escalate. Patients with complex, non-healing wounds will be increasingly cared for by the community care services who are already working under extreme pressure due to the additional demands made upon their services. The relatively recent development of community leg ulcer clinics and the

emergence of community wound care nurse advisors is an example of how community nursing is responding to the challenge of providing new patterns of health care. Alternative models of care are developing where specialist outreach nurses, rather than generic community nursing services, are employed by hospitals to give care based on specialist expertise. This approach may have the additional advantage of providing continuity of care and improving liaison between the acute and primary health care teams.

The passing of the Medicinal Products: Prescription by Nurses, Midwives and Health Visitors Act in the UK in 1992 has significant implications for the improvement of tissue viability services, as it potentially allows specific categories of community nurses to prescribe wound dressings and certain medicines from a limited list of products (RCN 1995). The profession is currently awaiting the results of an evaluation of the effectiveness of nurse prescribing commissioned by the Department of Health in 1994 and is hoping in the future to see an extension of nurses' prescribing rights and the adoption of a nationally accepted system through which community nurses can provide non-nurse formulary items through group protocols agreed with medical practitioners (RCN 1995). Patients who will particularly benefit from these developments are the elderly and those suffering from chronic disabilities.

New approaches to wound management

A greater understanding of the physiology of wound healing and tissue repair has resulted in the development of various innovative treatment approaches. The efficacy of these has not as yet always been scientifically demonstrated, so that currently most of these newer techniques are only available on a limited basis from specialist centres. There are many examples of innovations in wound management practice which include the use of: topical growth factors to accelerate healing and control scarring (Shah et al 1992); hyperbaric oxygen; tissue engineering techniques (Andeassi 1991); and new methods of culturing and grafting cells, to name but a few. All of these evolving treatments represent exciting progress within the field of tissue viability and may in the future become established practice as we strive to unravel the complexities of wound healing.

Nurses will always occupy a central role when caring for patients with compromised tissue viability and indications are that this role is set to expand and take on new impetus as the relationship between medical and nursing practice, particularly within the speciality of tissue viability, becomes less defined. This increase in professional responsibility brings with it new challenges, which can only be met by a sound theoretical basis of wound repair and an up-to-date knowledge of current developments in wound management. Continuing professional education aims to disseminate research findings and provide the opportunity for practitioners to examine their own clinical practice. Specialist programmes of study focusing on wound management are becoming available that integrate theory with clinical practice and enable participants from a variety of different settings to facilitate changes in wound management practice (Flanagan 1995).

Nurses have been instrumental in effecting changes in wound management practices over the years and in many cases are fostering the development of multidisciplinary wound management groups. These groups have spent an increasing amount of time and effort in the development of clinical practice guidelines for acute and chronic wound management; the impact of such documents on the quality of care has been significant. Only one certainty remains in a rapidly changing world and that is that the future of tissue viability services will always be dependent on collaborative professional practice.

Self-assessment 5 MINUTES

List three major influences that seem likely to affect the provision of tissue viability services in the future.

FEEDBACK

Your answer should have included the following points:

1. demographic changes in the population
2. health care reforms and subsequent changes in the delivery of services
3. wound healing research and development activity
4. increasing economic costs of chronic wound care
5. the extending role of the nurse.

Activity 20 MINUTES

Re-read Article 1 in the Reader (p. 134) in which Ellis describes the influences that history and politics have had on wound management services today. Describe at least six ways in which nurses can help to influence change.

FEEDBACK

Summarised below are some general principles that nurses can use to facilitate the management of change in clinical practice settings.

1. Recognise the value of the unique contribution that nursing makes to the management of patients with wounds.
2. Take responsibility for clinical decision making and recognise professional accountability.
3. Value the potential of nursing's power base when negotiating with members of the multidisciplinary team.
4. Recognise the importance of working collaboratively within the multidisciplinary team.
5. Be aware of the prevailing socio-political environment.
6. Develop your knowledge base and professional contacts.
7. Utilise current research to underpin clinical practice.
8. Be aware of your own limitations, but get involved.

SUMMARY

This section has briefly reviewed developments in the future provision of tissue viability services. In it you have learnt that:

- The hallmark of professional practice is accountability which is based upon the general public's trust and dependency on nursing care.

- Accountability requires the justification of clinical decision making and an exploration of an individual's own practice.

- The role of the clinical nurse specialist is complex and involves a combination of sub-roles including clinical practice, education, research, acting as an agent of change and patient advocate.

- The future provision of tissue viability services is influenced by a combination of factors such as demographic changes, technological advances in treatment modalities, economic constraints and the rapidly expanding role of nursing.

REFERENCES

Andeassi L 1991 Human keratinocytes cultured on membranes composed of benzyl ester of hyaluronic acid suitable for grafting. Wounds 3: 116–126
Barrown A 1983 The clinical nurse specialist as consultant. In: Hamric A B, Spross J (eds) The clinical nurse specialist in theory and practice. Grune & Stratton, New York

Caruso L A, Payne D F 1990 Collaborative management: a nursing practice model. Journal of Nursing Administration 20(12): 28–32

Dimond B 1990 Legal aspects of nursing. Prentice Hall, New York

Fenton M 1985 Identifying competences of clinical nurse specialists. Journal of Nursing Administration 15(12): 31–37

Flanagan M 1995 A contemporary approach to wound care education. Journal of Wound Care 4(9): 422–424

Hamric A B, Spross J 1983 The clinical nurse specialist in theory and practice. Grune & Stratton, New York

Hill S 1995 The problems tissue viability nurses have in advising their health authorities in the purchase of pressure relieving equipment. Journal of Tissue Viability 5(4): 127–129

James H 1994 Exploring the role of the tissue viability specialist nurse. Nursing Standard 9(6): 258–259

Medicinal Products: Prescription by Nurses, Health Visitors and Health Visitors Act 1992 HMSO, London

Ralph C 1990 Nursing management and leadership—the challenge. In: Jolley M, Allan P (eds) Current issues in nursing development. Croom Helm, Beckenham

Royal College of Nursing 1995 Community health care nurses, challenging the present, improving the future. RCN, London

Shah M, Foreman D M, Ferguson M W 1992 Control of scarring in adult wounds by neutralising antibody to transforming growth factor beta. Lancet 339: 213–214

Sims J 1991 When planning ahead avoids costly claims. Health Service Journal 101(5240): 16

Storr G 1988 The clinical nurse specialist: from the outside looking in. Journal of Advanced Nursing 2: 265–272

Tingle J 1991 Negligence: the new accountability. Nursing Standard 5(29): 18–19

Wiseman S 1990 Patient advocacy. AORN Journal 81(3): 754–762

Wright S 1991 The nurse as a consultant. Nursing Standard 5(20): 31-34

Reader

TREATING THE WOUNDED: GALEN OR NIGHTINGALE?

MR TAL ELLIS
Lecturer Nursing
University South Australia

As the twentieth century draws to a close, humanity continues to manifest its amazing curiosity, seeking more and more 'knowledge' in a never ending effort to unlock life's mysteries. The physical bases of life are dissected, spliced and reconstituted; the dimensions of the universe are probed, photographed and published; the depths of the oceans are mapped, drilled and tested; the Cartesian medical paradigm still penetrates, proctoscopes and postulates; and nurses, though supposedly free of their 'Sairy Gampish' image, continue to experience a 'two-pence and beer' attitude toward many areas of their practice, 'burning at the stake' as 'perpetrators of arcane rituals' and an attitude that their position is rightly and somehow, 'naturally', subordinate. How far we have come!!

It is surprising that in this age of information and discovery that these paradoxes should exist. Of course the over dramatisation contained in preceding statements serves merely to illustrate the point that in many practice settings nurses still feel powerless to fully realise their professional potential. (Flanagan, M. 1992) This is of particular concern when care is compromised in deference to the prevailing politico-social environment of the practice area. This is not meant to infer that nurses within this environment are providing poor care, far from it! Rather, it implies that nurses are sometimes unable to effectively assert their influence in key care planning areas. (Stein, L. Watts, D. 1990. Flanagan, M. 1992.)

The care of people experiencing integumentary deficit is one such area. It is a common contemporary experience that the surgeon/physician orders a wound care regimen which nurses then carry out. It is now becoming a more frequent occurrence that nurses know they are carrying out outmoded wound care practices but despite their best efforts are unable to convince the medical officer concerned to change approach. For example, there is a large body of evidence suggesting that the use of hypochlorite solutions is absolutely contraindicated.

Leaper et al, (1985) Thomas, (1991) Biley (1991) and many other leading researchers in the area of wound healing have published their findings extensively, demonstrating the damage to epithelium these solutions

cause. Despite this, Eusol is currently being used to treat wounds in Adelaide's (S.A.) major metropolitan hospitals. This phenomenon extends beyond the bounds of the acute care setting and into the community, aged care, rehabilitation, palliative and extended care areas. Considering that continuity of the integument is so important for health and 'care of the integument' such a clear and fundamental area of nursing activity, it is bewildering to think nurses should have so little direct influence on wound care.

Nurses face many challenges in practice and one of the greatest is living up to high professional standards when unable to effectively contribute to care related decisions. It is important they are able to participate in the health discourse of the 21st century and beyond, necessitating a high level of political activity in the present to ensure this occurs. This activity would ideally be at both the micro (ward, clinical setting) and macro (public health) levels and strategies implemented in kind. In turn, these strategies must effectively resolve issues, such as those relating to wound care, in a manner which upholds ethical principles and public health goals and yet be cognizant of the most effective political means of achieving this purpose.

An examination of history reveals that the issue over who is able to make decisions relating to care of a person's wound is a power-oriented one. Indeed it is clearly a manifestation of the continuing predominance of western medical philosophy where traditionally "Doctor knows best, nurse does what they order and the patient does what they're told'. Moreover, in the current socio-political climate there are many threats to this tradition as a whole, (Stein, L. Watts, D. 1990.), further fuelling a desire to maintain the status quo in relation to wound care.

It is important therefore that any strategy for change be implemented in a way which establishes a co-operative practice model and recognises the holistic, person-centred, multi-disciplinary nature of care.

The maintenance of an intact integument is essential as a human's first line of defence: both physical and microbiological. It follows then that humans have always treated integumentary lesions and indeed the very earliest of medical records indicate this was the case. (Bibbings, J. 1984) The Edwin Smith papyrus (Egypt, 1600 BC) provided evidence of the prevailing surgical opinion regarding the treatment of wounds. It recommended that following a wound to the head, which penetrates to the bone, a dressing of fresh meat should be applied for the first day and treated daily thereafter with lint smeared with grease and honey (Ibid). Other such applications included dung, the use of which was in fact quite widespread on the Indian sub-continent where its spiritual properties were prized (Ibid).

In other cultures the treatment of wounds was carried out according to various religious and health care philosophies and practiced by both men and women. Galen (Roman, AD 130-200), to many the 'father' of surgery, had a tremendous influence on the treatment of wounds, some of his practices having apparently stood the test of time. It is incredible to think that for over 1600 years the 'most advanced' medicine of cultures ranging from Arab to European was practiced according to his principles. He, of course, advocated the washing of wounds with oils, salt water and wine and the application of bread poultices. (Bibbings, J. 1984 pp 36) Interestingly, he and his followers advocated the notion of 'laudable pus' - that a wound had to develop pus in order to heal. This belief continued up until the mid 19th century when Semmelweiss, Pasteur, Lister and others questioned accepted notions and finally demonstrated the strength of the 'germ theory'. Antiseptics such as hypochlorites were introduced in this period in order to combat infection.

Of historical interest was the fact that Florence Nightingale did not actually support the 'germ theory'. Indeed, her notions of introducing light and air to wards, removing excreta from beneath beds and keeping the environment clean were revolutionary at the time. This radical thinking did not extend to the world of the microbe, however, as she preferred to seek the answer to disease elsewhere. Apparently in 1894 she said, "... not in bacteriology but looking into drains (for smells) is the thing needed." (Bibbings, J 1984) Nightingale did, however, have a firm belief in hygiene and practices such as regular hand washing and strict personal cleanliness were part of her doctrine. Also of note is the fact that as far as wound care was concerned Nightingale followed the medical officer's orders. (Wyndham, D. 1980).

The establishment of a militaristic structure for nursing by Nightingale was at the time a necessary event (Wyndham, D. 1980). The survival of the nurses in her charge actually depended on a deal made with a medical-military official. Nurses were being abused by soldiers so Nightingale protected them by only acting under the strict instructions of the medical superintendent: the soldiers could not then touch the women without being insubordinate and thus were more inclined to leave them alone. (Ibid) This modis-operandum was perpetuated by several other less noble factors. It is known that

Nightingale was an advocate for change in the status of women (Smith, F. 1980) and yet the prevailing male-dominated social paradigm caused the very 'profession' she initiated to be structured in kind. (Reverby, S. 1987) It was also believed that the care and ministering of the sick was a spiritual, self-sacrificing pursuit and therefore well suited to women. (Reverby, S. 1987)

These factors led to a situation where up to the 1960's nurses were unable to act without medical order in most areas of care, including wound care. It meant they were essentially powerless in the acute care areas and lost 'control' over midwifery. This powerlessness extended to the treatment of women generally where even in the home they were fed a diet of incredible mis-information. An extract from Virtue's Household Physician (circa 1930) supports this assertion:

> "Passions of a Nursing Woman.- Let the woman who nurses a young child be careful of her passions. An irritable disposition, giving rise to gusts of violent passion, may so alter the character of the milk as to throw the child into convulsions. Grief, envy, hatred, fear, jealousy, and peevishness, unfit the milk for nourishing the child, and often cause the child's stomach to be much disordered" (pp485)

The parallel is obvious: prevailing social attitudes influenced the conduct and structure of nursing care from the early developmental to modern period. (Wyndham, D. 1980) It further clarifies the reason nurses have generally been unable to influence decision-making in relation to wound care. The male-dominated medical profession not only had authority with respect to care but also was socially dominant in the ward context as the majority of nurses were and still are, women. (Stein, L. Watts, D. 1990; Wyndham, D. 1980) As this situation still exists, that is, the gender distribution, (Wyndham, D. 1980) it follows that at least some of the problems encountered by nurses are related to this almost 'traditional' power imbalance. In a sense it seems that nursing, despite the presence of men amongst its numbers, is characterised as female and its practitioners treated accordingly.

The masculine scientific paradigm, so pre-dominant throughout the last two hundred years, also reinforced the notion that empirical research was the only meritorious method of enquiry. As nurses were not in a position either educationally or occupationally, to perform such research, their knowledge-base was often categorised as 'folklore' or 'intuition'. (Matthews, J. 1984; Stein, L. et al, 1990) Despite Paracelsus' assertion that he had, "... learned from the sorceress all he knew" (Wyndham, D. 1980), nursing knowledge was not so esteemed by his contemporaries.

It is only relatively recently that nurses have been able to effectively research their practice and therefore a sceptical attitude persists in many health-care settings. This means that it is quite possible for well constructed and published research relating to wound care to be dismissed by physicians and surgeons as 'unscientific' and ignored. (Hicks, C. 1992).

The question of who directs care is certainly complex. Despite increased levels of responsibility and accountability within the professional context of nursing and other health professions, the medical officer's name still appears above the bed of most clients in acute hospitals. Whilst this form of patient allocation is reasonably efficient, it is certainly reminiscent of where the power balance lies in health care. The advent of Diagnosis Related Groupings, Case-mix and Functional Unit based funding may cause some re-arrangement in this area but the functional dominance of the medical profession is unlikely to diminish in the short term and therefore any strategy for changing nursing influence in the management of people with integumentary deficit will have to take this into account. (Hicks, C. 1992).

In order to bring about meaningful change in nursing practice it is evident that a great number of factors need to be addressed. In devising a plan of action to increase the influence of nurses in wound care it is important that it takes account of prevailing social attitudes, historical relationships, research approaches and the political nature of the environment in which the change is to take place. The strategy would also need to reflect nursing philosophy to ensure professional integrity and therefore, positive client-health outcomes. The multi-disciplinary nature of the health care team in the 90's must also be reflected in any change. This is worthy of note due to the levels of professional inter-dependence which exist even in the face of a power imbalance such as the one nurses face in relation to wound care.

Nursing, both in literature and in practice, supports a 'holistic approach' to care. Fundamental nursing texts such as those prepared by Brunner and Suddarth (1988), Roper, Logan and Tierny (1980), Beare and Meyers (1990) all make reference to 'holism' as a central feature of nursing care. This philosophical feature of nursing also permeates journal literature where literally thousands of works referring to holism have been published. (Literature search, 'Holistic care'. CINAHL, University S.A., May 1993). It follows then that nurses need to have some influence over wound treatment decisions in order to meet care goals adequately.

There is little doubt that the nurses' care 'brief' extends to the care of a client's integument. Hygiene related activities, turning, moisturising, assessing, applying medication to the skin and performing dressings are all common nursing interventions. Adopting a 'holistic' approach means looking at a host of factors influencing the state of a client's integument in order to assess the impact they may have on the healing of a wound. It is not just a matter of applying the right dressing but of treating the whole person in order to achieve re-establishment of integumentary continuity (Flanagan,M. 1992). Nurses need to appreciate they have the skills and knowledge to treat people with wounds and that it is well within their practice parameters to do so. If they truly wish to manage the care of a person 'holistically' they must adopt strategies which allow them to participate in the care related decisions.

Part of the difficulty experienced by nurses when treating wounds is that should an infection develop, anti-biotics need to be prescribed. In order for this to occur, medical intervention is necessary and it is often at this point that nurses 'lose' control over a client's wound care treatment. It is vital that nurses appreciate their ability to effectively assess and treat a client suffering from wound infection and that they do not have to relinquish care responsibilities merely because another health-care professional has been asked to contribute to the client's care. It is also vital they recognise their accountability and assess whether their input toward decisions affecting care/practice is equitable.

As previously mentioned, the change strategy needs to be cognizant of the prevailing socio-political environment. Health care is serviced by a multi disciplinary team in the 1990's and therefore the potential exists for rational discussion to take place between the parties concerned. If nurses are to exert appropriate influence on wound management principles and practice, then negotiation and utilisation of proper political processes should form the basis of their action (Clay,T. 1987). They need to recognise and realise their power-potential and utilise it in a way which enhances the service provided to the public, without compromising their own integrity or feeling in any way dissident (Marles, F. 1989; Clay,T. 1987).

It would serve no useful purpose for nurses to set themselves apart from the other health professions as this would lead to isolation and difficulties with practice (Game, A., Pringle, R. 1983). The nursing practitioner must work within the contextual political system to achieve firstly practice changes and perhaps changes to the system itself over time (Clay, T. 1987). An understanding of the nature of the system in which one practices is therefore essential to the development of change strategy, especially where other allied professions are working within and utilising the said system.

Nurses can establish a collegiate approach to the care of clients with integumentary deficit by empowering themselves. Employing the tools of education, research and practice expertise to underpin the communication skills they possess, nurses can assert their goals, ideas and knowledge in a way that is meaningful to themselves and to the other health care professionals contributing to care. This must take place in such a way as to lead others toward a truly multi disciplinary approach by example and away from the professionally ethnic model which often masquerades as multi disciplinary.

In the workplace nurses must utilise current research to underpin their practice. There is a wealth of quantitative, qualitative and anecdotal data in the medical and nursing literature which will provide support for practice changes. It is not enough to have simply "heard about this new dressing" - nurses must provide data for consideration by other members of the health care team. This is an appropriate means of entering a healthy, patient centred debate and helps to objectify the situation. There is less likelihood of threat to personal or professional integrity when strong empirical evidence is used as a basis for discussion. At the very least it will provide a catalyst for further informed debate and if the practice is not adopted, perhaps research may take place in an effort to support or refute the findings of others.

In relation to professional organisations, it is evident that nurses are already beginning to adopt appropriate political approaches to influencing wound management. The last five years have seen a number of special interest groups come into being. With the exception of Australian Capital Territory each state/territory of Australia has what is known as a Wound Care Association. These associations were largely started by nurses alone but have now grown into significant multi-disciplinary organisations. The West Australian Wound Care Association hosted the Inaugural Australian Conference on Wound Care in March 1993. Over five hundred national and international delegates attended and a majority of presentations, workshops and key-note addresses were given by nurses.

This high level of organisation and assertion has meant that nurses, with the other health professionals, now comprise a powerful political lobby group in relation to wound management. The inauguration of a national wound care association at the Australian International Wound Management Conference, Melbourne, 1994 will see the establishment of a multi-disciplinary group capable of influencing government departments directly, given the nature of its representation. This will have ramifications at the bed side as it will no longer be the care directives of one profession determining the allocation of resources in relation to wound care.

A feature of the power of this lobby group is the fact that wound care costs the Australian public hundreds of millions of dollars per year. Therefore, anything which is likely to reduce that cost and reduce bed occupancy as well would be well received in Parliament House. Nurses, by taking the lead in this sort of macro-organisational effort, are demonstrating to the public their abilities as a profession, as a community lobby and politically enabled group. This in turn enhances their reputation at the bedside and contributes to better patient outcomes through the improved delivery of care and better inter-professional discourse.

The improved care techniques and new knowledge must also be published so that undergraduate nursing students are able to continue the process of discovery, improvement and change. The nursing profession must, therefore, continue to build its own basis for practice in order to ensure the best care outcomes for the client are achieved now and in the future (Stein et al, (1990) pp26). Nurses can achieve a greater level of influence in wound management through the adoption of a sensible, well thought out and politically aware approach.

So is it to be Galen or Nightingale who directs wound management? With all due respect, the prospect of Galen and Nightingale working together to provide wound care presents one with a most unsavoury vision: can you imagine Galen ordering Nightingale to apply her lunch fare to a patient's wound in an effort to produce suppuration; Nightingale washing her hands between each application but all the while looking in drains for the suppuration's source! Perhaps not. Fortunately, through improvements in education and the social attitudes toward women, nurses today are faced with a totally different situation to that encountered by Nightingale.

The answer therefore, is neither and both. Ultimately all people who suffer a loss of integumentary continuity should be able to make their own informed care decisions (where they are capable). The primary care thrust of future health care planning and resource allocation is presently being embraced by the nursing profession in Australia and to this end, nurses should be leading the way in the management of people with wounds. Only through self empowerment will nurses effectively take their place in the multi-disciplinary health team of the 1990's and beyond.

BIBLIOGRAPHY

Beare, G., Meyers, J. (1990) Principles and Practice of Adult Health Nursing. Mosby Co, Missouri.

Benner, P. (1984) From Novice to Expert: Excellence and Power in Clinical Nursing Practice. Addison Wesley Co., New York.

Bibbings, J. (1984) Honey, lizard dung and pigeons' blood. Nursing Times, Nov 28, 1984, pp 36-38.

Biley, F. (1991) Eusol: There'll by no eulogy. Nursing, July 11-24, 1991. Vol 4, No. 37, pp. 21-37.

Brennan, S., Foster,M., Leaper, D. (1986) Antiseptic Toxicity in Wounds healing by secondary intention. Journal of Hospital Infection, No.8. pp263-267.

Bilton,T., Bonnett, K et al (1981) Power and Politics. Introductory Sociology. Macmillan Press London. pp170-173.

Brennan, S., Leaper, D. (1985) Antiseptics and wound healing. British Journal of Surgery, Vol 72. pp780-782.

Brown,K. (1987) Stand together. Nursing Times, Oct 21, Vol 83, No. 42. pp70.

Brunner, S., Suddarth, D. (1988) Textbook of Medical - Surgical Nursing. 6th ed. Lippincott Co. Phil, USA.

Bryant,R. (1982) Power in Nursing - the Australian scene in Jenkins, E. et al. Issues in Australasian Nursing. Churchill-Livingstone, Melbourne. pp197-202.

Clay, T. (1982) Nurses, Power and Politics. Heineman Nursing. London.

Cox, A., Furlong, P., Page, E. (1985) Power and the problem of contestability. Power in Capitalist Societies: Theory, Explanations and Cases. Harvester Press, London pp 26-44.

Dahl, R. (1957) The Concept of Power. Behavioural Science. No.2 pp201-205.

Ferguson,V. (1985) Two perspectives on power in Mason, D., Talbot, S. (1985) Political action handbook for nurses. Addison-Wesley Co. California.

Flanagan, M. (1992) Variables influencing nurses' selection of wound dressings. Journal of Wound Care, May-June, Vol 1 No.1 pp 33-43.

Game, A., Pringle,R. (1983) Sex and Power in Hospitals. The Division of labour in the health industry. Allen and Unwin, Sydney pp 94-118.

Green, GF. (1982) Patient rights: power and dependency. The Australian Nurses Journal, Vol 11, No. 8, March 1982. pp43-50.

Hicks, C. (1992) Of Sex and Status: a study of the effects of gender and occupation on nurses evaluations of nursing research. Journal of Advanced Nursing, Vol 17, pp 1343-1349.

Holden,P., Littlewood, J. (1991) Anthropology and Nursing, Routledge, London.

Kalisch,AP., Kalisch, BJ. (1987) The Changing Image of the Nurse. Addison Wesley Pub Co. Calif, USA.

Keen,J., Malby, R. (1992) Nursing power and practice in the United Kingdom National Health Service. Journal of Advanced Nursing, No. 17. pp 863-870.

Leaper, D., Brennan, S., Foster, M. (1985) The effect of antiseptics on the healing wound: a study using the rabbit ear chamber. Journal of Hospital Infection Vol 8, No 3, pp263-267.

Lorde, A. (1984) Age, race, class and sex: Redefining the difference in Lorde, A. Sister Outsider. Trumansberg, New York. pp 114-123.

Lukes, S. (1974) Power: A Radical View. MacMillan, London.

McIntosh, D. (1989) Grassroots lobbying. American Journal of Nursing. Nov, 1989. Vol 89, No 11. pp 1515-1516.

Marles, F. (1989) The Politics of Nursing in Victoria in 1987. Deakin University Press, Vic Aust.

Mason, D. (1990) Nursing and politics: A profession comes of age. Orthopaedic Nursing, Sep-Oct, Vol 9, No. 5.pp11-17.

Meyer, C., Writer, S. (1992) Nursing on the political front. American Journal of Nursing, October, 1992. pp56-64.

Newman, M. (1990) Toward an integrative model of professional practice. Journal of Professional Nursing, Vol 6, No 3, May-June. pp 167-173.

Pearson, A. (1986) Nursing Models and the multi-disciplinary clinical team in Kershaw, B. & Salvage, J. (1986) Models for Nursing. Wiley and Sons, Chichester.

Persons,C., Wieck, L. (1985) Networking: A power strategy. Nursing Economics. No.3, pp 53-57.

Reverby, S. (1987) A caring dilemma: Womanhood and nursing in historical perspective. Nursing Research. Vol 36, No. 1 pp 5-11.

Roper,N., Logan,W., Tierny, A. (1980) The Elements of Nursing. Churchill Livingstone, London.

Smith, F. (1980) Florence Nightingale, Reputation and Power. Croom Helm London. pp183-204.

Salvage, J. (1989) The Politics of Nursing. Heinmann Nursing, Oxford.

Schattschneider,EE. (1960) The Semi-sovereign people: A realists view of democracy in America. Holt, Rinehart, Winston New York.

Stein, L.,Watts, D.,Howell, T. (1990) Sounding board: the doctor - nurse game revisited. Lamp. October 1990. Vol 47 No. 9. pp23-26.

Thomas, S. (1991) Evidence fails to justify use of hypochlorite. Journal of Tissue Viability. Vol 1, No. 1, pp9-10.

Unknown author (Circa 1930) Care of Children and their diseases. Virtue's Household Physician, Vol 1.

Wilkes,G., Krebs, W. (eds) (1988) The Collins Concise Dictionary of the English Language. 2nd ed. Collins, London.

Wydnham, D. Sexism and Health Care in Windscuttle, E. Women, Class and History: Feminist perspectives on Australia, 1788-1978. Fontana, Melbourne. pp 558-581.

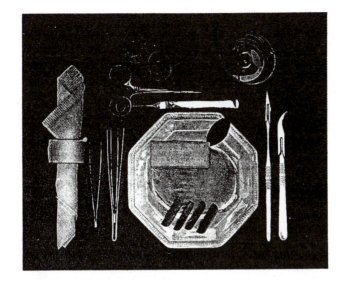

Nutrition and wound healing

A review of the role of macro- and micro-nutrients in injury response and wound healing, the effects of nutrient depletion and repletion on healing and recovery, and an examination of the process of nutrient assessment, delivery and evaluation

Contemporary knowledge of the role of nutrition in wound healing has expanded on several fronts. Nutritional factors have been shown to be prognostic of pressure sore development and wound-related complications; investigations in wound models, animal and clinical studies have demonstrated the adverse effects which nutrient deficiency can exert on healing, together with the beneficial effects of repletion. Nutritional support techniques, both enteral and parenteral, have also advanced to meet a complex range of requirements, but recently the research focus has shifted in an attempt to understand how the processes of inflammation and repair, both local and systemic, are regulated. Future innovations in nutrient support will arise from modulation of these processes to promote healing, reduce organ failure and maintain immuno-competence.

LOCAL AND METABOLIC EFFECTS OF NUTRIENTS IN INJURY

Glucose

Following injury, glucose provides a vital energy substrate for the cellular infiltrate of leucocytes and macrophages, both of which

S.M.G. McLaren, BSc. RGN, is director of undergraduate studies, Department of Nursing and Midwifery, University of Surrey, Guildford

have a high capacity for aerobic glycolysis and a crucial role in the production of factors which stimulate fibroblast growth and collagen synthesis. Goodson has shown extensive utilisation of glucose by fibroblasts in the synthesis of hexosamine sugars and proteoglycan polymers used in tissue repair[1]. Hyperglycaemia, resulting from the metabolic injury response, has long been considered an adaptive feature designed to meet increased wound requirements for glucose. It has been shown that these requirements can be considerable in severe injury. Wilmore found that wound glucose utilisation reached 175g per day in cases of 42% burns[2]. The increased energy requirement for tissue repair, combined with the effects of the metabolic injury response, can raise resting energy expenditure significantly. The rise is proportional to injury severity.

Efficiency of energy production from glucose depends on aerobic metabolism supported by an adequate red cell mass, wound angiogenesis, tissue perfusion and short intercapillary distances in granulating

tissue[3]. From observations made on experimental preparations of wounded muscle, Falcone and Caldwell[4] have suggested that, in part, the accelerated glycolysis found during healing is aerobic and is localised to the cellular infiltrate of leucocytes and macrophages that invade the wounded area. The purpose of the increased aerobic glycolysis linked to normal pyruvate oxidation is presumably to raise the concentrations of intermediate metabolites required for the biosynthesis of macromolecules during healing.

Fatty acids

Essential polyunsaturated fatty acids (PUFAs) are responsible for the structural and functional integrity of cell membranes, the production and release of membrane eicosanoids concerned with vascular and inflammatory responses and signal transduction through phospholipid-dependent second messenger pathways. Their role in the inflammatory response and tissue repair is of increasing importance. Recent interest has focused on the role of ω-3 and ω-6 PUFAs, derived from dietary fish and vegetable oils respectively, in relation to their effects once incorporated into the macrophage cell membrane. Metabolism of ω-3 PUFAs results in the formation of prostaglandin E_3 and leucotrienes, which both have vasodilatory and anti-inflammatory actions. In contrast, ω-6 PUFA metabolites include prostaglandins E_2 and I_2, which mediate the inflammatory response, platelet aggregation and vasoconstriction. PGE_2 is more immunosuppressive than PGE_3. Excessive PGE_2 production increases the activity of cytokines and depresses the T cell proliferation response. Cerra has suggested that increasing ω-3 PUFAs in the macrophage cell membrane by dietary manipulation could result in reduced incorporation of ω-6 PUFAs[5], thus reducing PGE_2 production and increasing the T cell proliferative response. This could, hypothetically, benefit clinical states where persistent inflammation is in part caused by activation of macrophages. However, optimum proportions of ω-3 and ω-6 PUFAs may be clinically significant in injury, trauma and sepsis to balance the effects of their metabolites.

Recent findings have shown that, in animal models, survival after peritonitis improved significantly when diets contained equal proportions of ω-3 and ω-6 fatty acids[6]. A clinical study by Gottschlich has suggested that ω-3 fatty acids incorporated in a dietary regimen for burns patients is of significant benefit in reducing wound infection[7].

Short chain fatty acids (SCFAs), which are the preferred energy substrate for colonic mucosa, also appear to be influential in the healing of colonic anastomoses. Butyrate and propionate stimulate mucosal proliferation by an undefined mechanism[8]. Koruda has shown, in animal studies, that when SCFAs are administered intravenously, improved bursting strength of colonic anastomoses results[9]. Similar results in postoperative wound healing are obtained by feeding rats on enteral diets supplemented by pectin, which increases SCFA production by the gut microflora[10]. No detailed studies on human subjects have been performed because neurotoxicity has been observed as a possible adverse effect.

Protein: experimental studies on dietary deficiency

The critical importance of protein in wound healing has been demonstrated in many investigations concerned with the impact of dietary deficiency. Effects of depletion include prolongation of the lag phase, with reduced fibroplasia, proteoglycan and collagen synthesis, angiogenesis and impaired remodelling in the presence of

hypoalbuminaemia[11]. If depletion is severe, oedema secondary to hypoalbuminaemia can develop, compromising healing by increasing diffusion distances for nutrients, resulting in decreased fibroplasia with risk of dehiscence[12]. A low protein intake compromises repair and callus quality following bony fracture.

Other effects of protein depletion have emerged from the investigations of Daly,[13] Irvin and Hunt,[14] and Ward,[15] which have confirmed that pre-operative dietary protein depletion in rodents compromises the healing of colonic anastomoses, as demonstrated by reduced bursting strength and reduced hydroxyproline content. Postoperative repletion studies with parenteral nutrition showed that optimal healing (increased colonic bursting strength, serum albumin and body weight) occurred when combinations of amino acids and dextrose were administered. It has been demonstrated in many investigations in animal and human subjects that a positive nitrogen balance promotes optimal healing[16].

However, a negative nitrogen balance is inevitable following the muscle catabolism which characterises the metabolic response to injury. Where the response is short, in animals which are well nourished with moderate injury indices, the majority of surgical wounds attain functional union during the period of negative nitrogen balance, the wound area having biological priority in terms of healing. However, this may not apply to all types of wounds since Delaney et al. have shown that very early postoperative feeding, with parenteral amino acid, lipid and dextrose combinations, exerted the most beneficial effects on anastomotic healing and weight gain in pre-operatively well-nourished rodents[17]. Delaying feeding until the third postoperative day, using either the same regimen or one comprising dextrose/vitamins only, produced impaired healing, most severely with the latter. Wound healing may be so sensitive to postoperative protein intake that, in certain wounds, even brief periods of inanition can adversely affect it.

Amino acids

Amino acids supply the structural components for wound healing; following trauma they provide a source for the synthesis of acute phase proteins required in the inflammatory process and are utilised as a metabolic fuel. Recent investigations have suggested an important therapeutic role for specific amino acids in promoting metabolic adaptation and wound healing[18,19].

In a wound, amino acids are required for

the synthesis of hexosamines, proteoglycan polymers, collagen, nucleic acids, cell skeletons and organelles and the structural proteins myosin, actin, collagen, keratin and elastin. All essential and some non-essential amino acids are required, some having a more significant role in reparative processes. The aminogram of a healing wound is altered from that seen in non-repairing tissue, demonstrating increased concentrations of proline, hydroxyproline, lysine, hydroxylysine, glycine, alanine and glutamine. Wounds are low in arginine because of the arginase released from dead macrophages, which converts it to ornithine. This, in turn, is utilised for proline synthesis. Both proline and lysine are incorporated into procollagen, then undergo hydroxylation before incorporation into collagen. Methionine and cysteine are both essential for fibroblast proliferation and collagen formation; cysteine being an important component of the terminal peptide of procollagen and necessary for disulphide bond formation in the tropocollagen helix[20].

One study demonstrated that impaired healing in protein-deficient animals is corrected following methionine repletion, demonstrated by reversal of lag phase slowing and accelerated fibroplasia[21]. Histidine also appears to be critical for healing, since Fitzpatrick and Fisher have found a reduction of wound-breaking strength in histidine-deficient animals which is reversed following repletion[22].

■ *Arginine.* Arginine significantly enhances reparative collagen synthesis as demonstrated by its hydroxyproline content in animal and human studies[23,24]. Arginine and ornithine both enhance wound-breaking strength, which correlates with increased collagen deposition in animal studies[25]. Protein metabolism is also significantly influenced by arginine in sepsis and stress. Daily administration of 30g arginine in human subjects undergoing surgery has resulted in improved nitrogen balance in comparison with controls[26]. Similar results were demonstrated by Daly and Reynolds in cancer patients undergoing surgery[27].

Beneficial effects of arginine on healing may also be derived from the metabolic pathway in macrophages and neutrophils, in which arginine is converted to citrulline and nitric oxide. Citrulline is subsequently utilised by fibroblasts for conversion to ornithine, proline and then incorporated into collagen. Nitric oxide is the endothelium-derived relaxing factor (EDRF) described by Palmer et al.[28]. Hypothetically, this could lead to microvascular haemodynamic changes favourable to wound healing.

Several *in vivo* and *in vitro* effects of arginine on immune function have been described. These have included enhanced T cell maturation, increase in thymic weight and stimulation of the peripheral blood mononuclear cell responses to antigens[29,30]. Observed *in vitro* effects have included induction of cytotoxic T cell function, natural killer cells[31]. Mechanisms of action of arginine on wound healing and immune function may be explained in part by its induction of growth hormone, prolactin, insulin and glucagon secretion[32].

■ *Glutamine.* Glutamine is categorised as a non-essential amino acid, but in trauma, injury and sepsis it is an essential nutrient for several reasons. Its molecular structure contains two readily mobilised nitrogen groups, hence its use as a vehicle for transfer of nitrogen between tissues. Following injury and sepsis, a rapid fall in the intracellular glutamine pool (mainly localised in skeletal muscle) and in plasma is seen. The decline is proportional to the injury's severity and is reversed later in the course of recovery[33]. The early decline is caused by the dramatic increase in glutamine requirements by macrophages, lymphocytes and fibroblasts at the injury site, where it is oxidised as a metabolic fuel[4]. Glutamine is also essential for purine and pyrimidine synthesis and is vital for lymphocyte proliferation in response to an antigenic challenge[34].

Other beneficial effects of glutamine, when administered exogenously, include an anti-catabolic effect on skeletal muscle by reducing glutamine efflux, thus sparing nitrogen and muscle wasting in catabolic states. The promotion of a positive nitrogen balance could benefit wound healing and further investigations are under way to substantiate this and other effects on clinical outcome[35].

■ *Ornithine-ketoglutarate (OKGA).* Leander and Furst have found that ornithine-ketoglutarate reduces nitrogen loss from muscle in patients receiving total parenteral nutrition (TPN)[36]. Mechanisms of action may include stimulation of growth hormone and insulin secretion. Its use in recovery from oropharyngeal resection has been suggested in a randomised controlled clinical trial by Pradoura et al.[37], where more rapid wound healing and a lower incidence of infections occurred in patients given OKGA-supplemented enteral nutrition.

Micronutrients

Zinc

The influence of zinc on wound healing resides in four actions: its stabilising effect on membrane structure and function, its role as a co-factor in enzyme systems, trophic effects on the immune system, and inhibitory actions on bacterial growth[38,39].

Zinc is an essential co-factor for the activity of more than 200 enzymes concerned in protein and nucleic acid synthesis, carbohydrate and lipid metabolism. Deficiency can therefore exert a considerable impact on all stages of healing. Following surgery, severe tissue injury, acute and chronic sepsis, zinc concentrations in plasma may rise initially. This is followed by a marked decrease and the appearance of zincuria; the decline in serum is related to the extent of tissue injury and catabolism. Interleukin-1 release probably accounts for these changes in the zinc profile which are also accompanied by a redistribution of zinc to the liver[40]. After routine surgery, the hypozincaemia is at its lowest level by six hours, following which it slowly returns to normal, provided that complications do not arise[41]. Clinically, the fall in serum after surgery can be reduced with zinc supplementation[42].

Effects of zinc deficiency on healing and the effects of repletion have been demonstrated in both animal and human studies. Wound healing in deficient rats occurred when oral supplements were given[43]. Hallboök and Lanner, in a study on patients with venous leg ulceration, found that oral zinc supplements were effective only when the serum zinc concentration was initially low[44]. More recently, Agren has investigated the effects of topically applied zinc oxide in a double-blind trial on patients with leg ulcers who had low serum zinc concentrations[45]. The group treated with zinc oxide demonstrated significantly greater epithelialisation and, in addition, infections and deterioration of ulcers were less common in zinc oxide-treated patients. Zinc oxide clearly has an important role in the local treatment of a zinc deficit. Slow topical administration of zinc oxide over extended time appears to be superior to rapid delivery with zinc sulphate, and no toxic effects have been reported with this form of treatment. The presence of zinc deficiency in some leg ulcer patients may reflect an underlying impairment in zinc metabolism[46].

Wound healing may also benefit from the antibacterial properties of zinc and its effects on immuno-competence. The antibacterial actions are mainly effective in Gram-positive organisms, where zinc causes bacterial aggregation and probably inactivation of enzyme systems[47]. Zinc deficiency exerts marked effects on all components of the immune system. In humans, these include lymphopenia, depressed T cell mitogenic responses and natural killer cell activity. These effects are reversed following zinc supplementation.

In summary, in venous leg ulceration, oral or topical zinc administration promotes healing in established deficiency states, but zinc excesses do not hasten healing[48]. Supplements can be of benefit in preventing depletion associated with severe injury and in patients on long-term parenteral nutrition careful monitoring of zinc status is necessary.

Copper

Copper is an intrinsic part of the oxidase system that aids cross-linkage between lysyl residues of collagen. The activity of the enzyme, lysyl oxidase, is reduced in copper deficiency[49]. Copper deficiency is rare, but individuals at risk of depletion include patients receiving long-term TPN, those suffering from malabsorption syndrome, protein-losing enteropathies and the nephrotic syndrome. Manifestations of deficiency include, in adults and children, a syndrome of anaemia, neutropenia and leukopenia. Skeletal demineralisation may also occur. No changes in serum copper levels were found in one study of patients undergoing surgery[50]. Hypercupraemia has been reported following severe injury, an effect probably induced by interleukin-1[40].

Iron

Significant iron depletion caused by dietary deficiency and chronic blood loss may cause hypochronic macrocytic anaemia, which can compromise healing through impaired oxygen transport[51]. Deficiency of iron could also affect collagen synthesis, since it is an essential co-factor for both lysyl and prolyl hydroxylase. Hypoferraemia is a feature of severe injury, sepsis and surgical stress, probably mediated by interleukin-1. It appears to represent a redistribution of iron in which the hypoferraemia prevails with normal or excess body iron stores, a normal serum transferrin and elevated ferritin. Replacement therapy using iron dextran is not thought appropriate or safe in this situation[50].

Vitamins

Vitamin C

The role of vitamin C in wound healing has been the subject of past controversy. It is an essential co-factor for the hydroxylation of proline and lysine before their incorporation into collagen, and deficiency results in a reduction in wound tensile strength. An increased incidence of wound dehiscence has been demonstrated in depletion states[52]. Depletion also impairs angiogenesis and increases capillary fragility. Another important function of vitamin C in relation to healing is its role in anti-oxidant defence. Oxygen free radicals generated in sepsis, ischaemia-reperfusion injury and during the inflammatory response can lead to collagen degradation, destruction of cell membranes by lipid peroxidation, disruption of cell organelles and enzyme systems[53]. Both vitamins C and E can break the chain reaction of free radical formation, limiting tissue damage and also exerting membrane stabilising effects[54].

The effects of vitamin C on immuno-competence are also particularly relevant to healing since it is necessary for the synthesis of complement and cell-mediated immune function. Supplements of vitamin C have been reported to increase T cell numbers and lymphocyte responsiveness in some subjects[55]. However, no depression of the immune response has been noted in experimentally deficient human subjects. Effects of megadose vitamin C on immune function are also conflicting[56,57].

In injury, sepsis and stress, increased utilisation and requirements for vitamin C have been noted, and the general consensus appears to be that supplements are necessary in seriously injured patients to prevent deficiency[48,58]. The benefits of vitamin C on the healing of pressure sores has been a contentious issue. An early study by Taylor suggested that the administration of large doses of ascorbate significantly enhanced the healing of pressure sores (demonstrated by a reduction in surface area) in a small, prospective, double-blind controlled trial[59]. Previous ascorbate status was assessed but not controlled in the study design. Results from other studies on the use of supplements in pressure sore and wound healing suggest that the maximum benefits are probably to be gained by using them in deficiency states, although opinion continues to be divided on the issue.

Vitamin B series
Vitamins of the B series play a key role in intermediary metabolism, where they are essential co-factors for enzyme activity. Implications of deficiency on the synthesis of macromolecules required for healing are therefore considerable.

Thiamine, riboflavin and pyridoxine are important co-factors for collagen cross-linkage[60]. Pyridoxine, pantothenic and folic acid are also important in immune defence. Aprahamian found that pantothenic acid supplementation improved the healing of aponeuroses in animals, but the precise mechanisms were unknown[6].

Vitamin A
The most important effects of vitamin A in relation to wound healing are as an essential co-factor for collagen cross-linkage and in support of epithelial proliferation and migration. The effects on epithelial proliferation and migration are achieved by actions on cell surface glycoproteins which affect adhesion[62].

Beneficial effects on the immune system include increased lymphocyte proliferation and natural killer cell activity[63]. Used topically on wounds with retarded healing, it also enhances epithelialisation[64] and can reverse the inhibitory actions of steroids. Greenwald has also found benefits of vitamin A on tendon healing *in vitro*[65]. Increased fibroblast maturation and collagen accumulation were the underlying mechanisms.

An increased requirement for vitamin A has been found following burns, when a decrease in the serum vitamin A concentration occurs. Vitamin supplements are commonly used in burns treatment and Kuroiwa has recently drawn attention to the need to determine the precise quantities of supplements required in different degrees of injury to reduce the risk of toxic effects[63].

Vitamin E
Vitamin E prevents lipid peroxidation of PUFAs in cell membranes by oxygen free radicals and hence has an important protective role in anti-oxidant defence and wound healing. An investigation by Powell found that administration of an α-tocopherol analogue significantly improved animal survival in sepsis[66], while Yoshikawa has demonstrated protective effects of vitamin E in gastric mucosal injury induced by ischaemia reperfusion[67]. The potential role of anti-oxidant free radical scavengers in the treatment of venous ulceration is currently under investigation[68].

CLINICAL STUDIES: WOUNDS AND NUTRIENT STATUS
In clinical studies, the relationship between nutritional status and wound healing has been focused on surgical populations, with a smaller number of investigations on pressure sores. Fig 1 outlines common effects of protein calorie malnutrition and their implications for wound healing.

The possibility that deteriorating nutritional status could influence the development of pressure sores was explored by Pinchcofsky-Devin and Kaminski[69]. In a prevalence survey of elderly patients, the overall incidence of malnutrition was 59%: when categorised, on the basis of predominantly biochemical variables, into mild, moderate and severe degrees of malnutrition, all the patients with pressure sores were found to be in the latter group. It was suggested that a severe deterioration in nutritional status was associated with the development of pressure sores. This may well be the case, but the possibility also exists that the loss of protein through the sore may have reduced the plasma protein concentration.

A number of studies in surgical populations have drawn correlations between pre-operative nutritional status and post-operative outcome, including healing and wound-related complications in addition to other indices of morbidity and mortality. A lower serum albumin has been consistently associated with a poor outcome in terms of wound-related complications[70].

Results of investigations into the effects of peri-operative nutritional support on postoperative morbidity and mortality are fraught with difficulties in interpretation, which were illustrated in a meta-analysis by Detsky et al.[71]. Comparisons between studies were difficult to make, owing to variations in criteria for patient selection, use of different nutritional support regimens, use of different or unclear end points and the use of small, non-randomised samples where the possibility of bias could not be excluded. The most common outcome measures used to report wound healing have included dehiscence, anastomotic failure and hydroxyproline content of wound implants and wound sepsis, but the criteria for sepsis are frequently not defined. Measurement of wound areas has seldom been included.

Mullen conducted a randomised trial of pre-operative TPN in patients with gastro-intestinal carcinoma[72]. Patients were assigned to control or intervention groups where the incidence of malnutrition (60%) was similar in both. One group received 10 days of pre-operative TPN, while the control group received the standard hospital diet providing 2 400kcal energy per day. The incidence of major complications (abdominal abscess, peritonitis, anastomotic leakage) was significantly lower in the parenteral nutrition group, as was the mortality. Unfortunately, the effects of malnutrition were not separately analysed for well-nourished and malnourished patients.

A randomised study by Heatley, also in patients with gastric cancer, evaluated the effects of a high energy/protein oral diet or the same diet supplemented by TPN for 7–10 days pre-operatively[73]. The groups were not significantly different regarding weight loss and serum albumin levels pre-operatively. No significant differences between the two groups were found in the incidence of anastomotic leakage; mortality was comparable in both groups, but the wound infection rate was significantly lower in the group that received parenteral nutrition in both normo-albuminaemic and hypo-albuminaemic subjects.

Benefits of both pre- and postoperative versus postoperative TPN were investigated by Mullen in patients undergoing major abdominal or intrathoracic surgery[74]. These groups of patients were again comparable in terms of diagnosis, age and nutritional status. Patients receiving combined pre- and postoperative support demonstrated a significantly lower mortality, incidence of wound dehiscence and fistula formation than those receiving only postoperative nutritional support.

Detsky et al. concluded from their meta-analysis that the incidence of major non-infectious complications (wound dehiscence, anastomotic leak, fistula) can be reduced in moderately to severely malnourished patients receiving pre-operative TPN[71]. Patients with mild degrees of malnutrition do not have a reduction in these complications compared with controls. There is a need to develop sensitive methods of nutritional assessment which will ensure that those patients who are at risk of developing wound healing problems are identified.

More recently, Buzby et al. have found a substantially higher infection rate in patients receiving pre-operative TPN (wound sepsis and pneumonia)[75]. The possibility of bacterial translocation from gut or seeding from catheter sepsis may explain this.

PROVISION OF NUTRITIONAL SUPPORT FOLLOWING INJURY

The primary aims of nutritional support are to maintain lean body mass and organ function, promote healing, improve immuno-competence and thereby reduce morbidity and mortality associated with a disorder and its treatment[76]. Essentially, the provision of support comprises a four-stage process. The apparent effects of giving support depend not only on how much and how well it is given but also on how depleted the recipient is. Thus, nutritional assessment to determine current status of

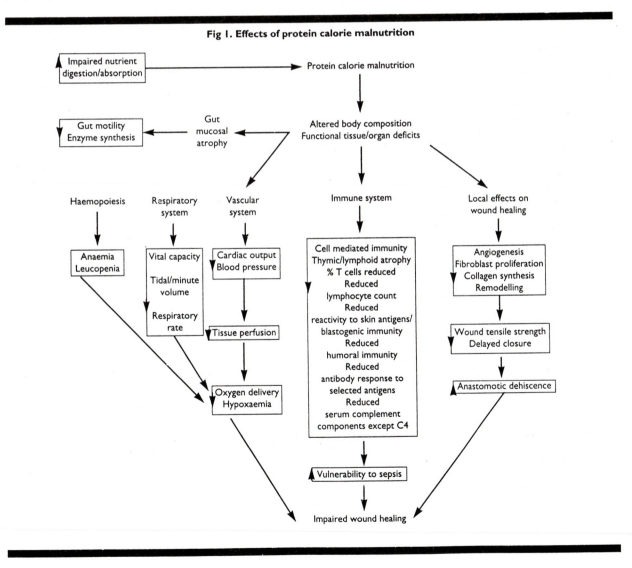

Fig 1. Effects of protein calorie malnutrition

body fuel stores and reserves is an important first stage. Determination of nutrient requirements is then necessary, taking into account metabolic status and severity of injury, sepsis or trauma. Decisions on the route of administration are determined by the functional status of the gastrointestinal tract and the absorptive capacity in relation to requirements.

Subsequent delivery of an appropriate enteral or parenteral regimen, which is adequate in terms of its macro- and micro-nutrient content, should be evaluated and readjusted during the period of support, including monitoring for potential adverse effects. The impact of an acute or chronic wound must be considered at every stage of the planning process, since many (burns or pressure sores, for example) can lead to depletion of protein reserve, and the presence of severe tissue injury and sepsis can initiate a metabolic response which alters nutrient requirements dramatically.

The wound site may influence the route by which nutritional support is delivered, and requirements for healing must be considered in formulating nutrient regimens. Although the promotion of healing is a primary concern, nutritional support must also be viewed in the context of an individual's diagnosis, therapy and response to treatment, all of which can affect nutritional status, requirements and the type and composition of the support selected.

Nutritional assessment

The aims of a nutritional assessment are to evaluate the adequacy of recent nutrient intake, to identify individuals who are malnourished, and therefore likely to develop wound-related problems and require support, and to evaluate by serial measurements the effectiveness of nutritional support. An impressive array of dietary, anthropometric, biochemical and physiological methods of assessment are currently available, but no single measure alone meets the criteria for the 'ideal' nutritional marker (one that is unaffected by non-nutritional factors, normalised by nutritional support and is consistently abnormal in patients with protein-calorie malnutrition)[77]. It is therefore necessary to carry out two or three investigations in parallel over a period of time and usually on a weekly basis to overcome the problems resulting from lack of specificity, sensitivity and difficulties in interpretation if one method only is used.

A central purpose of nutritional assessment is to identify individuals who are already malnourished or likely to become so

in order that nutritional support can be given to improve their outcome (that is, a reduced likelihood of morbid complications such as delayed wound healing and mortality). High-risk categories include elderly people, unconscious patients, individuals with gut, liver or renal disease and those with extensive pressure sores, burns, trauma, sepsis or those who are in the peri-operative period. An important question in relation to nutritional support in wound management is which tests are most suitable in the identification of malnourished patients who are likely to develop wound complications.

Dietary history

Traditionally, this is taken from the patient at an interview on admission and its purpose is to elicit information about eating habits, state of health and socio-economic background in relation to nutrition. Questions on eating patterns before and during illness, the presence of weight loss, anorexia, nausea, vomiting, dysphagia, dyspnoea, taste changes, impaired mobility and posture are all relevant to current nutritional status and future management. Information should also be obtained on drug therapy, since depression of macro- and micro-nutrient absorption can be an adverse effect of methotrexate, phenytoin and sulpho-namides (folate absorption), and 5-fluorouracil (thiamine absorption), with serious implications for wound healing.

Dietary surveys

These can provide very detailed information regarding dietary intake over time. A variety of methods can be used, including weighed food intakes, food diaries and dietary recall over periods ranging from 24 hours to one month. Burke and Bryson[78] have reviewed their merits and disadvantages. Recall methods may miss day-to-day or seasonal variations and can be subject to memory errors, while weighed food intakes are accurate but time-consuming and may reduce the aesthetic appeal of food by delaying meals. Once the type and quantity of foods consumed are obtained, daily energy and nutrient intake can be calculated using computerised standard tables of food composition[79]. Comparisons can then be made by consulting tables of recommended daily intakes and any deficits can be identified[80]. Care is required in making comparisons, for such tables apply to average values in healthy populations, and individuals whose intakes are marginally below the recommended level may not be

nutritionally at risk. However, intakes which are consistently less than 60% of the recommended value should be investigated further as a cause for concern.

Utilising the dietary recall method, Windsor et al. have demonstrated that pre-operative food intake exerts a significant impact on wound healing response as measured by hydroxyproline estimation in subcutaneous Goretex implants in patients undergoing elective bowel resections[81]. Patients with a history of reduction in food intake to at least 50% of normal in the week before surgery showed a significantly impaired healing response in comparison with those who maintained a normal intake. An interesting point to emerge from this study was that pre-operative food intake exerted a greater impact on healing response than loss from body fat stores and protein reserve. Maintenance of food intake up to the time of surgery was recommended to promote healing.

Physical examination: global assessment

Although a number of physical signs may indicate an underlying nutritional deficiency, they may also be manifestations of the underlying disease. A trained clinician may identify features of weight loss, muscle wasting, skin rashes and oedema symptomatic of malnutrition, in addition to the classic features of vitamin deficiency reviewed by Selhub and Rosenberg[82]. Detsky et al.[83] evaluated the accuracy of seven nutritional assessment techniques in predicting infection (including wound sepsis) in surgical patients. Predictive comparisons were made between the serum albumin, transferrin, creatinine height index, skin test antigen response, anthropometry and a subjective global assessment (SGA) comprising a dietary history, physical examination and functional assessment related to activities of daily living. The method which offered the best combination of specificity (0.72) and sensitivity (0.82) was the SGA.

Anthropometric indices

The anthropometric indices most commonly used are the thickness of skinfolds (thought to reflect fat stores) and limb muscle circumference or area (indicative of muscle mass). Estimates of fat stores are more accurately extrapolated from an average of skinfold measurements taken at six sites: triceps, biceps, sub-scapular, supra-iliac, thigh and calf. Interpretative problems are that the distribution of subcutaneous fat varies with age, sex, ethnic group, hydration status and the amount of fat measured. Muscle mass can be extrapolated by measuring mid-limb circumference in the arm, calf and thigh. It is derived from the following equation utilising the skinfold thickness:

Mid-arm muscle circ (cm) = arm circ (cm) − [0.314 x triceps skinfold thickness (mm)] (circ = circumference)

In the context of wound care, how useful are these measurements? Silberman has found anthropometric indices useful in monitoring acute trauma patients over long periods of time when it is not possible to obtain body weight[84]. Heymsfield has suggested that these indicators are used in conjunction with others in long-term monitoring[85], but the precise role of anthropometry in deciding which patients need nutritional support remains to be established.

Body weight

Estimations of body weight have played an important role in the nutritional assessment of surgical patients, since weight loss has shown good correlation with prognosis. Weight can be expressed with reference to a healthy population, for example, ideal body weight (IBW) for height, sex and frame size[86,87]. Measurements which are less than 80% IBW are considered a significant deficit[88]. The limitations of using reference tables have been emphasised under anthropometry. Percentage weight change:

$$\% \text{ weight change} = \frac{\text{usual weight} - \text{actual weight}}{\text{actual weight}} \times 100$$

and usual body weight:

$$\% \text{ usual body weight} = \frac{\text{actual weight}}{\text{usual weight}} \times 100$$

are particularly useful. Roy et al. demonstrated significant increases in the incidence of complications (including wound sepsis) where weight losses pre-operatively exceeded 6% usual body weight[89]. Seltzer et al. found a pre-operative weight loss of 4.5kg to be associated with a 19-fold increase in mortality[90]. In contrast, Windsor and Hill suggested that weight loss *per se* was not as significant in terms of prognosis as weight loss plus evidence of organ dysfunction[91]. In this study, a recent weight loss of >10% usual weight over three months combined with evidence of dysfunction in two or more organ systems was associated with a significant increase in

postoperative sepsis and hospital stay in comparison with a group who had suffered >10% weight loss with no organ impairment and a control group who had no evidence of weight change or organ dysfunction. Measurement of body weight clearly has an important value in the management of patients with surgical wounds. It is not a useful indicator of nutritional status in the presence of oedema, massive tumour growth or disease states associated with fluid overload.

Plasma proteins

Albumin, transferrin, retinol-binding protein and thyroxine-binding pre-albumin, which constitute part of the visceral protein reserve, are all synthesised by the liver. In malnutrition their serum concentrations decline because of a reduction in liver mass and protein synthesis. Table I gives their half-lives, body pool size, concentrations indicative of malnutrition, normal ranges in serum and the influence of non-nutritional factors on these. None entirely fulfils the criteria for an ideal protein marker (that is, short half-life, small body pool size, rapid rate of biosynthesis and being unaffected by non-nutritional variables).

Albumin, in particular, has a long half-life, large body pool size and is of use only in longer-term monitoring of nutritional status. All the plasma proteins decline during the metabolic response to injury, sepsis and trauma, which seriously limits their usefulness in many patients with wounds. Other factors which affect serum concentrations include transfer between intra- and extravascular compartments, losses in wound exudate (for example, burns) and the administration of blood products. However, albumin has been shown in several studies to provide an important and significant marker for postoperative morbidity (including wound complications) and mortality[90,92,93]. A low serum albumin on admission is also predictive of pressure sore development[94]. In patients undergoing postoperative intravenous nutritional repletion, both serum albumin and short half-life protein concentrations rise[95,96].

In summary, plasma proteins can be used to monitor the nutritional status of selected non-catabolic patients with wounds. The serum albumin concentration is a useful pre-operative marker of morbidity and mortality and, in conjunction with other parameters, can identify those at risk of developing pressure sores. In acutely ill catabolic patients, serum proteins cannot provide an indication of nutritional status, but they can be used to monitor the

metabolic response to injury. Repeated measurements can indicate when it has subsided and can be used to monitor nutritional status thereafter.

Nitrogen balance

Estimates of nitrogen balance provide one of the most valuable methods of determining whether an anabolic state has been achieved in response to nutritional support. A positive nitrogen balance is necessary for optimal wound healing to take place[16]. Balance is estimated over a 24-hour period by measuring nitrogen intake and losses in urine, taking into account additional losses (from wound fistulae, for example) and assuming a constant loss in hair, sweat, skin and faeces. Correction factors are available to allow for changes in blood urea, proteinuria and the fact that urinary area nitrogen comprises less than 100% of the total urinary nitrogen[97]. Consecutive measurements are usually made over three days for increased accuracy:

$$\frac{\text{nitrogen (g)}}{\text{balance}} = \frac{\text{protein intake (g)}}{6.25} - \frac{\text{urinary (g)}}{\text{nitrogen}} + 4g$$

Prognostic indices

Given the lack of specificity and sensitivity of single nutritional indices, Mullen and Buzby developed a prognostic nutritional index (PNI) which related the risk of postoperative morbidity and mortality to nutritional status on admission in patients undergoing elective surgery[98]. Nutritional parameters assessed were serum albumin (ALB), transferrin (TFN), triceps skinfold thickness (TSF) and delayed hypersensitivity (skin reactivity testing to three recall antigens, (DCH)).

Multivariate analysis with stepwise linear regression was used to develop the PNI.

$$\text{PNI\%} = 158016.6 \text{ (ALB)} - 0.78 \text{ (TSF)} - 0.2 \text{ (TFN)} - 5.8 \text{ (DCH)}$$

Patients at higher risk of morbidity (including wound-related complications) and mortality were those with a PNI >50%. The index was subsequently validated prospectively and a study by Smale used the PNI to investigate the effects of postoperative repletion on a group designated high risk (PNI >40%)[99]. A significant reduction in mortality and morbidity was demonstrated among those receiving six days pre-operative parenteral nutrition in comparison with high-risk patients who did not receive it. Jones has not found the PNI to be useful in predicting morbidity and mortality following acute abdominal trauma[100]. Clark has commented that indices of this kind can have only a good prognostic value in patients who are metabolically stable at pre-operative admission[101]. It is not of any use once the metabolic injury response is initiated and the components of the index are influenced by other variables. The skewed non-linearity of the PNI complications relationship also limits its use in assessing risk in individual patients[102]. Several PNIs have now been developed using a range of parameters. One of the most promising undergoing present validation is that of Ingenbleek and Carpentier, which combines two nutritional indices (plasma albumin and pre-albumin) with acute phase proteins in a prognostic inflammatory and nutritional index[103]. Preliminary results suggest that this may discriminate between nutritional and inflammatory causes of morbidity, which could have implications for management and may be relevant to patients with wounds.

Other parameters

An array of more sophisticated nutritional assessment techniques can give highly accurate measurements of body cell mass ([40]K isotope technique), and fat, skeletal and non-skeletal muscle (nuclear magnetic resonance, neutron activation analysis and ultrasonography). Currently their use is restricted to research settings.

Determination of nutrient requirements: injury and healing

Promotion of healing is dependent on the provision of a diet which meets individual requirements for energy and macro- and micronutrients.

Energy requirements following injury

Assessment of energy requirements after injury and during healing is imprecise. Resting energy expenditure must be considered, dependent on body size, age and sex, in addition to pyrexia, the metabolic response to injury and the demands of tissue repair. Energy needs vary according to injury severity and the magnitude of the metabolic response. The peak response can vary in duration from one or two days following routine surgery to several weeks after thermal injury. Indirect calorimetry and predictive equations are methods most commonly employed to calculate requirements for energy in metabolically stressed patients, neither of which offers absolute reliability and precision.

■ *Predictive equations.* A number of these have been developed from modifications of the Harris-Benedict equation used to determine resting energy requirements in healthy individuals of a given age, sex, height and weight. Predictive equations include weighting factors for injury which have been obtained from indirect calorimetry studies in patients subject to stress[104]. Correction factors can also be applied for average

temperature elevations, total burn surface area, caloric intake and total post-burn days[105,106]. Using indirect calorimetry as a standard, reports have varied enormously concerning the extent to which these equations overestimate, underestimate or closely correlate with actual requirements[107].

■ *Indirect calorimetry.* This determines energy expenditure by measuring gas exchange and estimating the respiratory quotient (ratio of CO_2 produced/oxygen consumed) during the oxidation of body fuels. Since measurements are made at brief intervals during the day, the estimate of resting metabolic energy expenditure (RME) obtained includes the altered requirements associated with injury but not allowances for the dynamic actions of food, periods of physical activity, intermittent pyrexia, or the energy increments necessary to achieve a positive balance for repletion. Corrections must be made to include these factors, such as multiplication of RME by 1.3 to determine the amount of non-protein calories[108].

Recently the estimates of energy requirements in catabolic states have been questioned. With the exception of thermal injury, it is thought unlikely that most patients require more than 40kcal per kg body weight per 24 hours, that is 2 000–2 500kcal per day or, in the case of burns, 3 500 – 4 500kcal per day[109].

In the critically injured, a minimal amount of energy in the form of carbohydrate equal

Table 1. Serum proteins: indicators of nutritional status

Serum proteins	Body pool size (per kg body weight)	Half-life	Normal ranges	Values suggesting severe protein calorie malnutrition	Non-nutritional factors affecting serum concentration
Albumin	5g	18 days	4.3-5 g/dl	<2.1 g/dl	Reduced during severe injury, liver disease, nephrotic syndrome, enteropathic states, intravenous fluids.
Transferrin	100mg	8 days	250–300 mg/dl	<100 mg/dl	Reduced during liver disease, trauma, infection. Increased during pregnancy, iron deficiency, hypoxia.
Retinol binding protein	2mg	12 hours	2.6-10 mg/dl	<1.5 mg/dl	Reduced during zinc deficiency, liver disease, hyperthyroidism, trauma, vitamin A deficiency. Increased during renal failure.
Thyroxine binding pre-albumin	10mg	2 days	16-36 mg/dl	<5 mg/dl	Reduced during liver disease, infection, stress, trauma.

to 150g glucose is needed, which cannot be replaced by fat. This is utilised by neural tissue, blood cells, the renal medulla and the wound. Additional energy should then be provided in equal proportions of carbohydrate or fat, since glucose resistance is usually present. It is becoming accepted practice to provide non-protein calories on a 50:50 basis for glucose and lipid, although 50–60% glucose is advocated in burns[110]. The use of fat in the shock phase of injury should be treated with caution, since it is poorly utilised and may result in detrimental elevation of plasma fatty acids.

Nitrogen

The extent of nitrogen loss during injury varies according to severity and the nutritional status before injury; less nitrogen is lost in depleted individuals. Evaluation of nitrogen status is usually made on the basis of nitrogen balance studies, but it is not usually possible to produce a positive balance in the catabolic phase of injury. In practice, nitrogen intakes usually approximate to 100–200mg nitrogen/kg body weight in the previously well-nourished and 200–400mg nitrogen/kg body weight in previously malnourished individuals. The ratio of energy to nitrogen is critical in sparing further losses, and it is usually possible to achieve nitrogen equilibrium by using a non-protein calorie nitrogen ratio of 150:1. In non-stressed, depleted patients, a similar approach can be used to calculate energy and nitrogen requirements, aiming for a positive nitrogen balance of approximately 5g per day and substituting a weight gain factor for an injury factor[104].

Micronutrients

A number of methods are available to determine vitamin status. They include biochemical estimations of serum or urine values and a number of functional assays. Reference values are available for recommended daily maintenance doses of most vitamins in normal, moderate and severe injury[111,112]. Methods are available for assessment of trace element status, but reference values for injury states are scanty.

Delivery of support: general considerations

Decisions on the route(s) by which nutritional support is delivered are governed by the extent to which the gut is functional and total energy requirements, which may be increased to the extent that use of the gut alone is inadequate in meeting needs. Important considerations here are that enteral feeding, to whatever extent possible, should be used to maintain gut mass and immunity and diminish the hazards of translocation. In burns, early enteral feeding appears safe and blunts the hypermetabolic response[113].

Combinations of enteral and parenteral feeding may be utilised in burns and other injuries; but if the gut is non-functional, then parenteral feeding is necessary. Adjunctive enteral tube feeding may be considered in some groups of patients who cannot ingest adequate amounts of food because of weakness or postoperative confusion. Bastow et al. found that in elderly postoperative patients with fractured femurs supplemental tube feeding exerted a positive impact on recovery, reducing the risk of morbid complications (wound and non-wound related) and mortality[114].

When refeeding chronically malnourished patients, care must be taken not to induce the 'refeeding syndrome,' which is associated with hypophosphataemia, confusion, coma and cardiac and ventilatory failure. This is caused by the dramatic compartmental shifts of phosphorus, potassium, magnesium and other substrates, which are induced by over-rapid repletion in situations where chronic starvation has already induced changes in these parameters. Preliminary correction of fluid and electrolyte balances with slower rates of repletion are recommended in the chronically malnourished individual[115].

Early initiation of nutritional support is recommended to prevent the development of significant nutritional deficits, and in catabolic patients this should occur when haemodynamic stability is achieved. The American Society for Parenteral and Enteral Nutrition suggests nutritional support (in relation to TPN) is necessary if a period of starvation in excess of five to seven days is anticipated in a well-nourished patient, but a more aggressive approach within one to three days should be used if a patient is malnourished[116]. Benefits of peri-operative feeding have been discussed earlier, which emphasise the advantages of pre-operative nutritional support in reducing morbidity and mortality.

The provision of nutritional support has many benefits but can also expose patients to mechanical, infective and metabolic complications. Careful monitoring is necessary to prevent substrate overload and osmotic, fluid and electrolyte disturbances associated with enteral or parenteral nutrition and to ensure that the nutritional support is effective. Outcomes in terms of nutritional and wound assessment criteria must be considered together.

MANAGEMENT OF NUTRITIONAL SUPPORT

If the aims of nutritional support are to be achieved, it is critical that the entire process of assessment, delivery and evaluation is managed effectively. The current state of the art is less than perfect. What are the problems?

Several surveys in recent years have suggested that protein-calorie malnutrition is a common, potentially serious and frequently unrecognised finding in acute and chronically sick adults, in a variety of institutional settings. The prevalence of the problem has been reported as ranging from 30 to 50%[69,95,117–120]. The exact number of malnourished individuals identified in these surveys who had also sustained an acute or chronic tissue injury was not always identified. However, some investigations were carried out exclusively on surgical populations, such as that by Bistrian et al.[93], while that of Pinchcofsky-Devin et al. linked the incidence of malnutrition with that of pressure sores[69]. Seltzer[90] and Grant et al.[121] have reviewed the adverse effects of malnutrition on recovery in terms of an increased risk of morbid complications, socio-economic costs and mortality.

Particular emphasis has been placed in this paper on the research evidence accrued from both experimental laboratory studies and clinical investigations, which have identified the adverse effects of specific nutritional deficiencies on wound healing, notably delayed closure, dehiscence and sepsis. Although some of the clinical evidence is not clear cut, an increasingly important therapeutic role for nutritional repletion in prevention and treatment of the consequences of nutritional deficiencies is emerging[17,71,122,123].

The high prevalence of malnutrition in the hospital population has been ascribed to a number of causes. The disease process may account for malnutrition on admission and subsequent deterioration of nutritional status thereafter; those affected need prompt nutritional support to improve the clinical outcome. However, in some situations, under-utilisation and inefficient management of nutritional support may be contributory factors[120,124]. Inadequate provision of enteral nutritional support to high-risk patients, failure to screen for or to diagnose protein-calorie malnutrition, and significant deficits between patients' actual energy intakes and requirements due, in part, to inadequate prescribing, were factors to emerge from these studies.

In the UK, a survey by Payne-James et al. found that only a small number of hospitals benefited from the presence of a multidisciplinary team to advise on nutritional support and appropriate use of peripheral parenteral nutrition, which is associated with fewer risks than central venous cannulation[125]. Other factors identified as contributing to poor nutritional support have included a lack of education on nutrition in the medical and nursing curriculum, unavailability of staff to supervise meals, conduct of medical investigations at mealtimes, lack of communication between staff involved in nutritional support and confusion over responsibilities in clinical decision-making[126,127].

A clear need has emerged to improve the practice and management of nutritional support and to identify the strategies by which this can be achieved. Payne-James et al. have advocated the inception of a multidisciplinary advisory group operating at national level to produce guidelines designed to improve current standards of practice, together with the formulation of nutrition support teams in health districts to provide a more balanced and coordinated service for hospital and community[125].

In the UK, the concept of a nutrition support team has recently grown in credibility and, it is to be hoped, will continue to do so as the role of nutrition is seen to be increasingly relevant to patient care. Advances in nutritional support now require the use of specialist equipment, innovative techniques, monitoring facilities and a range of scientific and clinical expertise which cuts across many professional boundaries. A team approach seems to be appropriate. General aims of such a team are envisaged to be provision for effective referral of patients who require support in hospital and community, operation of a nutrition advisory service, development of local standards of practice, education of health professionals and initiation of or involvement in research.

Preliminary reports have suggested that an effectively managed team can achieve substantial cost-effective improvements in nutritional support, reduce complications associated with parenteral and enteral feeding, and benefit the education of staff, formulation of policies and research[128-131].

In hospital and community settings, patients with acute and chronic wounds will always form a substantial proportion of those requiring nutritional support. The provision of optimal support to promote wound healing requires innovative research linked to multidisciplinary expertise and the machinery which translates benefits to the sharp end of patient care both effectively and safely. Perhaps the nutrition support team will break through some of the current barriers to efficient practice. Time will tell. ∎

REFERENCES
[1] Goodson, W.H. Wound healing. In: Condon, R.E. (ed.). Wound Healing in Surgical Care 2. Philadelphia: Lea and Febiger, 1985.
[2] Wilmore, D. Influence of burn wound on local and systemic responses to injury. Ann Surg 1977; 186: 444–458.
[3] Madden, J.W. Wound healing and wound care. In: Dudrick, S.J. (ed.). Manual of Preoperative and Postoperative Care. Philadelphia: W.B. Saunders, 1983.
[4] Falcone, P.A., Caldwell, M.D. Wound metabolism. Clin Plas Surg 1990; 17: 443–456.
[5] Cerra, F.B. Nutrient modulation of inflammatory and immune function. Am J Surg 1991; 161: 230–234.
[6] Peck, M.D. Composition of fat in enteral diets can influence outcome in experimental peritonitis. Ann Surg 1991; 214: 74–82.
[7] Gottschlich, M. Differential effects of three dietary regimens on selected outcome variables in burn patients. J Parenteral and Enteral Nutrition 1990; 14: 225–234.
[8] Sakata, T. Stimulatory effects of short chain fatty acids on epithelial cell proliferation in the small intestine. Br J Nutr 1987; 58: 95–103.
[9] Koruda, M. Effect of parenteral nutrition supplemented with short chain fatty acids on adaptation to massive small bowel resection. Gastroenterology 1988; 95: 715–720.
[10] Rolandelli, R.H., Koruda, M.J. Effects of enteral feeding supplemented with pectin in the healing of colonic anastomoses in the rat. Surgery 1986; 99: 703–707.
[11] Ruberg, R. Role of nutrition in wound healing. Surg Clin N Am 1984; 64: 705–714.
[12] Hunt, T.K., Zelderfeldt, B. Nutrition and environmental aspects of wound healing. In: Dunphy J.E., Van Winkle, W. (eds). Repair and Regeneration. New York: McGraw-Hill, 1969.
[13] Daly, J.M. Effects of protein depletion on strength of colonic anastomoses. Surg Gynae Obs 1972; 134: 15.
[14] Irvin, T.T., Hunt, T.K. Effect of malnutrition on colonic healing. Ann Surg 1974; 180: 765.
[15] Ward, M.W.N. Effects of subclinical malnutrition and refeeding on the healing of experimental colonic anastomoses. Br J Surg 1982; 69: 308.
[16] Rush, B.F. Positive nitrogen balance after abdominal operations. Am J Surg 1970; 119: 70–76.
[17] Delaney, H., Demetriou, A., Teh, E. et al. Effect of early post-operative support on skin wound and colon anastomosis healing. J Parenteral and Enteral Nutrition 1990; 14: 357–360.
[18] Cynober, L. Amino acid metabolism in thermal burns. J Parenteral and Enteral Nutrition 1989; 13: 196–205.
[19] Grimble, G., Payne-James, T., Rees, K. et al. Enteral nutrition: novel substrates. Int Ther Clin Mon 1989; 10: 2, 51–57.
[20] Williamson, M., Fromm, H. The incorporation of sulphur amino acids into the proteins of regenerating wound tissue. J Biol Chem 1955; 212: 705–712.
[21] Edwards, L., Dunphy, J. Methionine in wound healing during protein starvation. In: Williamson, M. (ed.). The Healing of Wounds. New York: McGraw-Hill, 1957.
[22] Fitzpatrick, D.W., Fisher, H. Carnosine, histidine and wound healing. Surgery 1982; 91: 56–60.
[23] Chyun, J.H., Griminger, P. Improvement of nitrogen retention by arginine and glycine supplementation. J Nutrition 1984; 144: 1687–1794.
[24] Barbul, A., Lazarou, S., Efron, D. Arginine enhances wound healing in humans and lymphocyte immune responses. Surgery 1992. In press.
[25] Rettura, G., Stratford, F., Levenson, S.M. Improved wound healing: anticatabolic and thymotrophic actions of supplemental ornithine. The 17th Mid-Atlantic Regional Meeting of the American Chemical Society. Washington, DC: American Chemical Society, 1983.
[26] Elsair, J., Poey, J., Issad, H. Effect of arginine chlorohydrate on nitrogen balance three days following routine surgery in man. Biomedical Express 1978; 29: 312–317.
[27] Daly, J.M., Reynolds, J. Immune and metabolic effects of arginine in the surgical patient. Ann Surg 1988; 208: 512–523.
[28] Palmer, R.M., Rees, D.D., Ashton, D.S. L arginine, the physiologic precursor for the formation of nitric oxide in endothelium dependent relaxation. Biochem Biophys Res Comm 1988; 153: 1251–1256.
[29] Barbul, A., Sisto, D.A., Wasserking, H.L. Arginine stimulates lymphocyte immune responses in healthy humans. Surgery 1981; 90: 244–251.
[30] Barbul, A., Efron, D., Shawe, T. Arginine increases the number of T-lymphocytes in nude mice. J Parenteral and Enteral Nutrition 1989; 13: 75.
[31] Moriguchi, S. Fundamental changes in human lymphocytes and monocytes after in vitro incubation with arginine. Nutrition Research 1987; 1: 719–729.
[32] Kirk, S., Barbul, A. Role of arginine in trauma, sepsis, immunity. J Parenteral and Enteral Nutrition 1990; 14: 2265–2295.
[33] Smith, R., Wilmore, D.W. Glutamine nutrition and requirements. J Parenteral and Enteral Nutrition 1990; 14: 945–985.
[34] Newsholme, E.A. Properties of glutamine release from muscle and its importance for the immune system. J Parenteral and Enteral Nutrition 1990; 14: 635–675.
[35] Roth, E., Karner, J., Ollenschlager, G. Glutamine: an anabolic effector? J Parenteral and Enteral Nutrition 1990; 14: 4, 130S–135S.
[36] Leander, U., Furst, P. Nitrogen sparing effect of ornicetil (R) in the immediate post-operative state. Clinical Nutrition 1985; 4: 43–51.
[37] Pradoura, J., Carcassone, Y., Spitalier, J.M. Double blind randomised trial of l-tormitrine alpha ketoglutarate enteral supplementation in operated patients with oropharynx cancer. Clinical Nutrition 1986; 5: (suppl.) 132.
[38] Bettger, W.J. A critical physiological role of zinc in the structure and function of biomembranes. Life Sciences 1981; 28, 1425–1438.
[39] Solomons, N.W. Zinc and copper. In: Shils, M.E. (ed.). Modern Nutrition in Health and Disease. Philadelphia: Lea and Febiger 1988.
[40] Dinarello, C.A. An update on human interleukin 1. J Clin Immunology 1985; 5: 287–296.
[41] Tengrup, I. Changes in serum zinc during and after surgical procedures. Acta Chir Scand 1977; 43: 195–199.
[42] Hallboök, T., Hedelin, H. Preoperative peroral zinc supplementation. Acta Chir Scand 1978; 144: 63–66.
[43] Lee, P. Zinc and wound healing. Surg Obstet Gynaecol 1976; 143: 549–554.
[44] Hallboök, T., Lanner, E. Serum zinc and healing of venous leg ulcers. Lancet 1972; 2: 780–782.
[45] Agren, M.S. Studies on Zinc in Wound Healing (Linkoping University Medical Dissertation No. 320). Linkoping, Sweden: Linkoping University, 1990.
[46] Hawkins, T., Marks, J.M., Plummer, V. et al. Whole body monitoring and other studies of zinc-65 metabolism in patients with dermatological disease. Clin Exp Dermatol 1976; 1: 243–252.
[47] Soderberg, T. Effects of zinc occlusive medicated dressing on the bacterial flora in excised wounds. Infection 1989; 17: 81–85.
[48] Hand, M. Anorexia. In: Lewis, L., Morris, M., Hand, M. (eds). Small Animal Clinical Nutrition III. Topeka, USA: Mark Morris Associates, 1987.
[49] Lindeman, R.D. Assessment of trace element depletion. In: Wright, R., Heymsfield, S. (eds). Nutritional Assessment. Oxford: Blackwell Scientific

Publications, 1984.

50 Shanbhogue, L.K., Paterson, N. Effect of sepsis and surgery on trace minerals.. *J Parenteral and Enteral Nutrition* 1991; **14:** 287–289.

51 Heughan, C., Grislis, G., Hunt, T.K. The effect of anaemia on wound healing. *Ann Surg* 1974; **179:** 163.

52 Schilling, J. Wound healing. *Surg Clin N Am* 1976; **56:** 859.

53 White, M.J. Oxygen free radicals and wound healing. *Clin Plas Surg* 1990; **17:** 473–484.

54 Weiss, S.J. Oxygen, ischaemia and inflammation. *Acta Physiol Scand* 1986; **548:** 9–37.

55 Penn, N., Purkins, L. Effect of dietary supplements with vitamins A, C, E, on cell-mediated immune function in elderly long-stay patients. *Age and Ageing* 1991; **20:** 169–174.

56 Kay, N.E. Human T cell function in experimental ascorbic acid deficiency. *Am J Clin Nutr* 1982; **36:** 127–130.

57 Anderson, R. The effects of increasing weekly doses of ascorbate on cellular and immune function. *Am J Clin Nutr* 1980; **33:** 71–76.

58 Pollack, S.V. Wound healing: a review. *J Derm Surg Onc* 1984; **5:** 614–619.

59 Taylor, T.V. Ascorbic acid supplementation in the treatment of pressure sores. *Lancet* 1974; **2:** 544–546.

60 Alvarez, O.M. Effects of dietary thiamine on intermolecular collagen cross-linking during wound repair. *J Trauma* 1982; **22:** 20.

61 Aprahamian, M. Effects of supplemental pantothenic acid on wound healing. *Am J Clin Nutr* 1985; **41:** 578–589.

62 Olson, J.A. Vitamin A, retinoids and carotenoids. In: Shils, M.E. (ed.). *Modern Nutrition in Health and Disease.* Philadelphia: Lea and Febiger, 1988.

63 Kuroiwa, A. Effect of vitamin A in enteral formula for burned guinea pigs. *Burns* 1990; **16:** 265–272.

64 Smith, K., Zarbiackas, L., Ditlake, R. Cortisone, vitamin A and wound healing. *J Surg Res* 1986; **40:** 120.

65 Greenwald, D. Intrinsic tendon healing *in vitro:* biomechanical analysis and effects of vitamins A and E. *Current Surgery* 1990; **47:** 440–443.

66 Powell, R.J. Effect of oxygen free radical scavengers on survival in sepsis. *Am Surgeon* 1990; **57: 2,** 86–88.

67 Yoshikawa, T. Vitamin E in gastric mucosal injury induced by reperfusion. *Am J Clin Nutr* 1991; **53:** 2105–2135.

68 Salim, A.S. The role of oxygen free radicals in the management of venous ulceration. *W J Surg* 1991; **15:** 264–269.

69 Pinchcofsky-Devin, G.D., Kaminski, M.V. Correlation of pressure sores and nutritional status. *J Am Geriatric Society* 1986; **34:** 435–440.

70 Mullen, J., Gertner, M., Buzby, G. et al. Implications of malnutrition in surgical patients. *Arch Surg* 1979; **114:** 121–125.

71 Detsky, A.S., Baker, J.P., O'Rourke, K. Peri-operative parenteral nutrition: a meta-analysis. *Ann Int Med* 1987; **107:** 195–203.

72 Mullen, J. Indications and effects of preoperative parenteral nutrition. *W J Surg* 1986; **10:** 53–63.

73 Heatley, R. Preoperative intravenous feeding: a controlled trial. *Postgrad Med J* 1979; **55:** 541–545.

74 Mullen, J.L. Reduction of operative morbidity and mortality by combined pre-operative and postoperative support. *Ann Surg* 1980; **192:** 604–613.

75 Buzby, G.P., Knox, L.S., Crosby, L.O. A randomised clinical trial of total parenteral nutrition in malnourished surgical patients. *Am J Clin Nutr* 1988; **47:** 366–381.

76 Dickerson, J.W.T.D., Lee. H. *Nutrition in the Clinical Management of Disease.* London: Edward Arnold, 1988.

77 Buzby, G., Mullen, J.L. Analysis of nutritional assessment indices. In: Wright, R., Heymsfield, S. (eds). *Nutritional Assessment.* Oxford: Blackwell Scientific Publications, 1985.

78 Burke, M., Bryson, E. Dietary intakes, resting metabolic rates and body composition in benign and malignant disease. *Br Med J* 1980; **1: i:** 211–215.

79 Paul, A., Southgate, D.A. *McCance and Widdowson's Composition of Foods (MRC Report No.297)*

(4th edn). London: HMSO, 1978.

80 Department of Health. *Dietary Reference Values for Food Energy and Nutrients for the UK* (Report No. 41). London: HMSO, 1991.

81 Windsor, J., Knight, G., Hill, G. Wound healing response in surgical patients: recent food intake is more important than nutritional status. *Br J Surg* 1988; **75:** 135–137.

82 Selhub, J., Rosenberg, I. Evaluation of vitamin deficiency states. In: Wright, R., Heymsfield, S. (eds). *Nutritional Assessment.* Oxford: Blackwell Scientific Publications, 1984.

83 Detsky, A., Baker, J., Mendelson, R. Evaluating the accuracy of nutritional assessment techniques: methodology and comparisons. *J Parenteral and Enteral Nutrition* 1984; **8:** 153–159.

84 Silberman, H. *Parenteral and Enteral Nutrition.* (2nd edn). Norwalk, Connecticut: Appleton and Lange, 1989.

85 Heymsfield, S.B., McManus, C. Anthropometric assessment of adult protein energy malnutrition. In: Wright, R., Heymsfield, S. (eds.). *Nutritional Assessment.* Oxford: Blackwell Scientific Publications, 1984.

86 Frisancho, A. New standards of weight and body composition by frame size and height. *Am J Clin Nutr* 1984; **40:** 809–819.

87 Grand Metropolitan Actuarial Tables. Height and weight tables. *Metropolitan Life Foundation Statistical Bulletin* 1983; **64:** 2–9.

88 Blackburn, G. Nutritional and metabolic assessment of the hospital patient. *J Parenteral and Enteral Nutrition* 1977; **1:** 11–22.

89 Roy, L., Edwards, P., Barr, L. The value of nutritional assessment in the surgical patient. *J Parenteral and Enteral Nutrition* 1985; **9:** 170–172.

90 Seltzer, M., Slocum, H., Betcher, E. Instant nutritional assessment: weight loss and surgical mortality. *J Parenteral and Enteral Nutrition* 1982; **6:** 218–221.

91 Windsor, J., Hill, G. Weight loss with physiologic impairment. *Ann Surg* 1988; **207:** 290–296.

92 Reinhardt, G.F. Incidence and mortality of hypoalbuminaemic patients and veterans. *J Parenteral and Enteral Nutrition* 1980; **4:** 357–359.

93 Bistrian, B.R., Blackburn, G.L., Halliwell, E. Protein status of general surgical patients. *J Am Med Assoc* 1974; **230:** 858–860.

94 Ek, A.C. Prediction of pressure sore development. *Scand J Caring Science* 1987; **1:** 77–84.

95 McEntee, G.P. The effect of parenteral nutritional support on cell mediated immunity. *Int Ther Clin Monitor* 1987; **8: 5,** 138–143.

96 Bourry, J., Milano, G. Assessment of nutritional proteins during parenteral nutrition in cancer patients. *Ann Clin Lab Sci* 1982; **12:** 158–162.

97 Hartley, T., Lee, H. A method of determining nitrogen balance. *Postgrad Med J* 1975; **51:** 441–445.

98 Mullen, J., Buzby, G. Prediction of operative morbidity and mortality by preoperative nutritional assessment. *Surg Forum* 1979; **30:** 80–82.

99 Smale, B.F. The efficacy of nutritional assessment and support in cancer surgery. *Cancer* 1981; **47:** 2375–2381.

100 Jones, T.N. Factors influencing nutritional assessment in abdominal trauma patients. *J Parenteral and Enteral Nutrition* 1983; **7:** 115–116.

101 Clark, R.G. Preoperative nutritional status. *Br J Clin Prac* 1990; **63:** 2–7

102 Meguid, M.M., Campos, A.C., Hammond, W.G. Nutritional support in surgical practice:. Part I. *Am J Surg* 1990; **159:** 345–359.

103 Ingenbleek, Y., Carpentier, Y.A. A prognostic inflammatory and nutritional index scoring critically ill patients. *Int J Vitamin Nutrition Research* 1985; **5:** 91–101.

104 Long, C. Energy requirements of the critically ill patient. In: Wright, R., Heymsfield, S. (eds). *Nutritional Assessment.* Oxford: Blackwell Scientific Publications, 1984.

105 Allard, J.P. Validation of a new formula for estimating energy requirements of burn patients. *J Parenteral and Enteral Nutrition* 1990; **14:** 115–118.

106 Goran, M. Estimating energy requirements in

burned children. *Am J Clin Nutr* 1991; **54:** 35–40.

107 Foster, G.D. Caloric requirements in total parenteral nutrition. *J Am Coll Nutr* 1987; **6:** 231–253.

108 Feurer, I.D, Mullen, J.L. Measurement of energy expenditure. In: Rombeau, S.L., Caldwell, M.D. (eds). *Parenteral Nutrition.* Philadelphia: W.B. Saunders, 1986.

109 Macfie, J. Towards cheaper intravenous nutrition. *Br Med J* 1986; **292:** 107–109.

110 Elwyn, D.H. Protein metabolism and requirements in critically ill patients. *Critical Care Clinics* 1987; **3:** 57–70.

111 National Academy of Sciences. *National Research Council Publication on Therapeutic Nutrition with Special Reference to Military Situations.* Washington, DC: National Research Council, 1951.

112 American Medical Association. Multivitamin preparations: a statement by the Nutrition Advisory Group. *J Parenteral and Enteral Nutrition* 1975; **3:** 258–262.

113 Dominioni, L. Enteral feeding in burns hypermetabolism: nutritional and metabolic effects of different levels of calorie and protein intake. *J Parenteral and Enteral Nutrition* 1985; **9:** 262–279.

114 Bastow, M., Rawlings, J., Allison, S.P. Benefits of supplementary tube feeding after fractured neck of femur. *Br Med J* 1983; **287:** 1589–1592.

115 Solomon, S., Kirby, D. The refeeding syndrome: a review. *J Parenteral and Enteral Nutrition* 1990; **14:** 90–97.

116 American Society for Parenteral and Enteral Nutrition Board of Directors. Guidelines for use of TPN in hospitalised patients. *J Parenteral and Enteral Nutrition* 1986; **10,** 441–445.

117 Bistrian, B.R., Blackburn, G.L., Vitale, J. Prevalence of malnutrition in general medical patients. *J Am Med Assoc* 1976; **235:** 1567–1570.

118 Willotts, H., Driscoll, J.J. Parenteral nutrition and nutritional assessment. *J Parenteral and Enteral Nutrition* 1978; **2:** 200.

119 Weinsier, R.L., Hunker, E.M., Krumdieck, C.L. Hospital malnutrition: a prospective evaluation of general medical patients during the course of hospitalisation. *Am J Clin Nutr* 1979; **32:** 418–426.

120 Sullivan, D., Chernoff, R., Moriarty, M. et al. Patterns of care: an analysis of nutritional care routinely provided to elderly hospitalised veterans. *J Parenteral and Enteral Nutrition* 1989; **13:** 249–254.

121 Grant, J., Custer, P., Thurlow, J. Current techniques of nutritional assessment. *Surg Clin N Am* 1981; **61:** 437–463.

122 Koruda, M., Rolandelli, R. Experimental studies on the healing of colonic anastomoses. *J Surg Res* 1990; **48:** 504–515.

123 Buzby, G.P. Peri-operative nutritional support. *J Parenteral and Enteral Nutrition* 1990; **14:** 197S–199S.

124 Abernathy, G. Heizer, W., Holcombe, B.J. Efficacy of tube feeding in supplying energy requirements of hospitalised patients. *J Parenteral and Enteral Nutrition* 1989; **13:** 387–391.

125 Payne-James, J., de Gara, C.J., Grimble, G.K. Nutritional support in hospitals in the UK: a national survey. *Health Trends* 1990; **22:** 9–13.

126 Dickerson, J.W.T., Wright, J. Hospital induced malnutrition. In: Holmes, S. (ed). *Nutrition in Nursing Practice.* Guildford: University of Surrey Publications, 1986.

127 British Nutrition Foundation. *Nutrition in Medical Education.* London: BNF Publications, 1983.

128 Puntis, J.N., Booth, I.W. The place of a nutrition care team in paediatric practice. *Int Ther Clin Monitor* 1990; **11:** 1232–1236.

129 O'Brien, D., Hodges, R.E., Day, A.T. Recommendations of a nutrition support team promote cost containment. *J Parenteral and Enteral Nutrition* 1986; **10:** 300–302.

130 Brown, R.D. Enteral nutrition support management in a university teaching hospital: team vs. non-team. *J Parenteral and Enteral Nutrition* 1987; **11:** 52–66.

131 Faubion, W., Wesley, J. Total parenteral nutrition catheter sepsis: impact of the team approach. *J Parenteral and Enteral Nutrition* 1986; **10:** 642–645.

Wound infection

A guide to detecting the presence of infection in wounds, with a discussion
of the most common bacteria species and prevention techniques

Skin wounds readily acquire bacteria because the presence of blood or serum at 37°C provides an excellent culture medium. Bacterial proliferation is further enhanced if devitalised tissue is also present.

The nature of bacteria detected in wounds depends on a variety of factors such as the workload of the treatment centre, the number and expertise of the staff, the arrangement of the treatment unit and the nature of the treatment provided.

Significance of bacteria in wounds
Wound bacteria may be transient, and detected on one occasion only or they may become established, and detectable on at least consecutive days. Established organisms often persist until the wound heals, unless there is therapeutic intervention[1]. Wounds colonised by non-pathogenic bacteria may more readily acquire pathogenic species[2].

A single bacteriological sample from a wound does not necessarily indicate that the wound is colonised, nor does it show whether the bacterial content is rising or falling; 10^5 bacteria per gram tissue is often considered a potentially infective level[2,3]. However, many wounds yield higher numbers, 10^7 to 10^8 per gram tissue, without exhibiting clinical signs of infection[4].

Diagnosis of wound sepsis is based on clinical criteria. Inflammation, together with peripheral cellulitis, is a typical sign; sometimes lymphangitis may also be present. When clinical infection has been diagnosed, treatment with suitable systemic antibiotics is desirable. Untreated wound infection may lead to lymphadenitis, bacteraemia, septicaemia and death.

Microscopy, culture and sensitivity of wound exudate will assist in prompt

J. C. Lawrence, PhD, CBiol, FBiol, is research director, Burns Research Group, Birmingham Accident Hospital, Birmingham

Infection

recognition of the offending organism, enabling prescription of the appropriate systemic antibiotic. Exceptionally, infection may be 'silent', with clinical evidence lacking until the patient shows signs of septicaemia. Bacteria may produce toxic metabolites, which can interfere with healing, or cause illness such as toxic shock syndrome.

Detection of bacteria
Perhaps the most effective way of sampling the bacterial flora of wounds is to obtain a specimen of the wound exudate: this is essential with deep wounds, because the infecting organism may be anaerobic. However, a commonly used and simple method is to rub a sterile swab over the wound surface, if the wound is moist. Using a standardised technique permits ap-

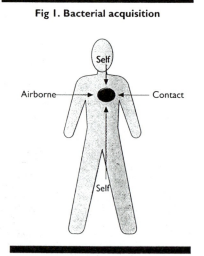

Fig I. Bacterial acquisition

proximate quantification; a dry wound may give a false impression of a low bacterial count.

The procedure for bacteriological sampling should include the following:

■ Two swabs should be taken from each wound at the time of sampling. Serum-tipped swabs supplied in sealed plastic tubes are used

■ Use of a cooked meat medium enables detection of anaerobes and also small numbers of bacteria that may not be revealed from the direct swab

■ Twist cap to break seal; remove swab and apply the tip to the wound surface, rub across the surface in a zig-zag manner, simultaneously rotating the swab between finger and thumb. Replace in tube and repeat the procedure with a second swab

■ One swab should be inserted into a cooked meat culture to about two-thirds of the container depth and the stick snapped such that the tip and part of the stick is left in the cooked meat container. This should be done as aseptically as possible; hold the cooked meat bottle in one hand and unscrew cap using index finger and thumb (if necessary loosen the cap first using both hands). The wooden stick usually breaks easily across the bottle rim

■ Clearly label both the cooked meat container and the unbroken swab with the patient's name, number, wound site and date

■ As far as may be practical keep used swabs as cool as possible. Cooked meat containers need protecting only from excessive heat.

No undue loss of bacteria occurs in such specimens over a 48-hour period provided that swabs are not exopsed to temperatures much above normal room temperature (about 20°C). Bacteria thrive in cooked meat medium and

CONTAMINATION

This five-year-old ulcer is heavily contaminated, but there is no sign of infection.

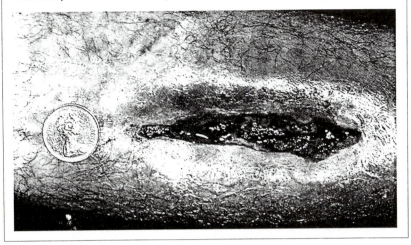

WOUND INFECTION

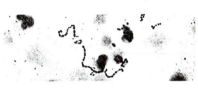

Streptococcus pyogenes: typical bead-like chains

DRESSINGS

Occlusive dressings protect the wound from environmental bacteria and reduce the level of airborne bacteria dispersal. Infection rates under occlusive dressings are significantly less than under traditional dry dressings.

TAKING A SWAB

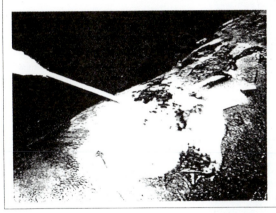

A sterile swab is rubbed over the wound surface of a burn injury, collecting exudate where possible. Surface swabbing of dry wounds can be assisted by the addition of culture medium or sterile sodium chloride 0.9%.

Swabs should be clearly labelled with the patient's name, number, wound site and date.

INTERPRETING RESULTS

NG = No growth (but there may be in liquid medium)

$\pm$ = Less than 30 colonies in zone 1 ($<10^5$ colony-forming units per gram of tissue)

+ = More than 30 colonies in zone 1 and growth just extending into zone 2 (about 10^6 colony-forming units per gram of tissue)

++ = Growth in zone 2 extending into zone 3 (about 10^6–10^7 colony-forming units per gram of tissue)

+++= Growth in zone 3 extending into zone 4 ($>10^7$ colony-forming units per gram of tissue)

Zone 5 enables separate colonies to develop in the event of growth being very dense.

CLEAN WOUND

Healthy granulation is visible in this scalp wound.

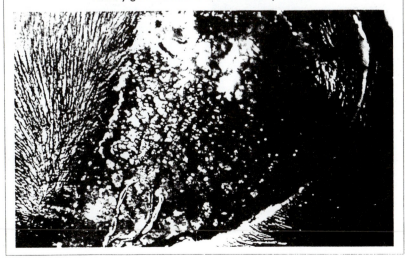

INCUBATION

The swab is inoculated onto an agar plate and into liquid culture medium to detect small numbers of bacteria that may be missed on plates. The swab is applied to zone 1, then successively spread, using sterile loops, to zones 2, 3, 4 and 5. After overnight incubation, bacterial growth is recorded.

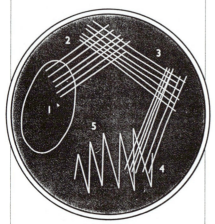

Below: *Staphylococcus aureus* on 4% blood agar plate

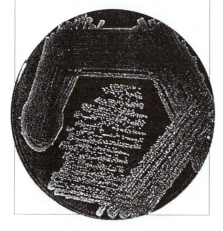

EFFECTIVE HAND HYGIENE

A simple but effective technique for hand disinfection

1. Take appropriate volume of antiseptic in the palm of one hand; rub hands together.
2. Interlace fingers while rubbing; move each palm over the dorsum of the opposite hand.
3. Interlace fingers palm to palm while rubbing.
4. Work knuckles of each hand into palm of opposite hand.
5. Rub each thumb with palm and fingers of the opposite hand.
6. Work fingertips of each hand into opposite palm.

Using aqueous solution, repeat three times before rinsing and drying with alcohol-based cleansers; repeat in sequence until hands are dry.

INFECTION

A burn infected with *Staphylococcus oureus* showing local cellulitis, septicaemia and bilateral lymphangitis

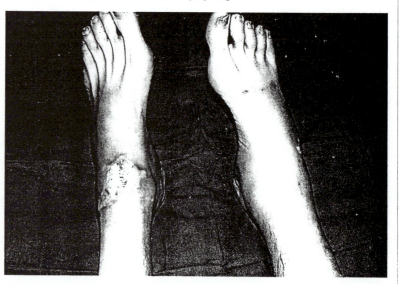

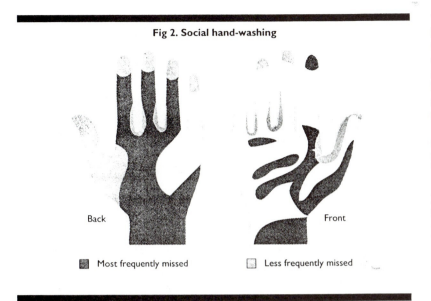

Fig 2. Social hand-washing

Back　　　　　　　　　　　Front

☐ Most frequently missed　　　☐ Less frequently missed

therefore no special precautions are needed. Investigation of a wound biopsy is an alternative method of overcoming the limitations of a superficial swab, but this invasive technique will inevitably disturb the wound.

All detected organisms should be identified, and antibiotic sensitivities obtained ('no growth' means 'no bacteria detected').

Routes of infection

Sources of a wide variety of bacteria are readily available and can reach skin wounds, or be dispersed from them by one or more main routes (Fig 1):
■ Self-contamination: for example, from the skin or gastrointestinal tract
■ Airborne contamination: for example, dust, skin squamae, water droplets
■ Contact: for example, clothing, equipment, helpers' hands.

Interrupting these routes provides the basis for infection control. Careful attention to sterility of equipment and a rigorous aseptic technique will minimise the risk of transferring bacteria by contact.

Irrigating wounds with antiseptics has little advantage over flushing with sodium chloride 0.9%[5], but antiseptics do have a role in disinfecting intact skin and the hands of health-care staff.

Hand hygiene

Hand-washing often misses important areas, especially the fingertips and thumbs[6] (Fig 2). A simple and effective technique has been devised to ensure thorough cleansing[7].

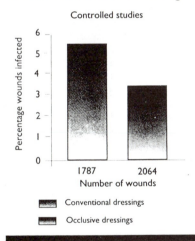

Fig 3. Wound infection rates under occlusive and non-occlusive dressings[12]

Controlled studies

Percentage wounds infected (y-axis: 0 to 6)

1787　2064
Number of wounds

▨ Conventional dressings
▨ Occlusive dressings

Airborne bacteria

Staff should be aware that significant airborne dispersal of bacteria can occur even from small wounds during dressing changes.

The level of bacteria dispersal is highest with dry dressings, but wet gauze dressings also liberate significant numbers of bacteria.

The problem can be markedly reduced by the use of hydrocolloids dressings, but this property has yet to be confirmed in other modern wound-care dressings.

The slow decline of airborne bacteria creates a potential cross-infection risk. This can be readily demonstrated by the use of settle plates.

The role of dressings

Dressings can provide antibacterial as well as physical protection to the wound. Traditional materials, such as cotton gauze and cotton wool, act as bacterial filters. However, once the exudate dampens the dressing, it ceases to provide any protection.

Applying an antibacterial substance at the wound interface may help to extend the life of the dressing, by containing bacteria[8-10].

Many modern dressings are occlusive, preventing environmental bacteria from reaching the wound[11]. Fears that such dressings would potentiate infection if used on colonised wounds have proved to be unjustified: infection rates under occlusive dressings are almost half those observed with traditional, non-occlusive dressings[12] (Fig 3).　■

REFERENCES
[1]Gilchrist, B., Reed, C. The bacteriology of leg ulcers under hydrocolloid dressings. Br J Derm 1989; 121: 337–344.
[2]Bornside, G.H., Bornside, B.B. Comparison between moist swab and tissue biopsy methods for quantitation of bacteria in experimental incisional wounds. J Trauma 1979; 19: 103–105.
[3]Pruitt, B.A. The diagnosis and treatment of infection in the burned patient. Burns 1984; 11: 79–81.
[4]Lookingbill, D.P., Miller, S.H., Knowles, R.C. Bacteriology of leg ulcers. Arch Derm 1978; 114: 1765–1768.
[5]Stringer, M., Lawrence, J.C., Lilly, H.A. Antiseptics and the casualty wound. J Hosp Infect 1983; 4: 410–413.
[6]Taylor, L.J. Evaluation of hand-washing techniques. Nurs Times 1978; 74: 2, 54–55.
[7]Ayliffe, G.A.J., Babb, J.R., Quorishi, A.H. A test for 'hygienic' hand disinfection. J Clin Path 1978; 31: 923–928.
[8]Lawrence, J.C. The treatment of small burns with a chlorhexidine-medicated tulle gras. Burns 1977; 3: 239–244.
[9]Lawrence, J.C. The bacteriology of burns. J Hosp Infect 1985; 6: 3–17.
[10]Mertz, P.M., Marshall, D.A., Eaglstein, W.H. Occlusive wound dressings to prevent bacterial invasion and wound infection. J Am Acad Derm 1985; 12: 662–668.
[11]Lawrence, J.C. Bacterial barrier properties of dressings. Pharm J 1990; 245: 695–697.
[12]Hutchinson, J.J., Lawrence, J.C. Wound infection under occlusive dressings. J Hosp Infect 1991; 17: 83–94.

BIBLIOGRAPHY
Dunn, L.J., Wilson, P. Evaluating the permeability of hydrocolloid dressings to multi-resistant Staphylococcus aureus. Pharm J 1990; 245: 248–250.
Sleigh, J.D., Timbury, M.C. Notes on Medical Microbiology (2nd edn). Edinburgh: Churchill Livingstone, 1986.
Selwyn, S., Ellis, H. Skin bacteria and disinfection reconsidered. Br Med J 1972; 1: 136–140.
Meers, P.D., Ayliffe, G.A.J., Emmerson, A.M. et al. Report on the national survey of infection in hospital. J Hosp Infect 1981; 2: (supplement).
Wilson, P., Burroughs, D., Dunn, L. Methicillin-resistant Staphylococcus aureus and hydrocolloid dressings. Pharm J 1988; 239: 184.
Lawrence, J.C. What materials for dressings? Injury 1982; 13: 500–512.
Lawrence, J.C. Infection control in burns. In: Bailliere's Clinical Anaesthesiology 1987; 1: 673–691.

Common problems in wound care: wound and ulcer measurement

Kathryn Vowden

Accurate measurement is an important part of wound assessment. Wounds vary considerably in their nature, shape and site. Many measurement techniques exist. It is important to choose the correct technique for a specific wound and to understand the degree of accuracy obtained from the measurements.

Kathryn Vowden is Clinical Nurse Specialist (Vascular) at the Bradford Royal Infirmary, Duckworth Lane, Bradford

The NHS guidelines for the assessment of skin ulcers (Morgan, 1987) identifies the need for objective, non-contact measurement. Quantitative methods to characterise the rate of wound healing are essential for evaluating the response to new wound therapies. Studies of wound healing have been hampered by the lack of objective methods of measurement that can safely and ethically be applied to humans (Ahroni et al, 1992). They also stress the inaccuracy of common ward practice which uses crude subjective or contact methods for estimating skin ulcer size.

Measurement serves three purposes (*Table 1*). The degree of accuracy demanded varies for each task and requires different measuring tools. The accuracy of

measurement of an area and/or volume of a wound will depend largely on the position of that wound and the technique used. For example, a wound on a convex surface will need a different approach from a wound on a concave surface, a cavity wound or an undermining wound or sinus (Ahroni et al, 1992). Irrespective of whether the shape of the cavity is good, all wounds will require some form of measurement (Bale, 1993). *Table 2* sets out the measurement techniques available.

Area measurement

Linear measurement

Most nurses do not have access to sophisticated measuring devices. The most common method of calculating area is by measuring the length and width of the wound. Although imprecise, linear measurements provide an objective basis for evaluating the overall wound dimensions (Bryant, 1992). They also allow calculation (*Figure 1*) of the area of the wound, although this can be inaccurate (Majeske, 1992; Morrison, 1992). Dealey (1994) acknowledges this inaccuracy and suggests that this method should only be used for regular-shaped wounds. Consistency in technique does improve accuracy.

Tracing

Open wounds can also be measured by tracing the perimeter onto a clear film or acetate (Dealey, 1994). This can be a simple transparent sheet with or without a grid. Two-layer versions are available. The tracing is made on the upper layer, and the lower layer, which has been in contact with the wound, and is then discarded. The next stage is to transfer the tracing to graph paper.

Majeske (1992) compared different methods of calculating area, including counting 1 mm squares within the perimeter of the tracing (*Figure 1*). She reported that this method can be incorporated into

Table 1. Purposes of wound measurement
To document progress in an individual wound as part of treatment and assessment
To assess the efficacy in terms of wound healing of a dressing or drug therapy
To predict healing time

Table 2. Wound and ulcer measurement techniques	
Contact	Tracing: overlays and contour
	Depth gauges
	Volume: moulding or liquid
Non-contact	Photography
	Stereophotogrammetry
	Video-image analysis
	Structured light
	Laser triangulation

clinical practice as it is easy to use and low in cost. Counting squares can, however, be tedious and time-consuming — it may take 10 minutes to calculate the area of a 70 cm² ulcer.

A hand-held planimeter is a quick, portable and accurate alternative method of calculating the area of an open wound (Majeske, 1992). A digitiser can partially automate the process but a computer is required to translate the wound edge to area (Stacey et al, 1991). Both are subject to human error during data entry (Anthony, 1985). *Figure 1* compares the results of wound area measurement using different techniques.

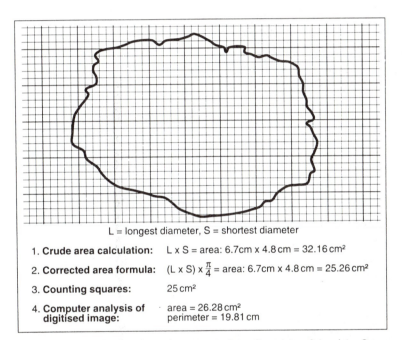

L = longest diameter, S = shortest diameter

1. **Crude area calculation:** L x S = area: 6.7cm x 4.8 cm = 32.16 cm²

2. **Corrected area formula:** (L x S) x $\frac{\pi}{4}$ = area: 6.7cm x 4.8 cm = 25.26 cm²

3. **Counting squares:** 25 cm²

4. **Computer analysis of digitised image:** area = 26.28 cm²
   perimeter = 19.81 cm

Figure 1. Acetate tracing of a venous leg ulcer transferred to 2 mm graph paper. Four area calculation methods are illustrated.

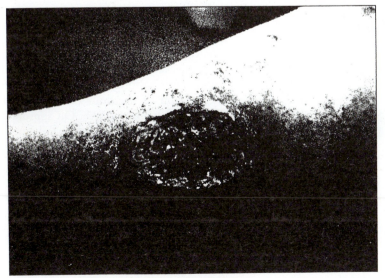

Figure 2a. Standard photograph including ruler.

Photograpy

Tracings and linear measurements involve wound contact. Photography provides a popular non-contact method of measuring area and healing. Comparable measurements can be obtained using both systems (Etris et al, 1994) (*Figure 2*). Information obtained from a series of photographs can also be used to evaluate colour changes and the condition of the wound bed.

However, standardised conditions must be used, including lighting, focal distance and camera angle (Ahroni et al, 1992; Boardman et al, 1994). Minns and Whittle (1992) reported fitting a frame to a Polaroid camera to give a constant focal distance and to help prevent change in the angle. Other cameras have a fitted measuring cord to predetermine the distance from the wound. Polaroid's HealthCam System camera produces a fixed focal length by aligning two light beams. Polaroid GridFilm allows the photographic image to be superimposed onto a grid (Wallace, 1994) which can be used to calculate wound area (*Figure 2b*). So far there are no comparative studies on the accuracy of what appears to be an effective method.

Volume measurement

Linear measurement

The techniques discussed so far are limited to biplanar (width and breadth) measurements and take no account of wound depth. Most wounds are on curved surfaces or over bony prominences and will therefore require a three-dimensional perspective (Frantz and Johnson, 1992). A sterile probe or gauge can be used to estimate the maximum wound depth (Covington et al, 1989; Thomas and Wysocki, 1990; Bale, 1993). This technique is clearly open to user bias (Covington et al, 1989).

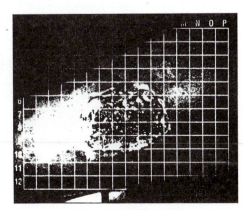

Figure 2b. Polaroid GridFilm image of same ulcer using Light-Lock focus system.

In 1989, Kundin developed the wound gauge for measurement of length, width and depth of a wound. By using a mathematical formula the area (area = length x breadth x 0.785) and volume (volume = area x depth x 0.327) of the wound can be calculated (Kundin, 1989). Thomas and Wysocki (1990) have demonstrated that although the wound gauge is as reliable as photographs and tracings in the evaluation of small wounds, it consistently underestimated the size of larger and irregular-shaped wounds.

Casting

To overcome the inherent inaccuracies associated with a single-point estimation of wound depth, attempts have been made to measure wound volume by filling the cavity. Berg et al (1990) measured the volume of saline needed to fill a wound to skin level under a film. Pories et al (1966), Resch et al (1988) and Covington et al (1989) measured the volume of a cast which can be stored to provide a permanent record.

These techniques have recently been reviewed by Plassmann (1995). Although more accurate than ruler-based measurements, the techniques are still subject to significant error. The cast formed by some dressings, e.g. Cavi-Care, can also be used to measure the volume of cavity wounds. However, these techniques are not very practical (Bryant, 1992; Johnson, 1993).

Photography, structured light and laser techniques

Photographic techniques can be enhanced to allow measurement of wound volume as well as area. Stereophotogrammetry pro-vides a three-dimensional picture from two photographs taken simultaneously from different angles. The images obtained can be measured (Dealey, 1994). Bulstrode et al (1986) have demonstrated that the results with such a camera system are 5–10 times more accurate than those obtained with direct tracing and simple photography.

Video systems provide area and volume measurement from a digitised, colour videogram (Smith et al, 1992). Extra data, such as maximum depth and perimeter, can also be calculated. In addition, the system can be used to quantify acetate tracings to give the area of an ulcer (Palmer et al, 1989; Ring, 1994).

Colour analysis is possible with this method and other photographic systems. van Riet Paap et al (1991), Mekkes et al (1993) and Boardman et al (1994) consider that the colour is more important than wound size when evaluating the cleansing and debriding effects of treatments, indicating the biological condition of the wound.

Plassman and Jones (1992) and Plassmann et al (1993) recorded a digital image of a series of parallel stripes of light projected onto the surface of a wound downloaded to a computer. A graphical representation of the wound was generated from this and the area and volume were calculated. Melhuish et al (1994a,b) used this technique to obtain serial measurements of wound area and volume. He noted that the results were dependent on the patient's positioning, thus a constant measuring routine is important.

A computer-generated, three-dimensional image of the wound (*Figure 3*) can also be produced by laser triangulation using a displacement image (Ibbett et al, 1994; Patete and Smith, 1994). As with all non-contact methods of measurement, errors are most commonly a result of the need to reconstruct the normal skin surface (Ibbett et al, 1994). Non-contact measurement tools cannot cope with undermining. The opening on the skin surface must be sufficiently large to allow illumination of the floor of the wound (Frantz and Johnson, 1992). On appropriately shaped cavity wounds, these techniques are more accurate than casting and ruler-based measurements (Plassmann, 1995).

Conclusions

When assessing a single wound, nurses require a quick, cost-effective method of documenting wound progress. This documentation is best obtained by a combination of tracing, photography and depth measurement. The more expensive

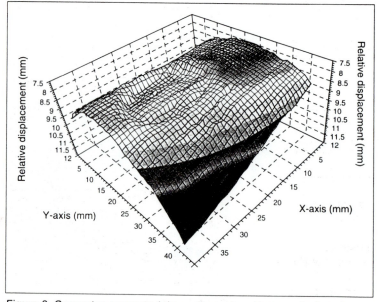

Figure 3. Computer-generated three-dimensional image of a leg ulcer.

research techniques of laser triangulation and stereophotography are more appropriate to comparative studies on wound healing and dressing assessment. Casting techniques have not been widely adopted as they are inappropriate for shallow simple wounds or undermined wounds from which the cast cannot be safely removed.

It is important to understand that the data may be interpreted in different ways. Gilman (1990) and Quinlan and Cooper (1994) have shown that different analyses of the same data can give conflicting results. Many studies rely on healing rates or a reduction in wound size to justify treatment (Quinlan and Cooper, 1994).

Clearly, an understanding of the methods of measurement used is necessary when reading research papers. It is difficult to standardise wound measurement as each situation requires a different technique. In order to critically evaluate and understand the findings of research studies on wound healing it is important to understand the limitations of the measuring systems used by the authors. 🄱🄽

Ahroni JH, Boyko EJ, Pecoraro RE (1992) Reliability of computerised wound surface area determinations. *Wounds: A Compendium of Clinical Research and Practice* 4(4): 133–7

Anthony D (1985) Measuring pressure sores. *Nurs Times* 81(29 May): 57–61

Bale S (1993) Wound assessment. *Surg Nurse* 6(1): 11–4

Berg W, Traneroth C, Gunnarsson A, Lossing C (1990) A method for measuring pressure sores. *Lancet* 335: 1445–6

Boardman M, Melhuish JM, Palmer K, Harding KG (1994) Hue, saturation and intensity in the healing wound image. *J Wound Care* 3(7): 314–9

Bryant RA (1992) *Acute and Chronic Wounds: Nursing Management.* Mosby Year Book, St Louis, Missouri: 75–809

Bulstrode CJK, Goode AW, Scott PJ (1986) Stereophotogrammetry for measuring rates of cutaneous healing: a comparison with conventional techniques. *Clin Sci* 71: 437–44

Covington JS, Griffin JW, Mendiius RK, Tooms RE, Clifft JK (1989) Measurement of pressure ulcer volume using dental impression materials: suggestion from the field. *Phys Ther* 69(8): 690–3

Dealey C (1994) *The Care of Wounds.* Blackwell Scientific Publications, Oxford: 76–80

Ertris MB, Pribbles J, LaBrecque J (1994) Evaluation of two wound measurement methods in a multicenter, controlled study. *Wounds: A Compendium of Clinical Research and Practice* 6(3): 107–11

Frantz RA, Johnson DA (1992) Stereophotography and computerised image analysis: A three-dimensional method of measuring wound healing. *Wounds: A Compendium of Clinical Research and Practice* 4(2): 58–64

Gilman TH (1990) Parameter for measurement of wound closure. *Wounds: A Compendium of Clinical Research and Practice* 2(3): 95–101

Ibbett DA, Dugdale RE, Hart GC, Vowden KR, Vowden P (1994) Measuring leg ulcers using a laser displacement sensor. *Physiol Measure* 15: 325–32

Johnson A (1993) Wound assessment. *Wound Management* 4(1): 27–30

Kundin JI (1989) A new way to size up a wound. *Am J Nurs* 89: 206–7

Majeske C (1992) Reliability of wound surface area measurements. *Phys Ther* 72(2): 138–41

Mekkes JR, Westerhof W, van Riet Paap E, Estevez O (1993) A new computer image analysis system designed for evaluating wound debriding products. In: Harding KG, Cherry G, Dealey C, Turner TD, eds. *Proceedings of the 2nd European Conference on Advances in Wound Management.* Macmillan Magazines, London: 4–7

Melhuish JM, Plassmann P, Harding KG (1994a) Circumference, area and volume of the healing wound. *J Wound Care* 3(8): 380–4

Melhuish JM, Plassmann P, Harding KG (1994b) Volume and circumference of the healing wound. In: Harding KG, Dealey C, Cherry G, Gottrup F, eds. *Proceedings of the 3rd European Conference on Advances in Wound Management.* Macmillan Magazines, London: 41–4

Minns J, Whittle D (1992) A simple photographic recording system for pressure sore assessment. *J Tissue Viability* 2(4): 126

Morgan DA (1987) *The Care and Management of Leg Ulcers — A Guide for Health Care Staff.* 2nd edn. Whitechurch Hospital, Cardiff

Morrison M (1992) *A Colour Guide to the Nursing Management of Wounds.* Wolfe Publishing, London: 28–30

Palmer RM, Ring EFJ, Ledgard L (1989) A digital video technique for radiographs and monitoring ulcers. *J Photographic Science* 37: 65–7

Patete P, Smith D (1994) Abstract: A non-invasive 3-dimensional diagnostic sound/laser imaging system for precise analysis of wounds. *Wound Repair and Regeneration* 2: 1, 88

Plassmann P (1995) Measuring wounds: a guide to the use of wound measurement techniques. *J Wound Care* 4(6): 269–72

Plassmann P, Jones BF (1992) Measuring leg ulcers by colour-coded structured light. *J Wound Care* 1(3): 35–8

Plassmann P, Jones BF, Ring EFJ (1993) Assessment of a non-contact instrument to measure the volume of leg ulcers. In: Harding KG, Cherry G, Dealey C, Turner TD, eds. *Proceedings of the 2nd European Conference on Advances in Wound Management.* Macmillan Magazines, London: 23–6

Pories WJ, Schear EW, Jordan DR et al (1966) The measurement of human wound healing. *Surgery* 59(5): 821–4

Quinlan D, Cooper PJ (1994) Endpoints in leg ulcer healing studies — is reduction in ulcer size a valid measure for proving treatment efficacy? (Poster: Wound Care 94 Conference, Harrogate)

Resch CS, Kerner E, Robson MC et al (1988) Pressure sore volume measurement: a technique to document and record wound healing. *J Am Geriatr Soc* 36: 444–6

Ring EFJ (1994) *Abstract: Electronic Imaging Techniques for Evaluating Peripheral Arterial Disease.* 18th European Conference on Microcirculation, Rome

Smith DJ, Bhat S, Bulgrin JP (1992) Video image analysis of wound repair. *Wounds: A Compendium of Clinical Research and Practice* 4(1): 6–15

Stacey MC, Burnand KG, Layer GT, Pattison M, Browse NL (1991) Measurement of the healing of venous ulcers. *Aust N Z J Surg* 61(11): 844–8

Thomas AC, Wysocki AB (1990) The healing wound: a comparison of three clinically useful methods of measurement. *Decubitus* 3: 18–25

van Riet Paap E, Mekkes JR, Westerhof EW (1991) A new colour video image analysis system for the objective assessment of wound healing in secondary healing ulcers. *Wounds: A Compendium of Clinical Research and Practice* 3(1): 41

Wallace P, ed (1994) *Polaroid Instant Record.* Wordpower Publishing, Welwyn

---

KEY POINTS

- **Measurement is an important part of wound assessment. Nurses require a quick, cost-effective method of documenting wound progress.**

- **Measurement techniques vary in their accuracy and applicability. It is important to realise this when choosing a measurement tool.**

- **Different answers can be obtained from the same data by changing the method of calculation.**

PRESSURE SORE RISK ASSESSMENT.

Introduction

For over 30 years the identification of risk factors has helped health professionals understand in more detail the complex aetiology of pressure sore formation, yet there is little evidence to suggest that the incidence of pressure sores or their treatment has dramatically improved. To prevent pressure sores, the risk status of an individual must be determined so that any predisposing factors can be reduced by early intervention. The most consistently cited factors contributing to pressure sore development include incontinence, inactivity, restricted mobility, nutritional status and mechanical factors such as friction/shear (Sparks 1993). Pressure sore risk assessment scales represent an attempt to determine an individual's risk status by quantifying a range of the most commonly recognised risk factors affecting the patient at a given time. This article describes some of the more commonly used risk assessment scales and attempts to evaluate their application to clinical practice.

Numerous risk assessment scales exist, but the reported sensitivity and specificity varies enormously. This variability is probably reflected in the differences in study methodology, clinical settings and patient populations. The ideal risk assessment tool needs to demonstrate good predictive value, high sensitivity and specificity and be simple to use (National Pressure Ulcer Advisory Panel 1989). **Specificity** is defined as the percentage of patients who do not develop pressure sores and were predicted not to, and **sensitivity** is the percentage of patients who develop sores and were predicted to do so (Polit and Hungler 1993). An ideal pressure sore risk calculator would be both 100% specific and 100% sensitive, however in reality this is not possible as sensitivity and specificity have an inverse relationship, one can only be improved at the expense of the other (Clark and Farrar 1992).

Despite limitations, risk assessment scales are a very useful and practical method of encouraging the systematic evaluation of individual patient's risk factors. However, because the general condition of a patient is not static, neither is their risk status, therefore re-assessement is necessary each time the patient's condition changes. Unfortunately the frequency with which such re-evaluation needs to be performed is undefined and will vary between difference practice settings. Thorough documentation of pressure sore risk assessment helps to ensure that nursing interventions are individualised and that continuity of the delivery of appropriate care is maintained. The use of risk assessment scales also facilitates clinical decision making by strengthening requests for pressure-relieving support systems.

The Norton Score

Norton et al developed the first recognised pressure sore risk assessement score in 1962 as a result of research into the largely unexplored area of pressure sore aetiology (figure 1). This now familiar rating scale was initially developed as part of a research project to monitor the most commonly occuring predisposing factors to pressure sore development. At this time, five risk factors were identified as being significant: general physical condition, mental state, activity, mobility and incontinence. Each is given a rating of between 1 and 4, the maximum patient score is 20, whilst the minimum is 5. A score of 14 was originally considered by Norton et al (1962) to be indicitave of risk status. However recent work by Clark and Farrar (1992) demonstrates that in their study, the threshold score discriminating between risk or risk free status should be more accurately re-defined as 13. Norton et al (1962) were able to demonstrate that pressure sore development in a group of 100 patients was significantly reduced when the Scale was used to predict risk status and early preventative intervention was implemented. They reported a sensitivity of 62.7%, a specificity of 69.9% and a predictive value of 38.9% when used on admission on elderly patients. Dealy (1989) compared the sensitivity and specificity of the Norton and Waterlow scores, although the Waterlow score appeared to be more sensitive, it was less specific. The Norton scale has been criticised on numerous occasions and its relevance to other clinical settings, in particular acute care environments has been questioned (Goldstone and Goldstone 1982). There are various reasons why this may be so, one being that this work needs to be considered within the context of time and the speciality in which it was developed; in the early 1960's it was relatively unusual for this patient group to be undergoing surgical procedures. So that the important influence of the immediate post-operative period on the development of presure sores was not taken into consideration.

Inter-rater reliability has also been demonstrated as a problem, it is now widely recognised that the rating criteria in each of the five sub-groups is generally too ambiguous for truly objective ratings. The Norton scale does not include nutritional status, which more subsequent risk assessment scales do, as Norton assumed that this important factor would be taken into consideration under the category of general physical condition. Despite various criticism, this scoring system is perhaps still the most familiar to practitioners, it's popularity, no doubt enhanced by it's ease of use. However it is regarded by many to be too simplistic and unable to accurately predict risk status in today's complex health care enviroment.

The Gosnell Scale

This scale (figure 2) was developed in 1973 in the USA (Gosnell 1973) and was based upon the earlier work of Norton (1962). Nutritional status was added as an assessment criteria and data concerning admission, discharge, medical disgnosis and demographic details were also included. Further additions to this rating scale were the inclusion of skin appearance, height, weight, vital signs and medications. Criteria guidelines were formulated for each of the possible rating scores as well as for any additional items on the scale. Gosnell identified that the additional factors of diastolic blood pressure below 60mmHg and a raised body temperature were significant in predicting pressure sore risk status, The original Gosnell Scale was revised in 1987 and again in 1988. The initial scoring of five risk factors - mental status, continence, mobility, activity, and nutrition were reversed so that the higher the score, indicated the greater risk of pressure sore development. The category describing skin appearance was expanded to include moisture, temperature, colour and texture. Other important modifications included the addition of a 24 hour fluid balance category. These changes resulted in a possible risk factor score of between 5 and 20: the higher the score, the higher the patient's risk status. The revised Gosnell score has since been evaluated positively in acute settings in the USA and it has been successfully incorporated into the admission procedure at many hospitals in the United States.

The Waterlow Pressure Sore Prevention Treatment Policy

The Waterlow Pressure Sore Prevention Treatment Policy (figure 3) was developed as a result of a pressure sore audit (Standing 1985). It was designed to be more than a risk assessment tool and offers guidelines on the selection and use of preventative equipment and dressings together with a pressure sore classification model which can help to improve consistency when grading and auditing tissue breakdown. This risk assessment scale was developed to be comprehensive enough to be relevant in both medical and surgical settings. The predisposing factors included in this rating scale are; build/weight, continence, skin type, mobility, sex, age and appetite. The additional of a special risk category which is sub-divided into tissure malnutrition, neurological deficit, major surgery/trauma and medication allows the carer to make a detailed assessment of these factors and if necessary award several scores within each of these categories in order to reflect accurately the patient's true risk status. It is therefore difficult to predict the maximum score possible for an individual patient, however a score of over 20 is recognised as being 'very high risk'. Scores of between 15-20 indicate 'high risk', whilst a score of over 10 indicates that the patient is 'at risk'. The predictive value of the Waterlow scale has been questioned, many claim that it over predicts risk status and for this reason its usefulness in some care settings has been questioned (Wardman 1991, Dealy 1989). In care of the elderly settings, many patients will be identified as at risk, having a score greater than 10, without a significant number going on to develop pressure sores. Indeed Clark and Farrar (1992) in a comparative study of risk assessment scales were able to demonstrate that 57% of patients who progressed from being risk free to at risk did not go on to develop sores. Waterlow designed this assessment tool to meet a variety of clinical situations and encourages those that use the scale to give feedback in order that this assesment tool can be developed further. A major advantage of this scoring system is that it differentiates between 'at risk', high risk, and 'very high risk' status and offers guidelines for the carer on general prevenatative and treatment guidelines which were updated in 1992 to include generic names of dressing products.

It is interesting to note that many carers using this score are in fact still working from the outdated version! The Waterlow Scale has done much to raise awareness of pressure sore prevention and offers practical guidelines for the management of patients, which explains it's popularity as a method of risk assessment. It remains at present the most widely used risk assessment tool in the UK.

The Braden Scale

The Braden risk assessment score was developed in America in 1986 by Braden and Bergstrom, who were reviewing nursing practices in nursing homes., The Braden scale consists of six predisposing factors; sensory perception, moisture, activity, mobility, nutrition and finally friction/shear. Included in this scoring system are specific assessment criteria for each of the risk factors described (figure 4), In both categories describing sensory perception and nutritional status, there is a second range of potential responses which improves reliability by reducing user ambiguity. The nutrition section is a good example of how specific this scoring system is without being too complicated. Carers are able to identify patients who are receiving tube feeds, parental nutrition, or simple intravenous support. The sections describing friction/shear and moisture recognise the importance of these factors in contributing to tissue breakdown and reminds the carer of relevant practical considerations. Most of the identified risk factors area awarded a rating of between 1 (least favourable) to 4 (most favourable) except friction/shear which can be given a maximum rating of 3. The maximum score possible is 23, indicating low risk status, whilst the minimum score is 6, indicating a high risk patient. Patients with a score of 16 or less were originally considered to be at risk of developing pressure sores. Subsequent studies suggest that t threshold score of 15 would increase sensitivity and specificity (Clark and Farrar 1992). However the validity of 16 as an indicator of risk status has been verified by Bergstrom (1987) in the intensive care setting, taking 16 as the cut-off score indicating risk, the reported sensitivity was 83% and specificity 64%. The Braden scale is used extensively in a variety of care settings in the USA and has generally demonstrated greater specificity and sensitivity than other risk assessment scales.

The Pressure Sore Prediction Scale

The Pressure Sore Prevention Score (PSPS) was initially developed in 1975 and published in 1987 by Lowthian (figure 5). It was first used in an orthopaedic setting and has since been implemented in a variety of clinical areas. The score constitutes the use of a simple 6-point questionnaire which asks the following key questions about the condition of the patient;

1)   Sitting up? (long time)
2)   Unconscious?
3)   Poor general condition?
4)   Incontinent?
5)   Lifts up?
6)   Gets up and walks?

For the first four questions, a definite 'no' answer scores nil, whilst a definite 'yes' scores 3 points; intermediate answers of 'yes or no, but' may be awarded a discretionary score of 1 or 2 and for the final two questions, a definite 'no', scores 2 points and a 'yes' scores nil. Although initially confusing this system is quickly understood even by inexperienced staff (Lowthian 1987). A score of 6 or more was considered by Lowthian to be indicitave of pressure sore risk. The questions 'sitting up' and lifts up' were based on research that indicated that prolonged periods of sitting in either bed or chair was a previously unrecognised causative factor important in the development of pressure sores. The answers to these six patient oriented questions can be easily ascertained by most carers, however objectivity can be increased further by using the 'category examples' (figure 3) which would be adaped relatively easily to include specific conditions/criteria relevant to specialist areas of practice. These 'category examples' are particularly useful whilst getting familiar with this scoring system for the first time. A valuable addition to this score is the inclusion of suggested patient support surfaces together with details of the pressure sore classification model used in conjunction with the PSPS which utilised a 0 to 5 grading system. PSPS admission scores have been shown to have a high degree of 'sensitivity', predicting between 86-89% of patients who subsequently developed pressure sores within 3 weeks of admission (Lowthian 1987, 1989), making the PSPS more successful in orthopaedic areas, than the Norton score is in care of the elderly settings. The findings of Clark and Farrar (1992) suggest that PSPS would be similarly effective in medical wards.

(fig1)   **NORTON SCALE**

NORTON RISK ASSESSMENT SCALE

		Physical Condition	Mental Condition	Activity	Mobility	Incontinent	TOTAL SCORE
		Good 4	Alert 4	Ambulant 4	Full 4	Not 4	
		Fair 3	Apathetic 3	Walk/help 3	Sl. limited 3	Occasional 3	
		Poor 2	Confused 2	Chairbound 2	V. limited 2	Usually/Urine 2	
		Very Bad 1	Stupor 1	Bed 1	Immobile 1	Doubly 1	
Name	Date						

Reprinted with permission, Norton D, McLaren R, and Exton-Smith AN: An investigation of geriatric nursing problems in hospital, 1962, reissue 1975, Churchill Livingstone, Edinburgh.

(fig 2)   **Gosnell Scale**

PRESSURE SORE RISK ASSESSMENT

I.D _____

Age _____ Sex _____

Height _____ Weight _____

Date of Admission _____

Date of Discharge _____

Medical Diagnosis:

Primary _____

Secondary _____

Nursing Diagnosis _____

_____

_____

Instructions: Complete all categories within 24 hours of admission and every other day thereafter. Refer to the accompanying guidelines for specific rating details.

DATE	Mental status	Continence:	Mobility:	Activity:	Nutrition:	TOTAL SCORE
	1. Alert 2. Apathetic 3. Confused 4. Stuporous 5. Unconscious	1. Fully controlled 2. Usually controlled 3. Minimally controlled 4. Absence of control	1. Full 2. Slightly limited 3. Very limited 4. Immobile	1. Ambulatory 2. Walks with assistance 3. Chairfast 4. Bedfast	1. Good 2. Fair 3. Poor	

Date	T	P	R	BP	Diet	Intake	Output	COLOR 1. Pallor 2. Mottled 3. Pink 4. Ashen 5. Ruddy 6 Cyanotic 7. Jaundice 8. Other	Moisture 1. Dry 2. Damp 3. Oily 4. Other	Temp 1. Cold 2. Cool 3. Warm 4. Hot	Texture 1. Smooth 2. Rough 3. Thin/ Transp 4. Scaly 5. Crusty 6. Other	No	Yes	Describe
	Vital Signs					24-Hour Fluid Balance		COLOR	GENERAL SKIN APPEARANCE			Interventions		

PRESSURE SORE RISK ASSESSMENT
MEDICATION PROFILE

Medication	Dosage	Frequency	Route	Date Begun	Date Discon.

© 1988 Davina Gosnell

Suggested flow sheets for monitoring data

GOSNELL SCALE

GUIDELINES FOR NUMERICAL RATING OF THE DEFINED CATEGORIES

Rating	1	2	3	4	5
Mental Status: An assessment of one's level of response to his environment.	**Alert:** Oriented to time. place. and person. Responsive to all stimuli. and understands explanations.	**Apathetic:** Lethargic, forgetful, drowsy, passive, and dull. Sluggish depressed. Able to obey simple commands. Possibly disoriented to time.	**Confused:** Partial and/or intermittent disorientation to transpulmonary pressure. Purposeless response to stimuli. Restless, aggressive, irritable, anxious and may require tranqualizers or sedatives.	**Stuporous:** Total disorientation. Does not respond to name, simple commands or verbal stimuli.	**Unconscious:** Nonresponsive to painful stimuli.
Continence: The amount of bodily control of urination and defecation.	**Fully Controlled:** Total control of urine and faeces.	**Usually Controlled** incontinent of urine and/or of faeces not more often than once. q 48 hrs. OR has Foley catheter and is incontinent of faeces.	**Minimally Controlled:** Incontinent of urine or faeces at least once q 24 hrs.	**Absence of Control:** Consistently incontinent of both urine and faeces.	
Mobility: The amount and control of movement of one's body.	**Full:** Able to control and move all extremities at will. May require the use of a device but turns, lifts, pulls, balances, and attains sitting position at will.	**Slightly Limited:** Able to control and move all extremities but a degree of limitation is present. Requires assistance of another person to turn, pull, balance, and/or attain a sitting position at will but self-initiates movement or request for help to move.	**Very Limited:** Can assist another person who must initiate movement via turning, lifting, pulling, balancing, and/or attaining a sitting position (contractures, paralysis may be present.)	**Immobile:** Does not assist self in any way to change position. Is unable to change position without assistance. Is completely dependent on others for movement.	
Activity: The ability of an individual to ambulate.	**Ambulatory:** Is able to walk unassisted. Rises from bed unassisted. With the use of a device such as cane or walker is able to ambulate without the assistance of another person.	**Walks with Help:** Able to ambulate with assistance of another person, braces, or crutches. May have limitation of stairs.	**Chairfast:** Ambulates only to chair, requires assistance to do so OR is confined to a wheelchair.	**Bedfast:** Is confined to bed during entire 24 hours of the day.	
Nutrition The process of food intake.	Eats some food from each basic food category every day and the majority of each meal served OR is on tube feeding.	Occasionally refuses a meal or frequently leaves at least half of a meal.	Seldom eats a complete meal and only a few bites of food at a meal.		

Vital Signs:	The temperature, pulse, respiration, and blood pressure to be taken and recorded at the time of every assessment rating.
Skin appearance:	A description of observed skin characteristics: colour, moisture, temperature, and texture.
Diet:	Record the specific diet order.
24-hour fluid balance:	The amount of fluid intake and output during the previous 24-hour period should be recorded.
Interventions:	List all devices. measures and/or nursing care activity being used for the purpose of pressure sore prevention.
Medications:	List name, dosage, frequency, and route for all prescribed medications. If A PRN order, list the pattern for the period since last assessment.
Comments:	Use this space to add explanation or further detail regarding any of the previously recorded data, patient condition, etc. OR Describe anything which you believe to be of importance but not accounted for previously.

© 1988 Davina Gosnell

(fig 3) WATERLOW PRESSURE SORE PREVENTION/TREATMENT POLICY
RING SCORES IN TABLE, ADD TOTAL. SEVERAL SCORES PER CATEGORY CAN BE USED

BUILD/WEIGHT FOR HEIGHT	★	SKIN TYPE VISUAL VISUAL RISK AREAS	★	SEX AGE	★	SPECIAL RISKS	★
						TISSUE MALNUTRITION	★
AVERAGE	0	HEALTHY	0	MALE	1	eg: TERMINAL CACHEXIA	8
ABOVE AVERAGE	1	TISSUE PAPER	1	FEMALE	2	CARDIAC FAILURE	5
OBESE	2	DRY	1	14 - 49	1	PERIPHERAL VASCULAR	
BELOW AVERAGE	3	OEDEMATOUS	1	50 - 64	2	DISEASE	5
		CLAMMY (TEMP ↑)	1	65 - 74	3	ANAEMIA	2
CONTINENCE	★	DISCOLOURED	2	75 - 80	4	SMOKING	1
		BROKEN/SPOT	3	81+	5		
COMPLETE/ CATHETERISED	0					**NEUROLOGICAL DEFICIT**	★
OCCASION INCONT	1	**MOBILITY**	★	**APPETITE**	★	eg: DIABETES, M.S, CVA, MOTOR/SENSORY	
CATH/INCONTINENT OF FAECES	2	FULLY	0	AVERAGE	0	PARAPLEGIA	4 - 6
DOUBLY INCONT	3	RESTLESS/FIDGETY	1	POOR	1		
		APATHETIC	2	N.G. TUBE/		**MAJOR SURGERY/TRAUMA**	★
		RESTRICTED	3	FLUIDS ONLY	2		
		INERT/TRACTION	4	NBM/ANOREXIC	3	ORTHOPAEDIC BELOW WAIST, SPINAL	5
		CHAIRBOUND	5			ON TABLE > 2 HOURS	5

SCORE	10 + AT RISK	15 + HIGH RISK	20 + VERY HIGH RISK

MEDICATION	★
CYTOTOXICS, HIGH DOSE STEROIDS ANTI - INFLAMMATORY	4

© J Waterlow 1991 Revised March 1992
OBTAINABLE FROM: NEWTONS, CURLAND, TAUNTON, TA3 5SG

REMEMBER : TISSUE DAMAGE OFTEN STARTS PRIOR TO ADMISSION, IN CASUALTY, A SEATED PATIENT IS ALSO AT RISK

ASSESSMENT: (See Above) IF THE PATIENT FALLS INTO ANY OF THE RISK CATEGORIES THEN PREVENTATIVE NURSING IS REQUIRED.
A COMBINATION OF GOOD NURSING TECHNIQUES AND PREVENTATIVE AIDS WILL DEFINITELY BE NECESSARY.

PREVENTION

PREVENTATIVE AIDS:
Special Mattress/ Bed: 10+ Overlays or specialist foam mattresses
15+ Alternating pressure overlays, mattresses and bed systems.
20+ Bed Systems: Fluidised, bead, low air loss and alternating pressure mattresses.
Note: Preventative aids cover a wide spectrum of specialist features. Efficacy in the 20+ area should be judged on the basis of independent evidence.

Cushions: No patient should sit in a wheelchair without some form of cushioning. If nothing else is available - use the patient's own pillow.
10+ 4" Foam cushion.
15+ Specialist Gel and/or foam cushion.
20+ Cushion capable of adjustment to suit individual patient.

Bed Clothing: Avoid plastic draw sheets, inco pads and tightly tucked in sheets/sheet covers, especially when using Specialist bed and mattress overlay systems. Duvet- plus vapour permeable cover

NURSING CARE:
General: Frequent changes of position, lying or sitting Use of pillows?
Pain: Appropriate pain control
Nutrition: High Protein, vitamins, minerals
Patient Handling: Correct lifting technique Hoists Monkey Pole Transfer devices
Patient Comfort Aids: Real sheepskins Bed cradle
Operating Table/ Theatre/A&E Trolley: 4" cover plus adequate protection
Skin Care: General Hygiene, NO rubbing. Correct lifting and positioning. Cover with an appropriate dressing

IF TREATMENT IS REQUIRED, FIRST REMOVE PRESSURE

WOUND CLASSIFICATION:			
BLANCHING HYPERAEMIA	STAGE 1	Is wound RED?	NO → YES • Semi-permeable film hydrocolloid sheet
NON-BLANCHING HYPERAEMIA	STAGE 2	Is wound RED, clean but not healed?	NO → YES • Hydrocolloid, alginate, hydrogel, Silastic foam (deep)
ULCERATION PROGRESSES	STAGE 3	Is wound YELLOW/ infected/inflamed?	NO → YES • Alginate, hydrogel, hydrocolloid
ULCERATION EXTENDS	STAGE 4	Infected?	NO → YES • Alginate ribbon on rope, non adherent topical antimicrobial dressing, polysaccharide paste
INFECTIVE NECROSIS	STAGE 5	Is wound Black/ Necrotic	NO → YES • Debride-surgical excision, hydrocolloid, hydrogel, enzymatic treatment

(fig 4)   **BRADEN SCALE**

FOR PREDICTING PRESSURE SORE RISK

Patient's Name _____   Evaluator's Name _____   Date of Assessment _____

SENSORY PERCEPTION ability to respond meaningfully to pressure related discomfort.	**1 Completely Limited:** Unresponsive (does not moan, flinch or grasp) to painful stimuli, due to diminished level consciousness or sedation **OR** limited ability to feel pain over most of body surface.	**2. Very Limited:** Responds only to painful stimuli. Cannot communicate discomfort except by moaning or restlessness **OR** has a sensory impairment which limits ability to feel pain or discomfort in 1 or 2extremities.	**3. Slightly Limited:** Responds to verbal commands, but cannot always communicate discomfort or need to be turned. **OR** has some sensory impairment which limits ability to feel pain or discomfort in 1 or 2 extremities.	**4. No Impairment:** Responds to verbal commands. Has no sensory deficit which would limit ability to feel or voice pain or discomfort
MOISTURE degree to which skin is exposed to moisture	**1. Constantly Moist:** Skin is kept moist almost constantly by perspiration, urine, etc. Dampness is detected every time patient is moved or turned.	**2. Very Moist:** Skin is often, but not always moist. Linen must be changed at least once a shift.	**3. Occasionally Moist:** Skin is occasionally moist, requiring an extra linen change approximately once a day.	**4. Rarely Moist:** Skin is usually dry, linen only requires changing at routine intervals.
ACTIVITY degree of physical activity	**1. Bedbound:** Confined to bed.	**2.Chairbound:** Ability to walk severely limited or non-existent. Cannot bear own weight and / or must be assisted into chair or wheelchair.	**3. Walks Occasionally:** Walks occasionally during day, but to very short distances, with or without assistance. Spends majority of each shift in bed or chair.	**4. Walks Frequently:** Walks outside the room at least twice a day and inside room at least once every 2 hours during waking hours.
MOBILITY ability to change and control body position	**1. Completely Immobile:** Does not make even slight changes in body or extremity position without assistance.	**2. Very Limited:** Makes occasional slight changes in body or extremity position but unable to make frequent or significant changes independently.	**3. Slightly Limited:** Make frequent though slight changes in body or extremity position independently.	**4. No Limitations:** Makes major and frequent changes in position without assistance.
NUTRITION *usual* food intake pattern	**1. Very Poor:** Never eats a complete meal. Rarely eats more than 1/3 of any food offered. Eats 2 servings or less of protein (meat or dairy products) per day. Takes fluids poorly. Does not take a liquid dietary supplement **OR** is Nil By Mouth and/or maintained on clear liquids or IV's for more than 5 days.	**2. Probably Inadequate:** Rarely eats a complete meal and generally eats only about 1/2 of any food offered. Protein intake includes only 3 servings of meat or dairy products per day. Occasionally will take a dietary supplement **OR** receives less than optimum amount of liquid diet or tube feeding.	**3. Adequate:** Eats over half of most meals. Eats a total of 4 servings of proteins (meat, dairy products) each day. Occasionally will refuse a meal, but will usually take a supplement if offered **OR** is on tube feeding or TPN regimen which probably meets most of nutritional needs.	**4. Excellent:** Eats most of every meal. Never refuses a meal. Usually eats a total of 4 or more servings of meat and dairy products. Occasionally eats between meals. Does not require supplementation.
FRICTION AND SHEAR	**1.Problem:** Requires moderate to maximum assistance in moving. Complete lifting without sliding against sheets is impossible. Frequently slides down in bed or chair, requiring frequent repositioning with maximum assistance. Spasticity, contractures or agitation leads to almost constant friction	**2. Potential Problem:** Moves freely or requires minimum assistance. During a move skin problem slides to some extent against sheets, chairs restraints or other devices. Maintains relatively good position in chair or in bed most of the time but occasionally slides down.	**3. No apparent Problem:** Moves in bed and in chair independently and has sufficient muscle strength to lift up completely during move. Maintains good position in bed or chair at all times.	

(fig 5)

PRESSURE SORE PREVENTION AID	**PSPS**				PRESSURE SORE PREDICTION SCORE (1988)

		No	No but	Yes but	Yes
*	Sitting up? (long time)	(0	1	2	3)
'A'	Unconscious?	(0	1	2	3)
	Poor general condition	(0	1	2	3)
	Incontinent?	(0	1	2	3)

		YES	Yes & No	NO	
*	Lifts Up?	(0	1	2)	**TICK SCORES WITH FELT PEN**
'B'	Gets up and walks?	(0	1	2)	

* 'A' & 'B' - QUESTIONS ON STATE OF PATIENT NOW :

SEE NOTES BELOW

USUALLY, A TOTAL OF 6 OR MORE MEANS DANGER

NOTES ON THE PSPS

Score your answers by how you begin each question: **a)** in part 'A' a 'YES' answer gives the greatest risk (3) while 'YES but' gives less risk (2) and 'NO but' gives a slight risk (1)
b) in Part 'B' a 'NO' answer gives the greatest risk (2) while 'YES and NO' gives somewhat less risk

Sitting up (long time)	-Propped up in bed for long periods means a definite 'YES' answer. Sitting in a chair can be risky, but wheelchairs are not as bad as ordinary chairs for sitting long. On admission decide nursing position to be used.
Unconscious ?	- Mental confusion may qualify as a 'No but' answer
Poor General	- Tis may be severe/sudden illness, or a long standing disability (eg Paralysis) . A lack of response to pain suggests a poor condition, as also does great age.
Incontinent?	- The main point is how often the patient is wet underneath: although poor bladder? bowel control may also mean that the skin is not healthy. On admission discover if patient was incontinent in the last two days.
Lifts up	- When possible the patient is asked to try, without help from anyone else to 'Lift up'. A 'YES' answer means that the patient does lift his pelvis clear of the bed (or seat) at the time of asking.
Gets up and walks ?	- A 'Yes' answer implies normal, or nearly normal walking.

NB Unusual circumstances (in your nursing station) may call for a slight change in the PSPS danger level (eg if many sores are starting, and are unexpected reduce the danger level to 5)

Pressure sores are not bound to happen even if the PSPS is very high

GUIDELINE FOR MAIN SUPPORT (BEDS) TO USE ACCORDING TO THE PSPS

PSPS LEVEL (no sudden change likely)	SUGGESTED MAIN SUPPORT
0 - 6	Confirming mattress alone (stretch mattress cover)
7 - 9	Confirming mattress plus some pillows and/or 'Soft' overlay (eg fluffy sheepskin beneath the bottom sheet) : and regular manual turning.
9 - 11	'Very Soft' overlay (eg criss-cross cut foam, about 10 cm thick, under the bottom sheet) and regular manual turning; or a reliable 'Large-cell' alternating pressure air mattress; or a reliable 'Low pressure' air mattress.
11 - 16	A 'Special' bed (eg a low air loss bed, or the 'Therapulse air bed). Some very high risk patients may need an air fluidised bed system.
	NB Patients with sores (grades 1 to 5) may need a 'Special' bed, even if their PSPS is very low, to allow their sores to heal.

CLASSIFICATION OF PRESSURE SORES

TYPE AND DESCRIPTION		GRADE
POTENTIAL SORES	...Inflammation with local heat, erythema, oedema and possible induration - more than 15 mm in diameter.	0
INCIPIENT SORES	...Blood under the skin or in a blister, or black (necrotic discolouration under the skin - more than 5 mm diameter; or clear blister/bullus more than 15 mm diameter.	1
SUPERFICIAL (OPEN SORES)	...A break in the skin (epidermis) which may include some damage to dermis but without black discolouration and more than 5 mm diameter.	2
MEDIUM (OPEN SORES	...Destruction of the skin (epidermis & dermis) without an obvious cavity, but possibly with black discolouration (possibly a slough) and more than 5 mm diameter.	3
DEEP (OPEN) SORES	..Penetration of the skin (epidermis & dermis) with a clearly visible cavity (with or without necrotic tissue) and more than 5 mm diameter at the service.	4
SINUS/BURSAL SORES	...Necrotic, possible infected and possibly supperating sore, more than 40 mm diameter overall, but with either not skin opening or less than 15 mm diameter.	5

PSPS CATEGORIES EXAMPLES (JAN 1994)

SITTING UP (long time)	Answer
a) Bedfast & nursed flat .... b) Only sits in a chair short periods ...... c) Does not sit for long periods (ambulant) ...	No
a) Sits in self-propelled chair (less than 10 hrs) but flat when in bed ...	No, but
a) Sits in self-propelled chair for 10 hrs or more b) Sits for short periods both in bed &in fixed chair	Yes, but
a) Propped up in bed - longish periods - most of the day ... b) Sits up both day and night ...	Yes

UNCONSCIOUS?

a) Fully conscious & orientated ... b) Fully conscious & slightly confused ...	No
a) Confused ... b) Withdrawn ... c) Semi-conscious at times ... d) Rousable-responds to commands or pain ...	No, but
a) Deeply unconscious, does not respond to pain	Yes

POOR GENERAL CONDITION?

a) Fairly good general condition ... b) Awaiting minor op ... c) Minor problem (mental or physical) ...	No
a) Recent op (under G.A) ... b) Some restriction of lower extremities ... . c) Minor sensory neuropoathy ... d) Periph. arterial disease ... e) Diabetic ... f) Arthritic ... g) Anorexic ... h) Pyrexial ... i) Hypotensive ... j) On steroids ... k) Chemotherapy ... l) Radiotherapy ... m) Elderly & thin or obese	No, but

POOR GEN. CONDITION? (continued)

a) Some injuries to lower half of body, but fair general condition ... b) Severe injuries (lower half) but no restriction of movement ... c) Well established chronic disease/disability ... d) Young paraplegic ... e) Active hemiplegic ... f) Elderly & on steroids ..	Yes, but
a) Limited mobility & great age ... b) Severe injuries - including legs/pelvis ... c) Seriously/critically ill ... d) Terminal (acute) illness .. e) Emaciated/cachetic ... f) Severe gen. infection ... g) Severe uraemia ... h) Multiple Pathology ... i) Iliac thrombosis ... j) Severe M.S. k) Hansen's disease ... l) Extensive loss of pain ... m) Recent paraplegic ... n) Quadriplegic ... o) On narcotics (for pain) .. p) Combined chemotherapy radiotherapy &or steroids	Yes

INCONTINENT?

a) No incontinence, & no 'accidents' recently ...	No
b) Indwelling cath./stoma, but no leaks/accidents	
a) Sometimes wets bed / spills urinal ... b) Occasional accidents with attached urinal ... c) Occasional leaks from indwelling catheter ... d) Occasional faecal incontinence ...	No, but

a) Small amounts & infrequent ... b) Urine only & infrequent . c) Faecal (infrequent) but some leaks (cath./urinal)	Yes, but
a) Continual dribble leak ... b) Frequent urine/faecal incontinence ... c) Doubly incontinent ...	Yes

LIFTS UP?

a) Lifts all of body clear of support ... b) Easily lifts pelvis clear ...	Yes
a) Can only lift pelvis with some effort & soon tires b) Seldom lifts self c) Can lift with help Lifts slightly - shuffles along support ...	Yes, but
a) Unable to lift pelvis ... b) Can neither help with lift, nor shuffle ...	No

GETS UP & WALKS?

a) Fully ambulant ... b) Slight impediment ... c) Uses aids with no difficulty ...	Yes
a) Has difficulty walking with aid ... b) Walks with help & encouragement ... c) Soon tires ... d) Can only walk to toilet ..	Yes & No
a) Bedfast ... b) Chairfast ... c) Stand & shuffles - with help & encouragement	No

This pressure sore prevention aid was developed at the Royal National Orthopedic Hospital (NHS) Trust, Stanmore, Middx

Conclusion

The inconclusiveness of studies examining the reliability and validity of the various pressure sore risk assessment tools adds to the confusion, making the choice of a definitive risk assessment score virtually impossible. To determine true sensitivity and specificity in vulnerable patients, would obviously be ethically unacceptable. It would appear that certain risk assessment scores are more suited to particular clinical settings and therefore the rigid choice of one specific scoring system across a particular health care facility is inappropriate and should be avoided. The work of Clark and Farrar (1992) goes on further to suggest that each clinical area using a risk assessment tool, should periodically identify the specific threshold score which achieves the best discrimination between those patients who develop sores and those who do not. They question the use of pre-printed score cards as they do not allow for variances in threshold scores to be recorded and further encourage discrepancies in overall accurace. Further work is required to adapt and develop appropriate risk assessment tools in specialist settings. Batson et al (1993) have begun work in this important area and have reviewed the use of risk score calculators in the Intensive Care environment.

The published literature generally suggests that many scoring systems over predict which patients will develop sores, this has great significance as it may lead to already limited resources being wasted on patients not actually requiring preventative intervention. The inability of many carers to appropriately re-evaluate risk status further compounds this issue, as even small improvements in a patient's condition may mean that the necessity for a particular type of pressure relieving mattress is no longer required. Many patients are inappropriately nursed on sophisticated pressure relieving systems for longer than necessary because risk status is not reviewed frequently enough, whilst others never benefit from such intervention due to scarcity of resources.

The greatest concern of all, is that in many instances lip service is paid to the use of risk assessment scores. Risk status is often only recorded as part of the routine admission procedure, evidence suggests that in many instances, a patient's risk status is rarely re-evaluated, whilst in many cases no preventative action is either documented or implemented. The incidence of pressure sores will only ever be reduced if health professionals are prepared to select an appropriate risk assessment tool, use it accurately and then implement relevant preventative/treatment strategies.

References

1.   BATSON (1993) The development of a pressure area scoring system for critically ill patients: a pilot study **Inten Crit Care Nurs, 9, 146-51**

2.   BERGSTROM N (1986) Adequacy of descriptive scales for reporting diet intake in the institutionalised elderly **J Nutrition Elderly 6, 1, 3-16**

3.   BERGSTROM N (1987) A clinical trial of the Braden scale for predicting pressure sore risk **Nurs Clin NA, 22, 2, 417-28**

4.   CLARK M & FARRAR S (1992) Comparison of pressure sore risk calculators. In: Harding KG, Leaper DL, Turner TD (Eds) Proceedings of the First European Conference on Wound Management **Macmillan, London**

5.   DEALEY C (1989) Risk assessment of pressure sores: a comparative study of Norton and Waterlow scores **Nursing Standard (supplement) 3, 27, 11-12**

6.   GOLDSTONE L A & GOLDSTONE J (1982) The Norton score: an early warning of pressure sores **J Advanced Nurs, 7, 419-26**

7.   GOSNELL D J (1973) An assessment tool to identify pressure sores **Nurs Res 1973: 22, 55-59**

8.   GOSNELL D J (1987) Assessment and evaluation of pressure sores **Nurse Clin NA 1987, 22, 2, 399-416**

9.   GOSNELL D J (1988) Pressure sore risk assessment part 2 : analysis of risk factors **Decubitus 2: 3, 40-43**

10.   LOWTHIAN P T (1987) The practical assessment of pressure sore risk **Care Sci Prac, 5, 4, 3-7**

11.   LOWTHIAN P T (1989) Identifying and protecting patients who may get pressure sores **Nursing Standard 4, 4, 26-29**

12.   NORTON D, McLAREN R & EXTON-SMITH A N (1962) An Investigation Of Geriatric Nursing Problems In Hospitals **National Corporation for the Care of Old People, London**

13.   POLIT D F & HUNGLER B P (1993) Nursing Research: principles and method (5th ed) **Lippincott, Philadelphia**

14.   SPARKS S M (1993) Clinical validation of pressure ulcer risk factor **Ostomy / Wound Man 29, 4, 40-50**

15.   STANDING J (1985) Somerset Health Authority Pressure Sore Survey **Somerset Health Authority, Taunton**

16.   GALVANI J F (1995) Update on surgical wounds **An International Forum on Wound Care; 3, 2: 36**

17   US NATIONAL PRESSURE ULCER ADVISORY PANEL (1992) Pressure ulcers in adults: prediction and prevention **Clinical Practice Guidelines 3. Public Health Service Agency for Health Care Policy and Research, Rockville, Maryland**

18   WARDMAN C (1991) Norton v Waterlow **Nursing Times 87, 13, 74-78**

Hypochlorites:
a review of the evidence

A literature review exploring the advice available
to practitioners on treating necrotic and sloughy wounds
with hypochlorites, with a guide to decision-making based
on the standard of liability in English civil law

D. Moore, RGN, ONC, RNT, RCNT, DipNEd,
is a lecturer in nursing studies,
Sussex and Kent Institute

A significant body of medical opinion still favours the use of hypochlorites for cleansing and debriding a wound that is necrotic or sloughy[1,2]. Problems arise, in practice, for nurses who are asked to use hypochlorites to treat necrotic and sloughy wounds. Failure to agree treatment always leads to nurse anxiety, which sometimes is resolved only through confrontation, subversion or ineffective practice. All these actions are detrimental to teamwork, and can mean the patient is not actively involved in decisions about treatment, which is essential for optimum wound care[3].

This review of the literature explores the physiology of the necrotic or sloughy wound and seeks to assess the quality of the advice that is readily available to the practitioner in the popular nursing press by evaluating the basic physiological studies upon which that advice was based. Finally, a guide to decision-making is offered, based on the standard of liability in English civil law, which may help those making decisions related to the use of hypochlorites.

DEVITALISED TISSUE AND ITS EFFECT ON WOUND HEALING

Wound healing is a multifaceted, imperfectly understood process comprising physical, psychological and social factors related to the patient and the way the wound is managed. Most wounds heal uneventfully[4], but this cannot happen in the presence of necrotic or sloughy tissue[5,6]. Where necrotic tissue becomes dehydrated, a brown or black leathery eschar develops[7]. Slough may present as white or grey soggy necrotic tissue[8]; a viscid yellow layer on a wound[9] that is anchored by the connective tissue[10]; or a complex mixture of

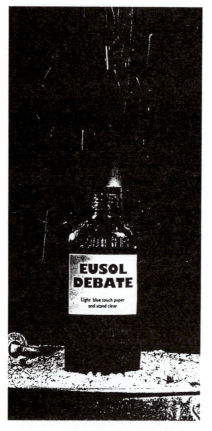

deoxyribonucleoprotein, serous exudate, leucocytes, bacteria and fibrin[7].

Slough or necrotic tissue is invariably locally infected in chronic wounds[11] which, in the compromised patient, might result in his developing a life-threatening septicaemia[9]. The mechanisms whereby infection is enhanced are such that it acts as a culture medium for bacterial growth[5,12–14]; it inhibits leucocyte phagocytosis of bacteria and their subsequent kill[14]; and limits the oxygen dependent functions of leucocytes[13,15]. It is essential that steps be taken to facilitate the process of debridement, wherein the dead

tissue sequestrates from the live, since the quality of this dictates the success of wound healing[16]. It would also seem reasonable to eliminate the presence of micro-organisms in order to proceed to the stage of fibroplasia. However, the role of bacteria in delaying healing is unclear at present[17]. It has been suggested that the presence of Gram-negative and anaerobic bacteria in necrotic pressure sores, are essential[18] for the first part of the healing process[11]. Where surgical excision[14] is not practicable, other means are sought, such as endogenous autolysis supported by the use of modern dressings, enzymes, physical techniques[19], antibacterial agents and chemical agents such as hypochlorites.

PHYSIOLOGICAL STUDIES RELATED TO CHLORINATED SOLUTIONS 1915–91

A chronological synopsis of research studies appears in Appendix 1.

The antiseptic properties of hypochlorites were first noted in the 1880s[20]. However, until the development of Surgical Soda Solution by Dakin in 1915 the commercially available antiseptics sometimes released chlorine and sometimes alkali, which were known to be irritating to tissues[21]. These antiseptics were both the inorganic hypochlorites and organic chlorine compounds such as chloramine-T[2], the latter having a slower action[22].

Hypochlorites as antimicrobial agents

The antimicrobial activity of hypochlorites depends on the stability of the chlorine which is affected by its concentration, pH, the presence of organic material, and light[22].

The lethal action of the solutions is thought to be due to the chlorination of any cell protein or enzyme systems by non-ionised hypochlorous acid[23]. It has been suggested that hypochlorites target the cell wall and enzymes together with the thiol groups, which comprise the sulphydryl groups of proteins in the cell[22], through a process of oxidisation.

Hypochlorites are capable of killing most bacteria and some fungi, yeasts, algae, viruses and protozoa, whereas they are less active against mycobacteria and relatively inactive against spores[23]. However, others say that hypochlorites, especially when buffered to pH 7.6–8.1, are a potent sporicidal agent and active against lipid and non-lipid viruses[22].

No reports of resistance to hypochlorites by microbial agents were found in any of the literature reviewed.

The bactericidal activity of hypochlorites has been demonstrated at varying levels of strength. Heggers suggested[24] that 0.025% was effective against Gram-positive and Gram-negative organisms after 30 minutes, whereas Lineaweaver[25] argued that 0.05% was needed to eliminate *Staphylococcus aureus* and Fader[20] found 0.1% ineffective against Pseudomonas.

The action of hypochlorites in the presence of organic matter

Hypochlorites are highly chemically reactive with organic matter, which thus leaves them with a very much reduced capacity to kill micro-organisms[10,22]. A 500-fold increase in strength was needed to eliminate *Staphylococcus aureus* in blood serum[21]. Fleming demonstrated that, in the presence of pus or serum, a titre of Dakin's solution 0.5% was reduced in under half a minute to 0.22% of hypochlorite, to 0.13% in five minutes and to 0.11% in 10 minutes. Similarly, he demonstrated that a titre of eusol 0.4% was reduced to less than 0.1% in five minutes[10].

Fleming found that it was not possible to eliminate bacteria in an infected wound by a single application of a hypochlorite, which further resulted in increased numbers of bacteria, since leucocytes are destroyed or immobilised by their actions[10]. These findings seem to have been confirmed in studies of leg ulcers[26], burns[27] and in a pig wound model using half-strength Eusol[28]. However, wound sterility was achieved in the granulating wound by irrigating first with normal saline, which removed the albuminous material, and then with eusol[10].

Hypochlorites as debriding agents

Hypochlorites are widely used to cleanse and debride wounds in plastic and general surgery[1,29–33]. Dakin suggested that the solution rapidly dissolved necrotic tissue when brought into contact with all parts of the wound as frequently as possible for considerable periods of time and suggested that a small wound would need 5–10ml of solution every two hours[21]. Taylor[34] found Dakin's solution lost its debriding properties at below 0.2% concentration. Fleming concurred that Dakin's solution dissolved cells but could not demonstrate any activity against connective tissue whereby slough adheres to tissue[10]. Bunyan[27] was the only person to suggest that hypochlorites differentiated between dead and live tissue. The debriding action of hypochlorites may be due to the agent necrosing superficial layers of healthy tissue, thus enabling separation to take place[35,36]. Thomas demonstrated that the quantities of hypochlorite needed to dissolve pus were unlikely to be applied in practice and therefore suggested that an alternative explanation must be sought[4,37,38]. It has been calculated that to remove 5g of slough from a small cavity would require 100 dressing changes[38].

Toxicity from hypochlorite agents
Irritancy
Dakin suggested that skin could be protected from the irritant properties of hypochlorites by using Vaseline on sound skin[21]. However, Bloomfield found some ward practice that took no account of this[39]. She elicited an irritant response in sound and abraded skin in rabbits, which typically showed moderate to severe erythema within four to five days. The *British National Formulary (BNF)* suggests that Eusol 0.25% and Dakin's solution 0.5% are too irritant to use for wound care[40].

Pain
A common complaint associated with hypochlorite treatment is pain[41]. Pain has been rated as unacceptable (11%), prolonged (24%) or occasional (64%)[39], while a small study found patients tolerated Eusol well in comparison to Varidase[42].

Delayed wound healing
Traditionally, Eusol has been attributed outstanding healing properties[21,27], which has been confirmed recently in healthy volunteers subjected to Eusol 0.1%[43]. However, in two comparatively rare human studies, Gorse and Messner[41] found statistically significant delayed healing in pressure sores treated with Dakin's solution 0.5%, and another author reported that for 10 patients treated with Eusol and paraffin the mean time for wound closure was longer, as was the hospital stay, when these were compared to the dextranomer-treated group[44]. In the latter study, reliability must be questioned with so small a sample.

Wound cell toxicity
Contradictory evidence was found for cytotoxicity of a hypochlorite at 0.5% to cultured human keratinocytes and basal cells in human cadaveric skin. Tatnall[45] found the agent to be 100% cytotoxic to the former, while another author[20] achieved 66% basal cell viability rate in the latter. Further, Tatnall[46] said a dilution of 1:1145 was needed for 50% survival of keratinocyte cells. Widely differing rates were cited at which hypochlorites will become non-cytotoxic to cultured fibroblasts[24,25,47,48,49]. Strengths ranged from 0.025%[24] to no safe concentration[47].

Fleming[10] found that leucocytes are killed immediately by eusol and chloramine-T 1% and their power to emigrate was impaired for 20 minutes, while another author suggested that a 90% impairment was seen at 0.025% with complete function returning only at 0.000 025%[47].

The tensile strength of rat wounds compared to normal saline-treated controls were found to be no different on day four using hypochlorite 0.5%[25], on day seven using chloramine-T 1%[50] or at all using hypochlorite 0.25 or 0.025%[24]. In the human wound one writer found no difference using hypochlorite 0.1%[43].

Epithelialising times in rat wounds were found to be slower using hypochlorite 0.5%[25] and delayed by two days using chloramine-T 1%[50] when compared to normal saline controls.

Damage to the microcirculation
Capillary shutdown and death was observed in the chambers of rabbits' ears together with a marked reduction in tissue perfusion. by application of eusol and chloramine-T 1%[51]. This is a much cited study, but the sample was two wounds only for each type of solution tested. Changes to the structure and function of capillaries, with clumping of red cells, blockages of fibrin platelet thrombi, together with cell damage, were found by Branemark[52].

Systemic effects of hypochlorite absorption
The Bartons cited an instance of uraemia caused by the application of hypochlorite packs and suggested that release of endotoxins from degrading bacteria could cause acute renal failure[16]. An instance of hypernatraemia resulting from Eusol substitute packs in a severely ill patient has also been described[53].

THE NURSING LITERATURE ON THE USE OF CHLORINATED SOLUTIONS 1984–91

The nursing journals which are easily available were searched in order to discover the kind of information which has been available to the non-specialist nurse.

Traditionally, nurses have not had access to laboratories and have had to depend on others' work. But there are signs that this is changing[28,43]. Therefore, the information. offered in the journal articles mainly depended on available medical experiments.

Hypochlorites as antimicrobial agents

Relatively few nurses explored the literature to discover the range of micro-organisms against which hypochlorites are effective[54,55]. Stewart[55] said hypochlorites were effective against Pseudomonas and Staphylococcus. Some authors[56,57] cautioned that Eusol and paraffin soaks could harbour bacteria, especially when they become sodden. Another writer[58,59] was concerned that indiscriminate use of chemical agents might result in bacterial resistance, although the writer found none recorded. Signs of clinical wound infection, as opposed to colonisation, have been discussed[5,55,60,61] and one author[5] reviewed the micro-organisms which are associated with it, or the chronic wound. Morison[12,13] pointed out that open wounds are invariably colonised by micro-organisms. Spanswick et al[54] applied the findings of Fader[20] to suggest that Eusol be syringed off after six minutes, although Fleming's experiments would suggest that the agent would be largely denatured by then[10].

No studies were found to support the view that paraffin, often added to Eusol, occluded oxygen and perhaps reduced the incidence of aerobic bacteria[55] and might also suffocate viable cells[55,62].

It was suggested that wound cleansing could be as well achieved by bathing[63] once or twice a day[64,65] or by showering[66]. However, it has been recommended that an aseptic technique was best in the hospital setting[12,13].

It was thought that Eusol was likely to be used in the treatment of Gulf war casualties owing to the danger of gas gangrene[57]. Fleming, however, showed that hypochlorite solutions act as an inhibitors only for *Bacillus welchii* and strongly favoured the gas-producing *Bacillus sporogenes* which produced large amounts of gas by the third day in the laboratory. His saline control, in contrast, did not produce gas until the eighth day[10].

The action of hypochlorites in the presence of organic matter

It has been suggested[55,61] that hypochlorites are rapidly inactivated in the presence of pus and by dressings, but few writers applied this concretely to practice. One author[67] mentioned the need to change dressings many times a day and another[68] suggested a two-hourly regime, but otherwise it was American nurses who recommended, as essential, that frequent wetting of the gauze sponges in the wound be carried out between dressing changes[69].

Hypochlorites as debriding agents

Hypochlorites, although not specific to dead tissue[67], are effective debriding agents[70], which many doctors and nurses still use[71] and find useful in the short term[67] of three to five days[72]. Others said they were not effective on eschar[61], taking weeks to separate from live tissue[72,73], but were more effective against soft slough[70,72] or the heavily infected wound[67]. One author[56] considered it too toxic for clinical use.

It has been argued that there was now evidence that hypochlorites could not be responsible for de-sloughing a wound and that autolysis and a moist wound environment were more likely to be the cause[61,66,74]. Mechanical debridement using normal saline[73] or water were seen to be a safer alternative to hypochlorites through flushing[66] or irrigation in some form[8], which could be a vital part of care for the sloughy wound[5].

Toxicity from hypochlorite agents
Irritancy

The advice by Dakin[21], and reinforced by the BNF[40], to protect surrounding skin with Vaseline was rarely specified[12,67]. Warning was, however, given that a moderate-to-severe irritant response might occur after four to five days[12,13,67]. since hypochlorites commonly damage skin[60] through maceration and bleaching[72].

Pain

Pain associated with the use of hypochlorites, was also relatively infrequently mentioned, yet nurses perform most of the dressings[75,76]. Indeed, some nurses use hypochlorites to soothe or reduce pain[62]. Morison[12] addressed the possible issue of pain associated with the prolonged use of Eusol, whereas pain was found by one author to be noticeably reduced by the newer dressings[64]. The only other references to pain being associated with

the use of hypochlorites were in an article in a specialist journal[77], one by a surgeon[1], two written by pharmacists[39,78], and one by an American nurse and doctor[41].

Delayed wound healing and cell toxicity

On the whole, extensive use was made of published studies when raising concerns over the potential toxicity of hypochlorites used in the open wound. One author[5] cautioned against transposing simple *in vitro* bactericidal studies to clinical use; otherwise the arguments for and against using *in vitro* and *in vivo* experiments to influence practice, with its infinitely more complex set of variables, were rarely found outside the medical journals. Studies were not evaluated critically for the benefit of the reader, therefore their merits or defects could not be judged.

Toxicity to local tissues

Citations were made from laboratory studies that showed hypochlorites were damaging[12,13,60,63,67,79]; destructive of the body's defences[62]; injurious to capillary flow[58,61,62,66,80,81]; and toxic to fibroblasts[12,13,61,67,80]. They were also said to be responsible for delayed collagen formation[12,13,55,56,62,81], prolongation of the inflammatory response[12,13,55,56] and delayed re-epithelialisation[12,13,61,81].

Systemic effects of hypochlorite absorption

Release of endotoxins as a result of using hypochlorites was widely cited in the literature[12,13,55,56,58,61,62,66,67,71,81,82]. One writer[62] cited coliforms as offending organisms and another[71] mentioned that endotoxin release could result from cell lysis in Gram-negative organisms. The Bartons[16] had suggested that bacteraemia or endotoxic shock could cause renal failure and lead to death. This has been cited as a clinical study[55], while Johnson[58] said that kidney damage was irreversible and Bale[72] cited Johnson[81] as stating that hypochlorites cause renal problems. However, the specific patient documented by the Bartons was shown to recover a blood urea of 5mmol/l from 25mmol/l 10 days after discontinuation of the hypochlorite treatment[16]. Hinchliff said[83] that acute renal failure was frequently reversible and Thomas found no other recorded instances of kidney damage from the use of hypochlorites[9]. No journal article cited hypernatraemia as a possible consequence of using Eusol substitute packs in the acutely ill person.

Table 1. A framework for decision-making applied to the use of hypochlorites in the open wound

Points to consider	Problem	Precautions to be taken against risk
Is the risk justifiable?	Known cytotoxic chemical [1-9]	Consider safer alternatives such as hydrogels, enzymes, hydrocolloids, polysaccharide paste
The degree of probability of harm	Hypochlorite is damaging to granulating tissue [10]	Should not be used on the clean granulating wound. Should not be used on the 'mixed' wound with islands of granulating tissue
	Hypochlorite delays epithelialisation [6,10]	Should not be used on the epithelialising wound
	No known resistance by micro-organisms	Preferable to topical antibiotics for cleansing

The magnitude of likely harm

	Prolonged inflammatory response [10]	Short-term use (three to a maximum of five days) [13]. Use non-woven gauze [16]
	Hyperthermia and burn [11]	Pressure relief by turning or use appropriate bed
	Localised oedema [12]	See points above and avoid addition of paraffin
	Local cell toxicity [1-9]	Consider strength. Dilute Eusol 0.25% at least 1:10[4]
	Reduced collagen synthesis [6,10]	Short-term use of three to five days and avoid granulating tissue
	Reduced microcirculation [12]	Pressure relief and do not use where vessels may be exposed
	Irritation and pain [13,14]	Short-term use: three to five days. Assess for pain at each dressing change and alter regime if necessary. Protect skin by polyurethane film or other waterproof protection
	Acute renal failure [11]	Monitor blood urea and abandon regime if rising
	Hypernatraemia [15]	Monitor plasma sodium when using Eusol substitute

The standard of skill expected of the practitioner

Knowledge:		The practitioner should have knowledge of the literature related to the use of hypochlorites in order to be able to foresee the consequences of the treatment and the resources available to inform practice such as a wound-care specialist, pharmacist or educationist
Effective practice:		The practitioner should prescribe a treatment regime to accord to the known properties of hypochlorites. Since Eusol is rapidly inactivated in the presence of necrotic tissue or slough and is followed by an increase in wound micro-organisms[3], ways must be found to supply a continuous or nearly continuous supply of the chemical to the wound at a non-cytotoxic yet bactericidal strength such as Eusol 0.025% which means diluting stock Eusol 0.25% 1:10[4]

Only the individual practitioner can take the decision to prescribe or treat a wound with a hypochlorite once all the factors relating to the patient have been weighed and assessed. The consequent actions will be judged on a 'balance of probabilities'.

References for decision-making framework
Synopses of studies may be found in Appendix I (apart from Barton and Barton (1981))

[1] Deas, J., Billings, P., Brennan, S. et al. The toxicity of commonly used antiseptics on fibroblasts in tissue culture. *Phlebology* 1986; 1: 205–209.

[2] Fader, R., Maurer, A., Stein, M. et al. Sodium hypochlorite decontamination of split-thickness cadaveric skin infected with bacteria and yeast with subsequent isolation and growth of basal cells to confluency in tissue culture. *Antimicrob Agents Chemo* 1983; 24: 2, 181–185.

[3] Fleming, A. The action of chemical and physiological antiseptics in a septic wound. *Br J Surg* 1919. 17: 25, 99–129.

[4] Heggers, J., Sazy, J., Stenberg, B. et al. Bactericidal and wound-healing properties of sodium hypochlorite solutions: the 1991 Linberg Award. *J Burn Care Rehab* 1991; 12: 5, 420-424.

[5] Kozol, R.A., Gillies, C., Elgebaly, S. Effects of sodium hypochlorite (Dakin's solution) on cells of the wound module. *Arch Surg* 1988; 123: 420–423.

[6] Lineweaver, W., Howard, R., Soucy, D. et al. Topical antimicrobial toxicity. *Arch Surg* 1985; 120: 267–268.

[7] Tatnall, F.M., Leigh, I.M., Gibson, J.R. Comparative study of antiseptic toxicity on basal keratinocytes, transformed human keratinocytes and fibroblasts. *Skin Pharmacology* 1990; 3: 3, 157–163.

[8] Tatnall, F.M., Leigh, I.M., Gibson, J.R. Comparative toxicity of antimicrobial agents on transformed keratinocytes. *Br J Dermatology* 1987; 117: (supplement) 32, 31–32.

[9] Thomas, S., Hay, N.P. Wound cleansing (letter). *Pharm J* 1985; 235: 206.

[10] Brennan, S.S., Foster, M.E., Leaper, D.J. Antiseptic toxicity in wounds healing by secondary intention. *J Hospital Infection* 1986; 18: 236-263.

[11] Barton, A., Barton, M. *The Management and Prevention of Pressure Sores.* London: Faber and Faber, 1981.

[12] Brennan, S.S., Leaper, D.J. The effect of antiseptics on the healing wound: a study using the rabbit ear chamber. *Br J Surg* 1985; 72: 780–782.

[13] Bloomfield, S.F. Eusol BPC and other hypochlorite formulations used in hospital. *Pharm J* 1985; 253: 153–157.

[14] Gorse, G.J., Messner, R.L. Improved pressure sore healing with hydrocolloid dressings. *Arch Dermatol* 1987; 123: 766–771.

[15] Thorp, J.M., Mackenzie, I., Simpson, E. Gross hypernatraemia associated with the use of antiseptic surgical packs. *Anaesthesia* 1987; 42: 750–753.

[16] Archer, H., Barnett, S., Irving, S. et al. A controlled model of moist wound healing: comparison between semi-permeable film, antiseptics and sugar paste. *J Exp Path* 1990; 71: 155–170.

Hyperthermic burn

Although many nurse writers cited from the Bartons[16] on the issue of burns, only one[61] mentioned the chemical burn that is caused to the tissues by use of hypochlorites, as shown by their use of thermography. Such burns caused further problems to the already damaged tissue[16].

STANDARD OF LIABILITY IN ENGLISH CIVIL LAW

The popular nursing press cited the physiological studies widely and gave consistent advice that Eusol is too toxic for widespread use. Nurses are now unhappy to use hypochlorites[84], their reluctance being linked to their legal obligations to the patient[63,71]. They therefore seek guidance from their code of conduct on exercising accountability[85]. Where disputes have arisen, nurses have claimed that they have a professional duty not to use hypochlorites[86], a point which Gilchrist suggested will have to be tested[87].

Bald statements in the nursing press that nurses break their code of conduct by using Eusol[88] raise anxiety without offering a means of resolution.

In English civil law the standard of liability[89] falls into three categories of seriousness; these are, in descending order, intention, recklessness and negligence, of which the latter may be inadvertent or advertent. Advertent negligence is that which is foreseen but not desired and is assessed against a fictitious person, the 'reasonable man', except in medical practice where 'standard practice' takes precedence. The factors which have to be taken into account are the degree of probability that damage will be done; the magnitude of the likely harm; the utility of the object to be achieved, the burden in time and trouble of taking precautions against the risk; and a requirement to show a certain standard of skill normally possessed by persons doing that work[89].

These factors are offered as a means of arriving at an informed decision as to whether hypochlorites might be an appropriate agent in clinical practice (Table I). However, it has to be recognised that: 'Nearly every human action involves some risk of harm, but every risky act will not necessarily result in liability. Care should be taken in respect of a risk that is reasonably foreseeable. Furthermore, foreseeability is a relative concept not to be scientifically tested'[89].

The degree of probability that damage will be done

The frequency of likelihood of occurrence is the determining factor in negligence[89].

The literature shows agreement that hypochlorites are damaging to granulating tissue[84,90,91] and epithelial cells[25,50]. Therefore there is no place for their use in the healing wound, although the probability of delayed wound healing from their use in practice is debatable. Hypochlorites have not been shown to become resistant to micro-organisms.

The magnitude of the likely harm

A formidable list can be compiled of potential adverse effects of hypochlorite application: delayed wound healing; prolonged inflammatory response; delayed epithelialisation; local cell toxicity; depressed collagen synthesis; reduced capillary flow; hyperthermia and burn; irritation and pain; localised oedema; renal failure; and hypernatraemia. Further, it has been suggested that overgranulation could be caused[2], or repression of this activity[90].

The utility of the object to be achieved

The literature, while accepting that there is still a body of medical opinion which prescribes hypochlorites, is predominantly in favour of using safer means to clean and deslough the open wound. Wound healing occurs in the presence of bacteria[92,93] and hypochlorites do not reduce the bacterial wound count[10,26]. They have not been shown intrinsically to be an effective debriding agent. Serious consideration needs to be given to exactly why they are used.

The burden in time and trouble of taking precautions against the risk

All reasonable precautions must be taken such as protecting the sound skin from hypochlorite contact by a thick layer of Vaseline, zinc and castor oil or applying a polyurethane film. Also, a full blood and platelet count to assess kidney function should be taken[16].

A meticulous assessment of the patient's pain should be taken, noting his/her feelings at every dressing change. Where pain is present, alternative treatments should be sought. Present knowledge would advise a time limit of three to five days for treatment[39], the use of a detailed wound assessment chart is recommended with perhaps the use of photographic records.

Requirement to show a certain standard of skill normally possessed by persons doing that work

Foreseeability may depend on the knowledge that a person ought to possess[89]. Care should be delivered to a standard equivalent to that offered by his or her professional peers.

To be effective, a hypochlorite should be applied every 10 minutes[10] or at least two-hourly[21]. This has a cost implication for both patients and resources. The latest research suggests that a bactericidal and non-cytotoxic strength of hypochlorites is 0.025%[24].

The nurse needs to be aware of and able to review the literature critically in order to foresee the consequences of her actions or identify such competent people as can advise her. Finally, when assessing for negligence the practitioner will be assessed on a 'balance of probabilities', with the burden of proof resting with the practitioner to show that she was not negligent according to the five criteria[89].

CONCLUSION

The literature search highlighted the lack of consensual findings in the physiological studies which examined the effects of hypochlorites on wound healing. Much of it comprised descriptive or methodologically weak studies[84]. The writer is not equipped to judge the validity and reliability of the use of the wound model for experimental purposes[94] but understands the problems of translating those findings to the infinitely more complex situation of the human wound[1,90].

Few studies, apart from those of Fleming[10] and Kozol[47], were found which examined the inhibitory effects of hypochlorites upon polymorphonuclear leucocyte chemotaxis, yet they are critical in promoting fibroplasia in addition to their internal debridement role[14]. Only Fleming[10] examined the time factor involved in leucocyte impairment after an application of a hypochlorite. Hypochlorites were shown to be cytotoxic at widely differing levels. If fibroblasts were damaged, why were wound tensile strengths ultimately not affected[24,25,43,50]? The study which revealed damage to the microcirculation[51] should be replicated to achieve statistical significance. Human comparative trials[41,44] are valuable because of their rarity, yet a total population of 35 patients treated with hypochlorite dressings does not constitute a statistically significant number upon which to change practice.

When their use of Eusol was questioned, were the irritated responses of surgeons[2] a symptom of a practice in decline or a deeper dispute about authority and autonomy? It is certainly a symptom arising from lack of first-rate experimental evidence[84].

In considering toxicity, the rate at which the agent acts on bacteria, leucocytes and the rate of destruction of the agent must be considered together[10]. Hypochlorites act quickly and are quenched almost immediately[10]. There is a need to discover whether Fleming[10] was correct in asserting a 10-minute period when bacteria are free to multiply after the extinction of the agent and before leucocyte recovery. In practice, this means providing a near continuous supply of fresh hypochlorite to the wound, which would be difficult and costly to implement.

For safe and effective practice, the nurse needs to know what strength of hypochlorite to use, how often to re-apply the solution and over what period of time. A replication of those of Fleming's experiments pertinent to today may be helpful.

The evidence presented in this literature search would seem to suggest that hypochlorites are too risky to use on a 'balance of probabilities' and, where multidisciplinary agreement can be gained, should be removed from the pharmacy shelves. However, it must be conceded that, until more clinical trial evidence is available, there may be a place in the treatment of the sloughy and necrotic wound for hypochlorites if the prescribing or treatment nurse is aware of the specialist body of knowledge that is emerging today in order to defend her actions against the criteria for negligence. To this end, the criteria used in civil law to assess possible negligence may be used. These can act as a framework for positive decision-making which should remove confrontational, subversive, inactive or ineffective nursing practice. ∎

REFERENCES
1 Porter, J.M. A review of dressing materials used for the treatment of raw areas in plastic surgery. J Tissue Viability 1991; 1: 2, 48–52.
2 Morgan, D. Chlorinated solutions: an update. J Tissue Viability 1991; 1: 2, 31–33.
3 Lawrence, C. Bacterial infection of wounds. Wound Management 1991; 1: 1, 13–15.
4 Thomas, S. Evidence fails to justify use of hypochlorite. J Tissue Viability 1991; 1: 1, 9–10.
5 Ayton, M. Infection control and infected wounds. Nursing Standard 1991; 5: 49, 30–32.
6 Torrance, C. The physiology of wound healing. Nursing 1986; 13: 5, 162–168.
7 Dressing Times. Dressing Times 1989; 2: 1.
8 David, J. Wound Management. London: Dunitz, 1986.
9 Thomas, S. Wound Management and Dressings. London: Pharmaceutical Press, 1990.
10 Fleming, A. The action of chemical and physiological antiseptics in a septic wound. Br J Surg 1919; 17: 25, 99–129.
11 Bliss, M. The management of pressure sores in elderly people. Dressing Times 1991; 4: 2.
12 Morison, M. Wound cleansing: which solution? Professional Nurse 1989; 4: 5, 220–225.
13 Morison, M. Wound cleansing: which solution? Nursing Standard 1990; 4: 52, 4–6.
14 Haury, B., Rodeheaver R. G., Vensko, J. et al. Debridement: an essential component of traumatic wound care. In: Hunt, T.K. (ed.). Wound Healing and Wound Infection: Theory and surgical practice. New York: Appleton-Century-Crofts, 1980.
15 Hohn, D.C. Host resistance to infection: established and emerging concepts. In: Hunt, T.K. Wound Healing and Wound Infection: Theory and surgical practice. New York: Appleton-Century-Crofts, 1980.
16 Barton, A. Barton, M. The Management and Prevention of Pressure Sores. London: Faber and Faber, 1981.
17 Ayliffe, G.A. Question and answer. J Hospital Infection 1990; 16: 173–174.
18 Pometan, J-P. The bacteriology of pressure sores. In Smith, T. (ed.). Highlights from the International Symposium on Wound Management, Helsingor, Denmark, May 27–28. Bussum, The Netherlands: Medicom Europe, 1991.
19 Fernandez, S. Prevention and treatment of pressure sores. Care: Science and Practice 1988; 16: 1, 17–21.
20 Fader, R., Maurer, A., Stein, M. et al. Sodium hypochlorite decontamination of split-thickness cadaveric skin infected with bacteria and yeast with subsequent isolation and growth of basal cells to confluency in tissue culture. Antimicrob Agents and Chemo 1983; 24: 2, 181–185.
21 Dakin, H.D. On the use of certain antiseptic substances in the treatment of infected wounds. Br Med J 1915; 2: 318–321.
22 Russell, L. A.D., Hugo, W.B., Ayliffe, G.A. Principles and Practice of Disinfection, Preservation and Sterilisation. Oxford: Blackwell Scientific Publications, 1982.
23 Reynolds, J.E.F. (ed.). Martindale: The extra pharmocopoeia. London: Pharmaceutical Press, 1989, p. 958.
24 Heggers, S. J., Sazy, J., Stenberg, B. et al. Bactericidal and wound-healing properties of sodium chlorite solutions: the 1991 Linberg Award. J Burn Care Rehab 1991; 12: 5, 420–424.
25 Lineaweaver, W., Howard, R., Soucy, D. et al. Topical antimicrobial toxicity. Arch Surg 1985; 120: 267–268.
26 Daltrey, D.C., Cunliffe, W.J. A double-blind trial of the effects of benzoyl peroxide 20% and Eusol and liquid paraffin on the microbial flora of leg ulcers. Acta Dermatovener (Stockholm) 1981; 61: 575–577.
27 Bunyan, J. The treatment of burns and wounds by the envelope method. Br Med J 1941; 2: 4200–4208.
28 Archer, H., Barnett, S., Irving, S. et al. A controlled model of moist wound healing: comparison between semi-permeable film, antiseptics and sugar paste. J Exper Path 1990; 71: 155–170.
29 Gummer, C. Milton and the treatment of burns. Pharm J 1986; 236: 181–185.
30 Elliott, D. Lab data should not overrule experience (letter). Hospital Doctor 1990; 10: 32, 10.
31 Langridge, C.J. Protest against misguided ban (letter). Hospital Doctor 1990; 10: 32, 10.
32 Ravishandran, G. Hypochlorite is valid on short-term basis (letter). Hospital Doctor 1990; 10: 31, 12.
33 Taylor, R. Eusol: alternatives are of little value (letter). Hospital Doctor 1990; 10: 31, 12.
34 Taylor, H., Austin, H. The solvent action of antiseptics on necrotic tissue. J Exper Med 1918; 27: 155–164.
35 Leaper, D., Simpson, R. The effects of antiseptics and topical antimicrobials on wound healing. J Antimicrob Chemo 1986; 17: 2, 135–137.
36 Leaper, D. Antiseptics and their effect on healing tissue. Nursing Times 1986; 82: 22, 45–47.
37 Thomas, S. Milton and the treatment of burns (letter). Pharm J 1986; 236: 128–129.
38 Dressing Times. Eusol revisited. Dressing Times 1990; 13: 1.
39 Bloomfield, S.F. Eusol BPC and other hypochlorite formulations used in hospital. Pharm J 1985; 253: 153–157.
40 BMA and RPSGB. British National Formulary (No.22). London: BMA and RPSGB, 1991.
41 Gorse, G.J., Messner, R.L. Improved pressure sore healing with hydrocolloid dressing. Arch Derm 1987; 123: 766–771.
42 Smith, M., Wilkinson, J., Leigh, A. et al. Report of a comparative study of the efficacy of Varidase Topical versus Eusol in the cleansing of leg ulcers. In: Rue, Y. (ed.). A Biological Approach to the Wound Healing Process: A clinical update. Oxford: Alden Press, 1987.
43 Fotherby, Y. M., Spanwick A., Gibbs, S. et al. Effect of various dressings on wound healing in healthy volunteers. J Tissue Viability 1991; 3: 68–70.
44 Goode, A. Infected wounds. Care: Science and Practice 1982; 1: 3, 4-7.
45 Tatnall, F.M., Leigh, I.M., Gibson, J.R. Comparative toxicity of antimicrobial agents on transformed keratinocytes. Br J Dermatology 1987; 117: (supplement) 32: 31–32.
46 Tatnall, F.M., Leigh, I.M., Gibson, J.R. Comparative study of antiseptic toxicity on basal keratinocytes, transformed human keratinocytes and fibroblasts. Skin Pharmacology 1990; 3: 3, 157–163.
47 Kozol, R.A., Gillies, C., Elgebaly, S. Effects of sodium hypochlorite (Dakin's solution) on cells of the wound module. Arch Surg 1988; 123: 420–423.
48 Deas, J., Billings, P., Brennan, S. et al. The toxicity of commonly used antiseptics on fibroblasts in tissue culture. Phlebology 1986; 1: 205–209.
49 Thomas, S., Hay, N.P. Wound cleansing (letter). Pharm J 1985; 235: 206.
50 Brennan, S.S., Foster, M.E., Leaper, D.J. Antiseptic toxicity in wounds healing by secondary intention. J Hospital Infection 1986; 18: 236–263.
51 Brennan, S.S., Leaper, D.J. The effect of antiseptics on the healing wound: a study using the rabbit ear chamber. Br J Surg, 1985; 72: 780–782.
52 Calver, R.F. Topical nutrition reviewed. Care: Science and Practice 1983, 12: 4, 20–23.
53 Thorp, J.M., Mackenzie, I., Simpson, E. Gross hypernatraemia associated with the use of antiseptic surgical packs. Anaesthesia 1987; 42: 750–753.
54 Spanswick, A., Gibbs, S., Ekelund, P. Eusol: the final word. Professional Nurse 1990; 5: 4, 211–213.
55 Stewart , A., Foster, M., Leaper, R. D. Cleaning v. healing. Community Outlook 1985; August, 22–26.
56 Simpson, G. Factsheet: assessment and choice. Community Outlook 1987; July, 16–18.
57 Turner, T. War wounds. Nursing Times 1991; 87: 5, 16–17.
58 Johnson, A. A time for change. Nursing Standard 1988; 2: 48, 34–35.
59 Johnson, A. Wound management: are you getting it right? Professional Nurse 1988; 3: 8, 306–309.
60 Bale, S. A holistic approach and the ideal dressing. Professional Nurse 1991; 6: 6, 316–323.
61 Dealey, C. Assessing wounds and selecting dressings. Nursing Standard 1990; 14: 27, (supplement 7) 8–9.
62 Saunders, P. Toilet cleaner for wound care? Community Outlook 1989; March, 11–13.
63 Turner, V. Standardisation of wound care. Nursing Standard 1991; 15: 19, 25–28.
64 Griffiths, G. Choosing a dressing. Nursing Times 1991; 87: 36, 84–90.
65 Rodgers, S. Using proper protocol. Nursing Times 1991; 87: 36, 76–80.
66 Ferguson, A. Best performer. Nursing Times 1988; 84: 14, 53–55.
67 Morison, M. Preventing delayed wound healing. Professional Nurse 1987; 2: 9, 298–300.
68 Sims, R., Fitgerald, V. Wound care in the community. Nursing 1986; 3: 6, 209–215.
69 Hadley, S.A., Black, V.L. Why use Dakin's solution? Am J Nursing 1988; 88: 3, 284–285.
70 Draper, J. Make the dressing fit the wound. Nursing Times 1985; 81: 41, 32–35.
71 Johnson, A. Wound care: packing wound cavities. Nursing Times 1987; 83: 36, 59–62.
72 Bale, S. Using modern dressings to effect debridement. Professional Nurse 1990; 5: 5, 244–248.
73 Morison, M. Priorities in wound management Part 1. Professional Nurse 1987; 2: 11, 352–355.
74 Biley, F. Eusol: there'll be no eulogy. Nursing 1991; 4: 37, 21–22.
75 Moody, M. Restrictive practices. Nursing Times 1988; 84: 2, 62.
76 David, J., Chapman, R.G., Lockett, B. An iInvestigation of the Current Methods Used in Nursing for the Care of Patients with Established Pressure Sores. Guildford: Univer-

sity of Surrey, Nursing Practice Research Unit, 1983.
[77] Millward, J. Assessment of wound management in a care of the elderly unit. *Care: Science and Practice* 1989; 7: 2, 47–49.
[78] Thomas, S. Pain and wound management. *Community Outlook* 1989; July, 11–15.
[79] Cutting, K.F. Wound cleansing. *Surgical Nurse* 1990; 3: 3, 4–6.
[80] Cameron, S., Leaper, D. Antiseptic toxicity in open wounds. *Nursing Times* 1988; 84: 25, 77–79.
[81] Johnson, A. Cleansing infected wounds. *Nursing Times* 1986; 82: 37, 30–34.
[82] Alderman, C. Wound infection: detection and treatment. *Nursing Standard* 1988; 2: 26.

[83] Hinchliff F. S., Montague, S. *Physiology for Nursing Practice.* London: Baillière Tindall, 1987.
[84] Farrow, S., Toth, B. The place of Eusol in wound management. *Nursing Standard* 1991; 5: 22, 25–27.
[85] United Kingdom Central Council. *Exercising Accountability.* London: UKCC, 1989.
[86] Tingle, J. Eusol and the law. *Nursing Times* 1990; 86: 38, 70–72.
[87] Gilchrist, B. Being accountable. *Nursing Times* 1989; 85: 26, 67.
[88] Swaffield, L. Quest for quality. *Nursing Times* 1990; 86: 12, 16–17.
[89] Cooke, P., Oughton, N. D. *The Common Law of Obligations.* London: Butterworth, 1989.

[90] Leaper, D. The use and abuse of antiseptics. *Wound Management* 1991; 1: 2, 4–5.
[91] Johnson, A. The case against the use of hypochlorites in the treatment of open wounds: a personal view. *Care: Science and Practice* 1988; 6: 3, 86–87.
[92] Gilchrist, B., Hutchinson, J. Does occlusion lead to infection? *Nursing Times* 1990; 86: 15, 70–71.
[93] Eriksson, G. Bacterial growth in venous leg ulcers: its clinical significance. In: Ryan, T.J. (ed.). *An Environment for Healing: The role of occlusion.* Oxford: Oxford University Press, 1985.
[94] Marks, R. The use of models for the study of wound healing. In: Ryan, T.J. (ed.). *An Environment for Healing: The role of occlusion.* Oxford: Oxford University Press, 1985.

Appendix 1: Physiological studies relating to hypochlorite solutions
(NB: Notes are personal observations)

1915 Dakin, H.[21]

On the use of certain antiseptic substances in the treatment of infected wounds.
Study: Laboratory experiments, bacterial, *in vitro* and human wounds. Described a way to stabilise hypochlorite through buffering the solution.
Microbial action of Dakin's solution. 0.5%: Staphylococci in serum killed at 1:1 500–2 000.
Action on body tissues: Assists in the rapid disolution of necrotic tissue. Rare instances of skin irritation observed.
Conclusion: Protect sound skin with Vaseline. Best to bring fresh quantities of NaOCl in contact with all parts of the wound as frequently as possible for a considerable period of time. Irrigate all wounds with 5–10ml solution every two hours using rubber tubes; large wounds may need 1–2 litres daily.
Note: Consider the practical applications of this for practice.

1918 Taylor, H.[34]
Austin, H.

Solvent action of antiseptics on necrotic tissue.
Study: *In vitro* using Dakin's solution and chloramine-T 0.2% to discover which is the essential factor in the solvent action of chlorinated solutions: the alkalinity; the nature or concentration of the chlorine solution used.
Results: (1.) Dakin's solution has the power to dissolve necrotic tissue and leucocytes. (2.) Chloramine-T 0.2% does not have this power and therefore is not a tissue solvent. (3.) The solvent action of Dakin's solution disappears at below 2%. (4.) The alkaline property assists effectiveness of the hypochlorite. Action of Dakin's 0.5% solution is enhanced as alkalinity increases.
Conclusion: Justifiable to stress the relatively great solvent action of Dakin's solution in contrast to the more stable chloramines.
Note: According to the authors, Eusol BPC 0.25% is not therefore a desloughing agent.

1919 Fleming, A.[10]

The action of chemical and physiological antiseptics in a septic wound.
Study: *In vitro* and war wound experiments and clinical observations.
Results: Staphylococci killed at 1:2 000 in blood serum. Hypochlorites fail to sterilise an infected wound or penetrate the tissue. A granulating wound could be sterilised by first irrigating with saline 0.9% followed by eusol 0.5% irrigation. Application of hypochlorites enhance bacterial growth because their action is extinguished from

NaOCl 0.5% > 0.13% in five minutes + > 0.11% in 10 minutes; eusol 0.4% > 0.1% in five minutes, whereas leucocytes were killed immediately and their emigration inhibited for 20 minutes. Little evidence found of hypochlorites dissolving slough, since they are ineffective on connective tissue and therefore recommended hypertonic saline as the most effective agent.
Conclusion: In estimating the value of an antiseptic it is necessary to 'study its effect on the tissues more than its effect upon the bacteria. . . It seems a pity that the surgeon should wish to share his glory with a chemical of more than doubtful utility.'
Note: Found a 10-minute lag time, after eusol and chloramine-T 1% ceased activity and before leucocytes recovered theirs, when bacteria multiplied unchecked. Does this explain the presence of bacteria found by Archer (1990), Daltrey (1981) and Bunyan (1941)? Demonstrated that normal saline was more effective in preventing actions of gas-producing spores than eusol or chloramine-T 1%.

1941 Bunyan, J.[27]

The treatment of burns and wounds by the envelope method.
Study: Burns and wounds. To find a way to improve burn treatment.
Results: Developed an electrolytic NaOCl which was used to wash wounds within silk sleeves. Used hypertonic salinated NaOCl (0.5%–0.25% w/v available chlorine) at 100°F for desloughing and isotonic levels (0.25% w/v available chlorine) for granulating tissue. Regime consisted of 20 minutes bathing three times daily. The wound was kept moist, warm and occluded. The wounds desloughed and healed well in spite of bacteria in sleeves.
Conclusion: Pain was relieved, primary infection controlled, secondary infection prevented and function restored. Primary shock not aggravated and secondary shock minimised.
Note: Observed that wounds healed in spite of bacterial presence and used many of the principles now known to promote rapid wound healing. Also see Fleming (1919), who recommended hypertonic saline for desloughing.

1981 Daltrey, D.[26]
Cunliffe, W.

A double-blind trial of the effects of benzoyl peroxide 20% and Eusol and liquid paraffin on the microbial flora of leg ulcers.
Study: Eusol and paraffin on 13 patients with leg ulcers dressed once daily.

Results: The wounds gained over six weeks: Pseudomonas, Streptococcus, Staphylococcus, Enterobacteria and Anaerobes.
Conclusion: Preparations helpful clinically in most patients, so mechanism of action deserves further thought.
Note: See Heggers (1991) who wondered why in vivo healing occurred despite known toxicity of NaOCl 0.25% to fibroblasts at that strength; also Archer (1990) and Fleming's (1991) explanation of why it might occur if NaOCl is infrequently applied.

1982 Goode, A.[44]

Infected wounds.
Report of a study: Report of a controlled randomised trial of dextranomer versus Eusol and paraffin. Ten patients after appendicectomy or bowel surgery, all on antibiotics, were allocated to each group. All the wounds were infected and were treated twice daily with ribbon gauze soaked in Eusol and paraffin or dextranomer. The predominant infecting organisms were Escherichia coli and Pseudomonas.
Results: Mean time to secondary closure was 11.6 days (Eusol group) to 8.1 days (p<0.05 Mann-Whitney U Test). Wound healing was the principal factor in deciding discharge from hospital which was delayed by 2.2 days in the Eusol group.
Conclusion: More research needed into the efficient management of established wound infection.
Note: A small study upon which to change practice. Information was selective since this was a report of the study, making independent judgement of reliability difficult.

1983 Fader, R.[20]
Maurer, A.
Stein, M.
Abston, S.
Hemdon, D
(US study)

Sodium hypochlorite decontamination of split-thickness cadaveric skin infected with bacteria and yeast with subsequent isolation and growth of basal cells to confluency in tissue culture.
Study: Investigated the ability to decontaminate skin while leaving sufficient epidermal cell viability to grow in culture. In vitro bactericidal assays were done on methicillin-resistant Staphylococcus aureus (MRSA), Pseudomonas aeruginosa and Candida albicans.
Results: At 0.1% NaOCl was found to eliminate Candida albicans in 10 minutes and be ineffective against MRSA and Pseudomonas aeruginosa. At 0.5% NaOCl was found to eliminate Candida albicans in one minute, MRSA in five minutes and Pseudomonas aeruginosa in six minutes. All leaving a basal cell viability of 66% at six minutes exposure to NaOCl. At NaOCl 0.5% cell viability decreased from 81% after one minute exposure to 33% after 10 minutes' exposure.
Conclusion: With the steady increase of antibiotic-resistant strains of bacteria, NaOCl may emerge again as a valuable topical antiseptic since no resistance to it has yet been recorded. The use of laboratory-grown tissue culture sheets to cover wounds may reduce the recovery time for burn patients significantly.
Note: Stock Eusol BPC 0.25% would not eliminate Pseudomonas. Compare cell viability and bactericidal rates with Heggers (1991), Kozol (1988), Lineaweaver (1985), Deas (1986) and Tatnell (1987).

1985 Bloomfield, S.[39]

Eusol BPC and other hypochlorite formulations used in hospitals.
Study: In vivo and in vitro experiments. Studied the stability of Eusol and other hypochlorite preparations; skin irritancy was tested on intact and abraded rabbit skins by applying five varieties of solution. All applied four times a day for five days (12 wounds in three rabbits); and surveyed incidence of irritancy to use of hypochlorite in 62 wards.
Results: Rabbit wounds and skin showed little or slight reaction to any of the strengths of hypochlorites in the first two days. At days three to five, the response increased so that moderate erythema was seen by fourth or fifth day. The ward survey responses were that 36% of wards recorded little or no irritation or pain and 64% of wards indicated pain sometimes or usually. Of these wards, 24% recorded occasional prolonged pain and 12% unacceptable pain.
Conclusion: This study found pain/irritation mainly associated with the wound rather than the surrounding tissue. Further work urgently needed.
Note: Nurses need to assess pain in relation to treatment at each dressing change and use the agent for not more than three days. See Dakin (1915).

1985 Lineaweaver, W.[25]
Howard, R.
Soucy, D.
McMorris, S.
Freeman, J.
Crain, C.
Rumley, T.
(US Study)

Topical antimicrobial toxicity.
Study: In vivo and bacterial studies comparing four topical antiseptics and four antibiotics; 0.5% NaOCl tested on 20 Sprague-Dawley rats by irrigating their wounds three times a day with 15ml of solution.
Results related to NaOCl: NaOCl 0.5% is100% toxic to fibroblasts; NaOCl 0.025% is 100% toxic to fibroblasts; NaOCl 0.005% causes no decrease in fibroblast survival and yet is still bactericidal. No significant decrease in tensile wound strength at days four, eight,12,16. Wound epithelialisation retarded at eighth and 16th days with NaOCl 0.5%.
Conclusion: Cytotoxicity, bacterial and in vivo experiments provide evidence for unsuitability of four commonly used antiseptics.
Note: Compare tensile strength of wound outcomes with Heggers (1991), Fotherby (1991) and Brennan (1986). Compare cytotoxic figures with Heggers (1991), Kozol (1988), Deas (1986) and Tatnell (1987).

1985 Brennan, S.[51]
Leaper, D.

The effect of antiseptics on the healing wound.
Study: In vivo using the rabbit's ear chamber (two chambers for each solution). Compared actions of antiseptics on granulating tissue. Eusol and chloramine-T 1% applied and then observed at one, five, 10, 30 minutes, 1hour and then daily.
Results: Eusol and chloramine-T 1% caused marked percapillary exudation. In the granulation tissue, blood flow ceased within seconds in all but largest vessels where sludging of blood cells was noted.
Tissue perfusion dropped from 46 > 0.5 in five minutes (saline control 40.5 > 42). Damage was permanent and took five days from Eusol and chloramine-T 1% application for new vessels to grow. Saline had little effect.
Conclusion: Eusol and chloramine-T 1% toxic to granulation tissue.

Note: It must be presumed that the Eusol was BPC stock strength 2.5%. Small study. Two chambers tested for each type of solution. See Brennan and Foster (1986) and Thomas (1986).

1986 Brennan, S.[50]
Foster, M.
Leaper, D.J.

Antiseptic toxicity in wounds healing by secondary intention.
Study: *In vivo*: 135 Sprague-Dawley rats divided into three groups: saline, chloramine-T 1% and chlorhexidine 0.05%. Forty-five Sprague-Dawley rats each had four wounds dressed once with 5ml chloramine-T 1%. and covered. On third, fifth, and seventh postoperative day 15 rats were killed and wounds examined and compared with saline controls.
Results: Increased inflammatory response in NaOCl wounds as shown by an increase in polymorphonuclear neutrophils. Day 3: Hydroxyproline (collagen ingredient) chloramine-T 1% < saline control (p < 0.002). Day 5: Hydroxyproline (collagen) chloramine-T 1% < saline control (p < 0.05).Day 7: Hydroxyproline (collagen) no significant difference. Fibroblasts were less numerous and well oriented than saline controls. Epithelialisation delayed by two days in chloramine-T 1% group.
Conclusion: Hypochlorites may adversely affect wound healing.
Note: The 5ml chloramine-T 1% was soaked in starch granules and applied once only, thereafter being kept moist by occlusive dressing. Fleming's work (1919) would suggest that the agent is quickly denatured.
Compare with wound tensile studies by Heggers (1991), Fotherby (1991) and Lineaweaver (1987). Compare delayed epithelialising times with Lineaweaver (1987).

1985 Thomas, S.,[49]
Hay, N.P.

Letter: Wound cleansing.
Study: *In vitro* experiment in which mouse fibroblasts were exposed to Milton 1 in 4 (0.25% w/v available chlorine).
Results: Eusol substitute toxic to cells down to levels of 0.005% and some cell damage detected at 0.0025%.
Conclusion: Hypochlorite is likely to affect adversely granulation and hence delay wound healing.
Note: Unreliable form of scientific communication upon which to base practice.

1986 Deas, J.,[48]
Brennan, S.,
Billings, P.,
Silver, I.,
Leaper, D.

The toxicity of commonly used antiseptics on fibroblasts in tissue culture.
Study: *In vitro*. Baby hamster kidney fibroblasts subjected to chloramine-T 2%, chlorhexidine 0.05%, povidone-iodine 10%, Savlodil 1.5%, hydrogen peroxide 10vols% and noxythiolin 5%.
Results: All solutions toxic to fibroblasts in stock concentrations. Chloramine-T 2% 100% cytotoxic at $0.02\% \times 10^{-3}$ (0.000 02%) and non-cytotoxic at 10^{-6} (0.000 000 02%).
Conclusion: Study is evidence for toxicity of antiseptics to cells needed for healing.
Note: Compare findings with Heggers (1991), Kozol (1988) and Lineaweaver (1985).

1987 Tatnall, F.M.[45]
Leigh, I.M.,
Gibson, J.R.

Comparative toxicity of antimicrobial agents on transformed human keratinocytes.
Study: *In vitro* study using human keratinocytes.

Cells subjected for 15 minutes to NaOCl 0.5%, povidone-iodine 4%, cetrimide 1%, hydrogen peroxide 3%, and three antibiotics.
Results: All antiseptics 100% toxic to cells while none of antibiotics were toxic at therapeutic concentrations.
Rank descending order of toxicity: NaOCl > cetrimide > povidone-iodine > hydrogen peroxide.
Conclusion: Care needed in selecting antimicrobial agents for wounds.
Note: See their 1990 study and compare these results with Fader (1983).

1987 Gorse, G.J.,[41]
Messner, R. ,
(US study)

Improved pressure sore healing with hydrocolloid dressings.
Study: *In vivo* human study comparing outcomes for 27 patients with 76 pressure sores treated with hydrocolloid dressings (HCD) changed every four days and 25 patients with 52 pressure sores treated with 0.5% Dakin's solution treated with a wet-to-dry dressing regime (WDD) three times daily. A sub-group of protein malnourished patients was included. Excessive necrotic tissue was mechanically debrided before entering the trial.
Results: A smaller proportion of the sores were healed or healing in the WDD group 69.2% > 86.8% (p = 0.026) during the study, even among the malnourished group, although no statistical significance was found in the mean days to resolution. Incompletely healed sores in the WDD group took significantly longer to heal completely. Where frequent assessment was necessary WDD was preferred, such as in complicated sores — grade 3 or over or infected.
Conclusion: WDD inferior to HCD in that fewer pressure sores improved or resolved; pain was a common complaint; WDD was more expensive in nursing time and materials.
Note: A valuable comparative study. Needs replicating to enhance reliability using NaOCl 0.25% which is the more usual agent used in the UK. Compare results with Fotherby (1991) and Daltrey (1981). Note the cost element.

1987 Thorp, J.M.,[53]
Mackenzie, I.,
Simpson, E.

Gross hypernatraemia associated with the use of antiseptic surgical packs.
Study: A case history related to an acutely ill patient with gas gangrene where a Eusol substitute was used for wound packing.
Results: Patient developed hypernatraemia which was attributed to the systemic absorption of the chemical, since the water balance was positive and there was no enteral sodium input.
Note: This case highlights the potential for absorption of chemicals systemically and the need to monitor sodium levels if a Eusol substitute is dispensed by pharmacy.

1988 Kozol, R.A.,[47]
Gillies, C.,
Elgebaly, S.
(US study)

Effects of a hypochlorite (Dakin's solution) on cells of the wound module.
Study: *In vitro* wound chambers used and rabbit peritoneal neutrophils, bovine pulmonary artery endothelial cells and rabbit skin fibroblasts exposed to Dakin's solution of various strengths for 30 minutes or one hour.
Results: Leucocyte migration: > 90% inhibited at NaOCl 0.025%–0.000 25%. Return of leucocyte chemotactic function at 0.000 025%

strength. This was tested and found to be a functional response rather than owing to cell damage. In contrast to leucocytes, injury was found to fibroblasts and endothelial cells from NaOCl 0.025% or 0.0025% after 30 minutes' exposure, with total destruction at NaOCl 0.025%.

Conclusion: There is no safe concentration of Dakin's solution in the open wound.

Note: This study offers the most toxic results from NaOCl. For comparative fibroblast toxicity levels, see Heggers (1991), Kozol (1988), Deas (1986) and Lineaweaver (1985). For comparative leucocyte damage, see Fleming (1919). This study elicited irritated responses from US surgeons (Raffensperger (1989) and Barese and Cuono (1989) in *Arch Surg* 1989; **124**:.133–134.

1990 Archer, H.,[28]
Barnett, S.
Irving, S.
Middleton, K.
Seals, D.

A controlled model of moist wound healing: comparison between semi-permeable film, antiseptics and sugar paste.

Study: *In vivo* pig wound model used. Three pigs each had 12 wounds. First pig: six OpSite (controls) plus six sugar paste. Second and third each: four OpSite, two half-strength Eusol, two povidone-iodine 0.8%, two chlorhexidine 0.2% and Irgasan DP300 (0.2%). 5ml antiseptic applied on to five layers of gauze day one, three, and five.

Results: Of the four wounds treated with Eusol 0.125%: at days three and five: a heavy mixed growth of micro-organisms was cultured, and the mean pH of wound exudate was 7.6. Three wounds healed completely, one had a 33% deficiency with trapped cotton fibres and a cellular reaction. Trial problems: insufficient funds for more pigs, 48-hour gaps in re-applying Eusol.

Conclusion: Fibres from the gauze were shown to become trapped in immature repair tissue and initiate the 'foreign body' inflammatory response. Eusol is often applied through such a medium. Heavy mixed growth of micro-organisms found in the Eusol wounds which failed to inhibit healing. Authors suggest that use of antiseptics in the regular treatment of wounds can be harmful.

Note: The 48-hour gaps in applying Eusol must invalidate the wound-healing results. However, the study highlights the effects of gauze fibres (often an adjunct of Eusol treatment) in delaying wound healing through the 'foreign body' reaction. Researchers: infection control specialist, pharmacist, microbiologist, two researchers in plastic surgery.

1990 Tatnall, F.M.,[46]
Leigh, I.M.
Gibson, J.R.

Comparative study of antiseptic toxicity on basal keratinocytes, transformed human keratinocytes and fibroblasts.

Study: *In vitro* comparison of cytotoxicity of: NaOCl, chlorhexidine and hydrogen peroxide, all at therapeutic concentrations.

Results: All antiseptics 100% cytotoxic to all cell types (P < 0.005). Descending rank order of toxicity: NaOCl > hydrogen peroxide > chlorhexidine. To achieve 50% cell survival NaOCl 0.5% was diluted 1 145 times.

Conclusion: Findings support concerns related to using antiseptics in the open wound; in particular, when culture grafting is planned where their use is contraindicated.

Note: Compare toxicity levels with those of Fader (1983).

1991 Heggers, S.J.,[24]
Sazy, J.,
Stenberg, B.,
Strock, L.,
McCauley, R.,
Hemdon, D.
(US study)

Bactericidal and wound-healing properties of sodium hypochlorite solutions.

Study: *In vitro* and *in vivo* investigation to find a therapeutic concentration of NaOCl that is antiseptic and non-toxic to tissues. *In vitro*: range of micro-organisms subjected to buffered and unbuffered NaOCl at 0.25%, 0.025%, 0.0125% and 0.007%. *In vitro*: mouse fibroblasts assayed for cytotoxicity of NaOCl dilutions at 0.25%, 0.025% and 0.125%, at 10-, 20-, and 30- minute intervals. *In vivo* toxicity assay on 104 Sprague-Dawley rats each with three dorsal wounds bolstered with gauze to irrigate wounds four-hourly with NaOCl 0.25%. and 0.025%. Control: buffered saline (n = average 32 for each group).

Results: Bacterial index: at pH 7.5 NaOCl 0.25% bactericidal within 30 minutes and 0.025% (buffered or unbuffered p< 0.05). NaOCl at 0.0125% was not bactericidal to Gram-negative micro-organisms.Toxicity to fibroblasts: cell death in 10 minutes at NaOCl 0.25% with viability demonstrated at NaOCl 0.025%. Wound tension strengths: little/no difference between the NaOCl solutions at 0.25% and 0.025% and the normal saline controls.

Conclusion: The fibroblast toxicity assays were consistent with those of Lineaweaver (1985), while those of Kozol (1988) were rejected. Authors consider whether, as Fleming (1919) had suggested, there was some wound protective substance or mechanism which neutralised the toxicity of NaOCl, since their experiments showed that NaOCl 0.25% *in vivo* showed no detriment to healing yet were toxic to *in vitro* fibroblasts.

NB: the bactericidal and non-toxic strength is 1/10 of stock BPC NaOCl 0.25%. Best protocol in that wounds were irrigated four-hourly, yet still not as recommended by Dakin (1915) or consistent with the findings of Fleming (1919). Compare bactericidal yet non-cytotoxic findings with Deas (1986) and those discussed. Compare tensile wound strengths with Fotherby (1991), Lineaweaver (1987) and Brennan (1986).

1991 Fotherby,Y. M.,[43]
Spanswick, A.,
Gibbs, S.,
Barclay, C.,
Potter, J.,
Castleden, M.

Effect of various dressings on wound healing.

Study: *In vivo* human trephined wounds in eight healthy subjects aged 21-42 years; 16 wounds on forearms. Comparison between healing of: NaOCl 0.1% and normal saline (daily gauze dressing) and Granuflex, and Op-Site over 9–11days.

Results: Complete healing occurred in all wounds from 12-13 days onwards. Of the four NaOCl-dressed wounds, one erythematous reaction occured and healing rates compared equally with saline and OpSite. Granuflex wounds took longer to heal.

Conclusion: No detrimental effect on wound healing in healthy adults when using NaOCl 0.1% (BPC concentration is 2.5%). Newer dressings showed no particular advantage.

Note Daily dressings not an effective test of NaOCl activity (see Fleming (1919), Dakin (1915)) and therefore an ineffective protocol. (Letter from ConvaTec re Granuflex suggested that trephined wounds cannot be compared to chronic wounds (Hutchinson, J. (1991). *J Tissue Viability* 1991; 1: 4, 120.).

Journal of Tissue Viability Vol 5 No 2

Compression Bandaging for Venous Leg Ulcers

Andrea Nelson
Department of Nursing, University of Liverpool

HISTORICAL OVERVIEW

Hippocrates, described the use of bandages in the treatment of leg ulcers and varicose veins in the first century B.C.[1]. He identified bandaging as a skill and reported that his students had to be dissuaded from showing off their skills. In the first century AD it was believed that ulcers were the exits for vile humours which descended to the leg following standing. Healing these ulcers would lead to the humours being forced back up the leg towards the body, causing madness. Avicenna (980-1037) went so far as to recommend the breaking down of any ulcers that did heal and this belief persisted into the nineteenth century[2].

Soldiers in the first world war used non-elastic, lace-up gaiters, first described in the 17th century, to prevent their legs from becoming fatigued during marches. Elastomeric bandages made with rubber were first employed in the late 19th century in the management of varicose veins.

MODERN COMPRESSION PRODUCTS

Synthetic elastomeric fibres such as Elastane and Lycra (Dupont) have been incorporated into modern bandages, which are now light, strong, conformable and washable. Modern elastic bandages can be woven or knitted and are designed to provide prescribed levels of compression as defined by performance-based standards[3].

Bandages can be used for many purposes - dressing retention, support, and compression. However, their most significant role is in the treatment of venous ulcers. In 1805 The Edinburgh Medical and Surgical Journal[4] reported that;

'Ulcers on the leg form a very extensive and important class of diseases..... The treatment of such cases is generally looked upon as an inferior branch of practice; an unpleasant and inglorious task where much labour must be bestowed, and little honour gained'.

The care of ulcers remains an unglamorous branch of practice, but with improved diagnostic techniques, bandages, dressings and education, today's practitioners can achieve healing in the majority of cases.

WHAT CAUSES VENOUS ULCERS?

The return of blood from the leg is aided by the foot and calf muscle pumps. Contraction of the calf muscle compresses the deep veins and blood is propelled towards the heart, retrograde flow being prevented by one way valves. On relaxation of the calf muscle, the deep veins are filled by blood from the superficial system, via connecting veins. One way valves in the perforating and superficial veins prevent transmission of the high pressures in the deep veins to the weak walled superficial system. High pressure in the superficial system leads to distension of the veins, seen as varicosities. Venous ulcers are often described by patients as 'varicose ulcers' due to their association with varicose veins. In fact, venous ulcers may arise due to damage of the superficial venous system resulting in varicosities, the deep venous system secondary to thrombosis, or the communicating veins which connect the two systems. In each case, however, the calf muscle pump, which propels blood back towards the heart, is compromised. This results in high pressure and venous hypertension in the superficial system which is transmitted to the capillaries.

Investigations of patients with venous ulcers have suggested theories to account for the deposition of fibrin in the tissues and the sequestration of white blood cells in the capillaries[5,6]. The final result of these changes is venous hypertension, caused by incompetent or occluded venous valves.

EFFECT OF COMPRESSION ON VASCULAR FUNCTION

Starling's Law describes how graduated compression reduces ambulatory venous hypertension and reverses oedema, (Figure 1) and this is borne out experimentally[7]. Graduated compression also relieves discomfort, heals venous ulcers and prevents their recurrence[8]. Used inappropriately, however, it can lead to skin damage[9], therefore thorough assessment is essential before applying a compression bandage[10].

CURRENT PRACTICE: COMPRESSION AND LEG ULCER HEALING

Epidemiological studies suggest that some treatment regimes used in the community leave 50% of ulcers unhealed after 9 months[11]. Moffatt et al found that healing rates after 3 months in the community were 22% prior to the setting up of community leg ulcer clinics rising to 55% in their first 3 months[12]. Healing rates of 60-80% in 3 months published by specialist clinics are significantly better[13,14], and there may be many reasons for this, eg;

1) improved organisation of services with easy referral and improved access
2) education and training of nurses in assessment and treatment
3) provision of diagnostic equipment and services such as vascular surgery and dermatology
4) effective use of high compression bandaging regimes.

Surveys of leg ulcer care show that many patients are not receiving appropriate treatment regimes, with retention and

Journal of Tissue Viability Vol 5 No 2

Figure 1: Starling's Law

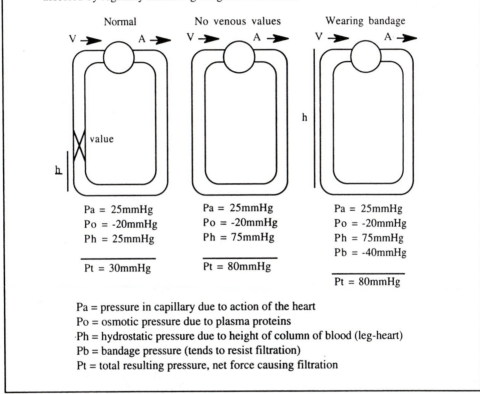

This relationship suggests two ways of reducing Pt;

- Bed rest: When venous valves are incompent, Pt increases with the distance between the feet and the heart. Reducing this distance, by lying flat, or elevating the feet to the level of the heart, will reduce the formation of oedema.
- Compression: When Pt is greater than 30-40mmHg, tissue fluid is not completely reabsorbed by the lymphatic vessels and oedema forms. Applying a graduated compression bandage reduces tissue filtration and hence oedema formation. This can be assessed by regularly measuring the girth of the limb.

Normal	No venous values	Wearing bandage
Pa = 25mmHg	Pa = 25mmHg	Pa = 25mmHg
Po = -20mmHg	Po = -20mmHg	Po = -20mmHg
Ph = 25mmHg	Ph = 75mmHg	Ph = 75mmHg
		Pb = -40mmHg
Pt = 30mmHg	Pt = 80mmHg	Pt = 80mmHg

Pa = pressure in capillary due to action of the heart
Po = osmotic pressure due to plasma proteins
Ph = hydrostatic pressure due to height of column of blood (leg-heart)
Pb = bandage pressure (tends to resist filtration)
Pt = total resulting pressure, net force causing filtration

support bandages being used, with only a small proportion of venous ulcer patients receiving compression bandaging - as little as 25% in one survey[15]. Furthermore, studies of nurses' bandaging skill shows the poor performance of most nurses[16,17]. Trials comparing different bandaging regimes show the superiority of high compression regimes over the cotton crepe regimes[18,19,20], although there is, at the moment, no evidence to recommend one high compression bandage regime over another[21].

Achieving healing requires assessment to exclude non-venous causes and then selection and application of an appropriate bandage; dressing selection appears to be of secondary importance.

The ideal compression bandage can be defined by its pressure profile, i.e., the magnitude, distribution and duration of the pressure achieved. In order to obtain the ideal pressure profile, an appropriate bandage (or combination of bandages) must be applied correctly. Nurses often choose an inappropriate bandage for applying support or compression[22]. The ability of a bandage to provide compression is determined by its construction, and described by Laplace's Law.

Elastic compression bandages, when stretched, have a tension within them due to the presence of elastomeric fibres. The force required to stretch the bandage is equal to the tension within the bandage. If one stretches two commonly available elastomeric bandages (e.g. a very high compression bandage such as elastic web bandage BP, and a high compression bandage such as Setopress (Seton) or Tensopress (Smith and Nephew)) one can feel the difference in the force required to extend a 10 cm section of the bandage to 15 cm. The tensile force generated in the elastomeric fibres when extended causes a pressure on the limb according to Laplace's Law when applied to bandages;

**Pressure is proportional to bandage tension and
inversely proportional to limb radius
or P=kNT/R**

(where k is a constant, N is the number of layers of bandage, T is the tension in the bandage and R is the radius of curvature of the limb)

Considering each of these factors in turn;

Layers of bandage

Two layers of bandage provide twice as much pressure as 1 layer. This is a particularly important relationship for bandage application as it dictates that there should be a constant number of layers of bandage up the leg (usually 2).

Tension

A high compression bandage can provide a high tension and thus a high pressure. Compare the force required to stretch a retaining bandage such as Slinky (Cuxson Gerrard), with that required to stretch a compression bandage. The tension in the bandage is produced by the nurse extending the bandage.

Limb radius

Given a constant tension and number of layers along the leg, a bandage will produce a higher pressure on a small limb than on a large limb. An analogy is the discomfort felt when carrying a heavy bag. The pressure or discomfort is greater if the load is spread over a small area, eg a finger, than if it is taken by the whole hand. This relationship implies that a bandage applied to a normal shaped leg, at constant tension and 50% overlap will produce a higher pressure at the ankle than at the calf.

The ideal compression bandage (or regime) can be described with reference to the following characteristics.

MAGNITUDE OF PRESSURE

The required magnitude of pressure at the ankle varies according to the pathology and the clinician's preferences. The pressure needed to counteract venous hypertension has been calculated to be around 30 mmHg at the ankle, reducing towards the calf[23]. There is still discussion on the precise levels of sub-bandage pressure required, and those recommended by Stemmer et al[23], are for example, up to 40% higher than those in the UK Drug Tariff[24], (Table 1). This difference may be a reflection of the preference for higher pressures in some countries, and of the different techniques used to measure the compression: the Hohenstein technique in Europe, the Hatra method in the UK and the Instron method in the United States[25].

Ankle pressures of around 40 mmHg have, in clinical studies, produced healing rates of 54-74% in 12 weeks[13,14]. It is still not clear, however, whether there is an optimal pressure for the healing of leg ulcers and whether this varies with arterial or venous pathology

DISTRIBUTION OF PRESSURE

In order to decrease venous hypertension due to the hydrostatic pressure within the superficial veins, the pressure should be graduated, being greatest at the ankle and gradually decreasing up the leg[26]. Laplace's Law, shows that the pressure on a limb will be greatest at its smallest radius of curvature. Therefore the shape of the leg helps achieve graduated pressure without varying the bandage tension. The bandage tension must be kept constant all the way up the leg until the widest part of the calf is reached, thereafter the bandage should be relaxed slightly in order to avoid a tourniquet effect below the knee. If the leg does not increase in diameter towards the knee, then the extension must be decreased from the ankle to the calf to achieve the necessary graduation. There is no recommended degree of graduation for bandages, but the standards for stockings require that the calf pressure is less than 70% of the ankle pressure[3].

DURATION OF PRESSURE

A bandage, once applied, should stay in place until the dressing requires removal, usually up to 7 days later. High compression elastomeric bandages have been monitored over this period and been found to sustain their compression[13,27]. Modern non-elastic bandages may require frequent re-application in the initial stages of treatment, as these cannot 'follow-in' when oedema is reduced and the leg volume decreases.

Extending crepe bandage straightens the bandage fibres and as the recoil is poor the tension is short lived. These bandages do not maintain their pressure well over time[28,29] and need frequent, ie daily, re-application.

PATIENT FACTORS: COMFORT & COMPLIANCE

In order for a well applied bandage to be effective it must be tolerated and worn continually by the patient. Compliance with treatment may be helped by an explanation of the importance of wearing the bandage, and by increasing the bandage pressure gradually. Some centres use multi-layered regimes in which the top layer is removable (eg a shaped tubular bandage) so that the patient may reduce the compression slightly in the evening, if necessary, and reapply the top layer again first thing in the morning. Patients may be labelled as 'non-compliant' if they remove their bandages. As

Table 1: Recommended ankle pressure (mmHg)

Clinical indications	Drug Tariff	Stemmer et al
Superficial or early varices	14-17	18-21
Moderate varices, ulcer treatment and prevention, mild oedema	18-24	25-32
Gross varices, post thrombotic syndrome, gross oedema, ulcer treatment and prevention	25-35	36-46
Severe lymphoedema		35-50

Journal of Tissue Viability Vol 5 No 2

nurses' bandaging techniques are so variable, however, the patient may be justified in removing a bandage which is exacerbating the venous insufficiency, rather than ameliorating it.

APPLICATION FACTORS: EASE OF USE, AVAILABILITY, COST

Bandages with surface markings indicating desired overlap and extension are available which may help nurses apply bandages effectively.

Restriction of bandage availability on the community Drug Tariff means that nurses cannot obtain shaped tubular bandages, some compression bandages and padding materials. There are effective high compression bandages available to the community nurses but they may be more effective if used with padding materials, as there is increasing awareness that parts of the leg need to be protected from the high compression which is required along the rest of the leg for healing to occur. This can be achieved with foam and orthopaedic wadding.

The cost-effectiveness of bandages depends on their effectiveness, whether they are reusable and the unit cost. Lycra-based bandages can be washed and re-used up to 20 times, thus greatly reducing cost. Modern, inelastic bandages are also washable.

BANDAGE SELECTION

Thomas[30] tested bandages to determine their ability to apply and sustain pressure and classified them according to the level of pressure generated on the ankle of an average leg.

- **Retention bandages** are designed to keep dressings in place, and are very conformable but exert very little pressure on a limb.
- **Support bandages** prevent the formation of oedema, and support joints. They are minimally extensible. Crepe bandages are support rather than compression bandages.
- **Compression bandages** can apply and sustain pressure on a limb. They have been further classified as light, moderate,

high and extra high compression bandages according to the magnitude of pressure generated on an average limb. (Table 2) The layered regimens use combinations of compression bandages to achieve around 40 mmHg at the ankle.

APPLICATION

Compression bandages can be harmful if they are not applied appropriately and in the correct way[9], and there is evidence that nurses' bandage application is poor[16,17]. It is essential that a bandaging technique is used which results in a graduated pressure from the ankle to the knee. A simple spiral technique, with 50% overlap, can be used with all bandages and instructions are included with most. A 'figure of eight' technique will produce higher pressures than the spiral and therefore this method should not be used with high compression bandages[31]. It is important to be able to assess one's technique by referring to the checklist below[32].

ASSESSING YOUR OWN BANDAGING

Ideally, bandaging technique should be assessed by measuring the sub-bandage pressure. However, pressure measuring devices are expensive, and do not provide all the information necessary to determine whether the bandage has been correctly applied. Assess your own technique by looking at bandage placement, overlap, extension and the effect of the bandage on the leg.

(i) Bandage placement

This should be inspected immediately after application and before removal. The bandage must extend from the base of the toes to the tibial plateau. Leaving out the foot in the hope that the patient will be able to wear his or her shoes will lead to oedema of the foot, which will make the wearing of usual footwear difficult or impossible. Oedematous skin is also particularly vulnerable to pressure damage.

The heel should be checked to ensure there are no gaps in the bandage. If the bandage becomes displaced during wear it can be secured with surgical tape.

The bandage should extend as high up the lower leg as possible, so that the knee can be bent without the bandage being affected. Check this after application by placing your hand on the bandage behind the knee while asking the patient to bend their knee.

(ii) Bandage overlap

In order to ensure a constant number of bandage layers along the leg, the overlap must also be consistent. An overlap of 50% will result in two layers of bandage up the leg, and this is the most commonly used overlap. If a 10 cm bandage is applied with a 50% overlap, then there should be 5 cm between edges of successive bandage layers. Use a measuring tape to measure the distance between bandage edges. Bandages of different widths should be placed so that the distance between bandage edges is 1/2 of the bandage width. Check the bandage width using a measuring tape as the bandage may

Table 2: Thomas's classification of bandages

Class	Example
1 Retention	Slinky, Stayform, Tensofix
2 Support	Crepe BP, Elastocrepe
3a Light compression	J-Plus, K-Crepe
3b Moderate compression	Veinopress, Granuflex Adhesive Compression Bandage
3c High Compression	Setopress, Tensopress
3d Extra high compression	Bilastic Forte, Blue line webbing

Journal of Tissue Viability Vol 5 No 2

be wider or narrower than indicated in the packaging. Instead of using a measuring tape, a quick check can be done by folding a small section of the bandage in two and comparing the width of this section with the distance between edges.

(iii) Bandage extension

The amount of bandage extension should be recommended by the bandage manufacturer, kept constant up the leg and only reduced slightly above the calf. If an extension guide is used, e.g. Setopress (Seton), use a measuring tape to check that the markers are all the same size along the bandaged leg. Bandages without extension guides can be marked and assessed in a similar way;

1 Mark a bandage along an edge or the centre line at 10 cm intervals using a marker pen
2 Apply the bandage, with marks visible, in a spiral with 50% overlap
3 Measure the distance between successive marks at the ankle, gaiter and calf.
4 Calculate the bandage extension thus; Extension (in percent) = 10x (new distance-10)
   eg if new separation of marks =13 cm,
   extension = 10x(13-10) = 10x3 = 30%,
   or: if new separation of marks = 15 cm,
   extension = 10x(15-10) = 10x(5) = 50%
   The extension should remain the same or decrease at sites further up the leg,

e.g. extn. @ calf = 50%   extn. @ calf = 30%
     extn. @ gaiter = 50% OR extn. @ gaiter = 40%
     extn. @ ankle = 50%   extn. @ ankle = 50%

A common mistake is overextending the bandage at the top of the leg, or applying more layers here, resulting in the production of a tourniquet.

LOOKING AT THE LEG

On removing the bandage one can often see puffy areas where oedema has formed. This indicates that there was insufficient pressure here, either due to too few layers of bandage or not enough bandage tension. Red or broken areas indicate that the pressure has been excessive at that point. It is important to establish whether skin damage is localised in vulnerable areas, or widespread. Strategies for minimising pressure damage include flattening the area by using padding, and reducing bandage extension. If the patient is removing the bandage due to pain or discomfort, one should firstly review assessment and then treatment.

Reduction in the area of ulceration is an indication that the bandage is effective, whereas lack of progress within 1-3 months should prompt reassessment of diagnosis and treatment. Finally, it is likely that an effective bandage will give the patient relief from the symptoms of venous insufficiency and therefore asking the patient to rate their pain and comfort will also provide feedback on bandage application.

SUMMARY

Compression bandaging is the single most important element in the treatment of venous leg ulcers. Nurses may be wary of applying high compression to limbs as they are aware of the consequences of inappropriate compression. However, once a thorough assessment (including full medical history, urinalysis, and inspection of the limb and ulcer), indicates that there is no sign of arterial disease, then treatment with a compression bandage should be commenced.

Effective compression therapy depends on the selection of a bandage, or combination of bandages, which can apply and sustain pressure on the leg. Support bandages are not suitable. Effectiveness also depends on application technique, which can be assessed by direct measurement or by use of a checklist; both in conjunction with frequent and regular ulcer re-assessment.

Address for Correspondence

Ms Andrea Nelson, Dept Nursing, University of Liverpool, PO Box 147, Liverpool L69 3BX

References

1 Adams EF. The genuine works of Hippocrates. Sydenham Press 1949.
2 Underwood M. A treatise upon ulcers of the legs. Mathews 1783.
3 British Standards Institution, British Standard Specification for Graduated Compression Hosiery. BS6612 London: The Institution 1985.
4 The Inquirer. What are the comparative advantages of the different modes for the treatment of ulcerated legs? *Edinburgh Medical and Surgical Journal* 1805; **1**: 187-193.
5 Browse NL, Burnand KG. The cause of venous ulceration. *Lancet* 1982; **2**:(**8292**): 243-5.
6 Coleridge-Smith PD, Thomas P, Scurr JH, Dormandy JA. The cause of venous ulceration: a new hypothesis. *BMJ* 1988; **296**: 1726-7.
7 Burnand KG, Pattison M, Layer GT. How effective and long lasting are elastic stockings. *Phlebology '85* 1986.
8 The Alexander House Group. Consensus paper on venous leg ulcers. *Phlebology* 1992; **7(2)**: 48-58
9 Callam MJ, Ruckley CV, Dale JJ, Harper DR. Hazards of compression treatment of the leg: an estimate from Scottish surgeons. *BMJ* 1987; **295**: 1382.
10 Gibson B. The nursing assessment of patients with leg ulceration. *Nursing Management* 1995; 27-34.
11 Callam MJ, Ruckley CV, Harper DR, Dale JJ. Chronic ulceration of the leg: extent of the problem and provision of care. *BMJ* 1985; **290**: 1855-6.
12 Moffatt CJ, Franks PJ, Oldroyd M, Bosanquet N, Brown P, Greenhalgh RM, McCollum CN. Community clinics for leg ulcers and impact on healing. *BMJ* 1992; **305**:1389-92.
13 Blair SD, Wright DD, Backhouse CM, Riddle E, McCollum CN. Sustained compression and healing of chronic venous ulcers. *BMJ* 1988; **297**: 1159-61.
14 Callam MJ, Harper DR, Dale JJ, Brown D, Gibson B,

Prescott RJ, Ruckley CV. Lothian and Forth valley Leg Ulcer Healing Trial, Part 1: Elastic versus non-elastic bandaging in the treatment of chronic leg ulceration. *Phlebology* 1992; **7(4)**:136-41.

15 Cullum NA, Last S. The prevalence, characteristics and management of leg ulcers in a UK community. *2nd European conference on advances in wound management* 1993.

16 Millard LG, Blecher A, Fentem PH. The pressure at which nursing staff apply compression bandages when treating patients with varicose ulcers. *Phlebology '85* 1986.

17 Logan RA, Thomas S, Harding EF, Collyer G. A comparison of sub-bandage pressures produced by experienced and inexperienced bandagers. *J Wound Care* 1992; **1(3)**: 23-26.

18 Northeast ADR, Layer GT, Wilson NM, Browse NL, Burnand KG. Increased compression expedites venous ulcer healing. *Paper presented at RSM Venous Forum* 1990.

19 Duby T, Hoffman D, Cameron J, Doblhoff-Brown D, Cherry G, Ryan T. A randomised trial in the treatment of venous leg ulcers comparing short-stretch bandages, 4-layer system and a long stretch paste system. *Wounds: A compendium of clinical research and practice* 1993; **5(6)**: 276-279.

20 Gould DJ, Campbell S, Harding EF. Short-stretch bandages vs. long-stretch bandages in the management of chronic venous leg ulcers. *Phlebology* 1993; **8(1)**: 43.

21 Cameron J, Poore S, Duby T. A comparative study of two bandage systems. *3rd European conference on advances in wound management* 1993:168-169.

22 Magazinovic N, Phillips-Turner J, Wilson GV Assessing nurses' knowledge of bandages and bandaging. *J Wound Care* 1993; **2(2)**: 97-101.

23 Stemmer R, Marescaux J, Furderer C. Compression treatment of the lower extremities particularly with compression stockings. *The Dermatologist* 1980; **31**: 355-65.

24 National Health Service, *Drug Tariff*. London: HMSO 1989.

25 Stolk R, Salz P. A quick pressure determining device for medical stockings based on the determination of the counter pressure of air filled leg segments. *Swiss Med* 1988; **10(4a)**: 91-96.

26 Sigel B, Edelstein AL, Savitch L, Hasty JH, Felix WR. Type of compression for reducing venous stasis. A study of the lower extremities during inactive recumbency. *Arch Surg* 1975; **110**: 171-5

27 Sockalingham S, Barbenel JC, Queen D. Ambulatory monitoring of the pressures beneath compression bandages. *Care Science and Practice* 1990; **8(2)**: 75-79.

28 Raj TB, Goddard M, Makin GS. How long do compression bandages maintain their pressure during ambulatory treatment of varicose veins? *Br J Surg* 1980; **67**:122-4.

29 Dale JJ, Callam M, Ruckley CV. How efficient is a compression bandage? *Nursing Times* 1983; **79(46)**: 49-51

30 Thomas S. Bandages and bandaging: The science behind the art. *Care Science & Practice* 1990; **8(2)**: 56-60.

31 Barbenel JC, Sockalingham S, Queen D. In vivo and laboratory evaluation of elastic bandages. *Care Science and Practice* 1990; **8(2)**: 72-74.

32 Nelson A. The art and science of bandaging. *Nursing management* 1995: 75-88.

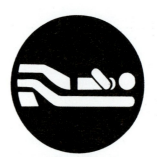

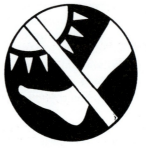

Caring for your legs

An Expert guide for people living with leg ulcers

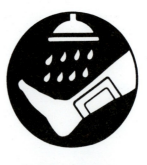

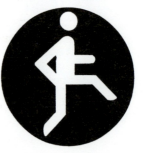

ConvaTec

Introduction

With almost half a million people in the UK alone suffering from venous leg ulcers, there is a growing medical interest in this painful and distressing condition.

This leaflet explains the cause of leg ulcers and provides an insight into the basics of modern treatment.

By listening to the advice of your doctor or district nurse and following the guidelines set out in this leaflet, you can minimise the distress that leg ulcers may cause and help ensure a better quality of life.

What causes venous leg ulcers

Venous ulcers are the most common type of leg ulcer and are usually the result of poor circulation in the veins of your legs.

Veins are the blood vessels that carry blood back to the heart and, in your legs, this usually means flowing upwards.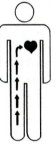

Every time your leg muscles move they help pump the blood uphill while a series of valves stop the blood from flowing backwards. If these valves are damaged, blood flows back down the legs when the muscles aren't moving.

If this goes on for years without treatment, veins become stretched and fluid can leak out causing swelling of the legs. You may also notice areas of darkened skin on the legs. Eventually, the legs may become itchy and irritated. At this stage a leg ulcer could appear.

If you have had a venous leg ulcer, it is probably the result of an injury to your veins that occurred years earlier.

Other causes of leg ulcers

It is important to seek expert medical advice from a doctor or nurse before considering any treatment yourself. They will be able to tell you the cause of the ulcer and identify any underlying problem that requires medical attention.

Causes of leg ulcers

- Diseases of the veins
- Diseases of the arteries
- Diabetes
- Physical injuries
- Diseases of the blood
- Infection of the blood
- Inflammatory diseases (such as arthritis)
- Pressure on the veins during pregnancy

How to care for <u>venous</u> leg ulcers

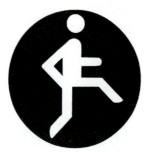

Remember to exercise.
If you're able, walking is good exercise as it helps the circulation. Otherwise, exercise by moving your ankles up and down regularly while you are sitting in a chair. Your district nurse may also recommend stretching exercises.

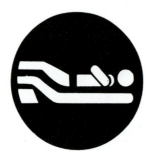

Elevating your legs.
During the day, sit your feet on a stool. At night, raise the foot of the bed or put cushions under the mattress.

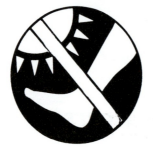

Protect your legs. The skin of the legs is easily damaged - take care. Do not scratch your legs, avoid sunburn and exposure to cold or excessive heat, e.g. sitting with your legs directly in front of an open fire.

IMPORTANT: Never consider treating yourself for leg ulcers, always consult your doctor or district nurse.

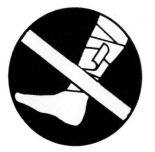

Wear appropriate elastic support on the leg.
Correctly fitted support stockings, tights, or bandages will help heal the ulcer and prevent new ones. Your district nurse or doctor should decide the most appropriate support for you. These should always be replaced when they become loose-fitting.

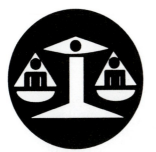

Control your weight.
This is good for your general health as well as for your legs. Eat plenty of protein, fresh fruit and vegetables. Avoid fatty, sweet and starchy foods.

Comfortable footwear.
Always wear footwear that is comfortable, does not create pressure or rub against the skin.

Take care of your feet.
Make sure toe nails are properly cut as they can cause sores if left uncut. Your doctor or chiropodist can advise you on proper footcare.

Early warning signs of <u>venous</u> leg ulcers

One of the early signs for people prone to venous leg ulcers can be swelling of the legs. Varicose veins can also be another early sign.

Itching, any sign of a rash or eczema, or darkening of the skin around the ankle may also be warning signs that an ulcer may occur. Should you notice any of these signs, contact your doctor or district nurse as soon as possible.

Things to avoid with leg ulcers

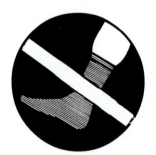

Avoid obstructing the veins. Do not wear tight socks, girdles or garters. When sitting down, take care not to allow the edge of the chair to press into the backs of your legs. You should also avoid crossing your legs while sitting.

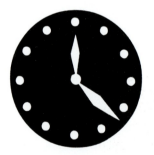

Do not sit or stand for long periods of time. If you have to stand a lot, try moving your toes inside your shoes, bend and straighten your knees from time to time and shift your weight from foot to foot.

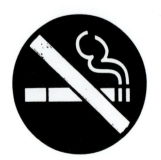

Do not smoke. Smoking actually reduces blood flow and can slow down the healing process. For this reason, it is very important to try to stop smoking if you have leg ulcers.

Helping the healing process

As a result of poor circulation, venous leg ulcers may take a long time to heal. And, even a small cut or graze could develop into a venous ulcer because poor circulation can slow down the natural healing process.

For years it was thought that a wound must be allowed to "breathe". Many of us have probably removed a plaster or bandage to let the wound dry up. Surprisingly, however, this can actually slow down the natural healing process because the growth of new skin is slowed by the hard scab that is formed.

Years of research has shown that keeping a wound moist and warm actually encourages healing as the body's natural defence and repair processes work best in moist, warm conditions.

This has led to the development of hydrocolloid dressings such as Granuflex* These dressings form a protective barrier to prevent infection while creating the ideal conditions for healing. And, as the ulcer is kept close to body temperature, it heals faster. Not only is the ulcer kept moist and warm but because air is kept from reaching the ulcer, the re-growth of the small blood vessels necessary for healing is actually encouraged. You may also find these dressings make living with leg ulcers more comfortable.

Living with leg ulcers

Many people will suffer from leg ulcers for years. Unfortunately, there is no magic cure but science has already provided some of the answers.

The use of modern dressings have resulted in faster healing of leg ulcers. More convenient, comfortable and cosmetically acceptable dressings make living with leg ulcers that much easier. It is even possible to shower and bathe with modern, waterproof dressings.

If you have a leg ulcer, you should follow the instructions of your doctor, district nurse or practice nurse but remember that these people can only do so much. By following the advice in this leaflet and helping yourself, you can make a difference.

Assessments

Level 2 assessment

This assessment is in the form of 3000–3500 word essay (excluding references, diagrams and appendices). The essay is in two parts:

PART A

1. Begin your essay by selecting a patient in your care who is requiring (or has recently required) wound management. Briefly describe the patient and the nature of the wound. Your description should be no more than 500 words.

2. Next, examine how physiological processes have contributed to the wound aetiology or to the healing process, making use of the relevant literature to support your arguments.

Part A of the essay should be no more that 1500 words.

PART B

In this part of your level 2 assessment you will continue to use the same patient as in Part A. This part of the essay is an analysis of particular aspects of this patient's wound management.

1. Begin Part B by selecting **three** elements of the wound assessment process from the following list:

   - intrinsic factors affecting wound healing
   - extrinsic factors affecting wound healing
   - nutritional assessment for wound healing
   - wound classification
   - wound measurement techniques
   - quality of life for people with wounds.

Give reasons/justifications for why the three elements you have selected are relevant to your chosen patient.

2. Next, drawing on relevant research findings, explore the interrelationship between the three elements of wound assessment which you selected (e.g. element one relates to element two; how does the second element relate to the first and third?).

3. Conclude your essay by exploring how your chosen elements of wound assessment influenced decisions that were made about the way this patient's wound was managed. Include in this conclusion your suggestions about how good wound assessment can influence the provision of a high quality wound management service using the appropriate literature to support your arguments.

LEVEL 2 ASSESSMENT—MARKING GRID

	Max.	Your marks	Min.	
Appropriate patient is clearly identified with brief description of the nature of the wound	10		0	Patient has not been clearly identified and/or is not appropriate to this essay No evidence of a description of the nature of the wound
Part A of the essay demonstrates exploration of how physiological factors contribute to the wound aetiology and/or its healing	20		0	Superficial exploration of how physiological factors contribute to the wound or its healing
Part B of the essay demonstrates clear identification of three relevant elements of wound assessment for the chosen patient and there is evidence of the justification of the choice of elements	10		0	Superficial or no identification of three key elements of wound assessment; or fewer than three elements identified. No justification for choice of elements
Clear and comprehensive analysis of how the three key elements of wound assessment selected are interrelated	25		0	Superficial or unclear analysis of how the three key elements selected are interrelated
Comprehensive analysis of how the three key elements of wound assessment influenced wound management decisions	25		0	Superficial analysis of how the key elements of wound assessment influenced wound management decisions
Essay is logically developed within word limit (+/− 10%) and is correctly referenced using a recognised referencing system	10		0	Essay is illogical, not within word limit and/or there is no evidence of the use of a recognised referencing system

Level 3 assessment

Nurses who wish to be assessed at level 3 should submit the following assessment which should be 3500–4000 words in length (excluding references, diagrams and appendices).

The level 3 assessment is in two parts:

Part A

1. Begin Part A by selecting one aspect of wound management practice in your place of work (e.g. management of patients with fungating wounds; leg ulcer management; complex surgical wounds; infected wounds—to suggest just a few possibilities).

2. Discuss current practices in your place of work related to the way your selected type of wound is managed.

3. Critically evaluate current practices against national or local guidelines for managing these types of wounds, technological advances and research evidence. Your evaluation of practice must draw conclusions about the extent to which current practice in your place of work reflects established guidelines, technological advances and research evidence. Any conclusions drawn must be justified and defended. You may wish to make recommendations for future practice.

Part A of your essay should be approximately 2000 words in length.

Part B

In this part of your assessment you will use the same aspect of wound management as you used in Part A.

In this part of the essay, however, you will be exploring the role of the specialist tissue viability nurse in relation to that aspect of wound management.

1. Select any **three** components of the role of tissue viability specialist nurse from the list below:

   • giving direct specialist care
   • advising/acting as consultant to other health care professionals
   • promoting health in patients
   • leadership
   • acting as patient advocate
   • managing resources
   • setting/monitoring standards
   • influencing policy
   • teaching
   • supporting staff
   • facilitating change
   • research and audit activities.

2. Critically examine, using current research findings, how the three role components of the tissue viability specialist nurse which you selected can enhance and improve practice related to the aspect of wound management you identified in Part A of this essay. For example, if you examined fungating wounds in Part A of this essay, how do your three components of the tissue viability specialist role enhance and improve practice related to fungating wounds?)

3. Conclude your essay by reflecting on how a tissue viability specialist enhances the quality of wound management services.

Part B of your essay should be approximately 2000 words.

LEVEL 3 ASSESSMENT—MARKING GRID

	Max.	Your marks	Min.	
An appropriate aspect of wound management practice has been selected	5		0	Aspect of wound management practice is not evident or is not appropriate
Comprehensive description of current practices related to the selected aspect of wound management	15		0	Superficial description of current practices or description is not related to the selected aspect of wound management
Part A demonstrates a comprehensive critical evaluation of current practices against local/national guidelines, technological advances and research evidence	20		0	Part A critical evaluation is superficial or uncritical with inadequate or no comparison of practice with local/national guidelines, technological advances and research evidence
Critical evaluation in Part A includes conclusions drawn and justification for these conclusions	15		0	Part A critical evaluation does not include any conclusions and/or they are not justified
In Part B three components of the role of the tissue viability specialist nurse are selected	5		0	Fewer than three components of the role of the tissue viability specialist nurse selected
Critical examination of the role of the tissue viability specialist nurse clearly demonstrates how such a specialist can contribute to the aspect of wound management selected	20		0	Superficial examination of the role of the tissue viability specialist nurse and/or how a specialist nurse contributes to the aspect of wound management selected
Conclusion to Part B demonstrates how a tissue viability specialist nurse may enhance the quality of a wound management service	10		0	Little or no evidence of how a tissue viability specialist may enhance the quality of a wound management service
Essay is logically developed within word limit (+/− 10%) and is correctly referenced using a recognised referencing system	10		0	Essay is illogical, not within word limit or incorrectly referenced/no recognised referencing system evident

Index